Physical Medicine and Rehabilitation

Stroke Rehabilitation

Guest Editor:

Robert W. Teasell, BSc, MD, FRCPC
Associate Professor and Acting Chair
Department of Physical Medicine and Rehabilitation
University of Western Ontario
Chief, Department of Physical Medicine and Rehabilitation
London Health Sciences Center
London, Ontario
Canada

Volume 12/Number 3
HANLEY & BELFUS, INC.

October 1998
Philadelphia

STATE OF THE ART REVIEWS

Publisher: HANLEY & BELFUS, INC.
210 South 13th Street
Philadelphia, PA 19107
(215) 546-7293
(215) 790-9330 (Fax)
Web site: http://www.hanleyandbelfus.com

PHYSICAL MEDICINE AND REHABILITATION: State of the Art Reviews is included in *BioSciences Information Service, Current Contents, ISI/BIOMED,* and *Cumulative Index to Nursing & Allied Health Literature.*

PHYSICAL MEDICINE AND REHABILITATION: State of the Art Reviews   ISSN 0888-7357
Volume 12, Number 3   ISBN 1-56053-281-5

PHYSICAL MEDICINE AND REHABILITATION: State of the Art Reviews is published triannually (three times per year) by Hanley & Belfus, Inc., 210 South 13th Street, Philadelphia, Pennsylvania 19107.

POSTMASTER: Send address changes to PHYSICAL MEDICINE AND REHABILITATION: State of the Art Reviews, Hanley & Belfus, Inc., 210 South 13th Street, Philadelphia, PA 19107.

The 1998 subscription price is $78.00 per year U.S., $88.00 outside U.S. (add $30.00 for air mail). Single copies $34.00 U.S., $37.00 outside U.S. (add $10.00 for single copy air mail).

Physical Medicine and Rehabilitation: State of the Art Reviews
Vol. 12, No. 3, October 1998

STROKE REHABILITATION

Robert W. Teasell, BSc, MD, FRCPC

CONTENTS

It is well established that stroke is a major contributor to mortality and morbidity worldwide. Though death due to stroke has been declining over the past 20 years, this may be changing. The author reviews the rates of stroke and recovery following stroke, including how stroke is tracked and health-related quality of life post-stroke.

This chapter provides an overview of the recent advances in the treatment and prevention of acute strokes from diverse causes. Risk factors for stroke, surgical prevention, and medical management of symptomatic patients are covered. The authors describe the pharmacologic agents currently in use for the treatment of vascular risk factors and the technologic advances in noninvasive imaging modalities, such as magnetic resonance imaging, that have made it possible to visualize acute strokes. The role of tissue plasminogen activator (TPA) is also discussed.

Disability following stroke varies according to the degree of neurologic recovery, the site of the lesion, the patient's premorbid status, and the environmental support systems. The authors describe the clinical consequences and recovery of stroke based on the anatomic regions of the brain that are affected.

This article summarizes current evidence pertaining to the relation between stroke and seizures or epilepsy and examines issues of relevance to clinicians dealing with this patient population. Risks, timing of seizure occurrence in relation to stroke, stroke type, stroke in children, and treatment are all covered.

Robert W. Teasell, Marc McRae, and Hillel M. Finestone

Aspiration following stroke is a common and serious source of morbidity. It can lead to pneumonia, sepsis, and death. The authors detail the incidence of dysphagia and aspiration, diagnosis of suspected aspiration with videofluoroscopic modified barium swallow (VMBS), aspiration pneumonia, and aspiration management including dietary modifications and nonoral feeding. Future issues are also addressed.

Hillel M. Finestone and Linda S. Greene-Finestone

Nutritional and dietary issues play fundamental roles in the rehabilitation of stroke patients. The past decade has brought to light new information regarding the high prevalence of undernourished stroke patients and subsequent adverse outcomes. The chapter outlines nutritional assessment and focuses on specific nutritional and dietary concerns of stroke patients and strategies for treatment.

Michael John Borrie

Urinary incontinence following stroke is common and is a predictor of poor functional recovery. However, it is not a necessary consequence of stroke. The author illustrates how accurate history, physical examination, and residual urine tests will pinpoint the pre- and poststroke factors contributing to incontinence, resulting in better treatment. Different management techniques are discussed including approaches to voiding, pelvic floor exercises, cystometry, and pharmacologic therapy.

K. J. Miller, S. J. Garland, and G. F. Koshland

The authors review the traditional rehabilitation interventions for stroke patients that focus on the symptoms of abnormal synergistic movement and spasticity. The rationale and efficacy of specific facilitatory techniques are covered. In addition, the authors discuss recent trends such as the importance of muscle-strengthening techniques in stroke patients and the increased emphasis on motor learning principles. The forced-use paradigm is presented.

Robert W. Teasell and Marc McRae

Hemiplegia is a common sequela of stroke, and a painful hemiplegic shoulder often results. Good shoulder function in stroke patients is a prerequisite for successful transfers, maintaining balance, performance of activities of daily living, and effective hand function. Causes and management of hemiplegic shoulder pain are addressed, and spasticity and sustained hemiplegic posture as the likely causes are discussed.

J. B. Orange and Andrew Kertesz

This chapter provides an overview of the studies that examine the usefulness of language therapy for aphasia. The different levels of usefulness (i.e., efficacy, effectiveness, efficiency) and the important methodologic challenges of conducting studies on the efficacy of language therapy for aphasia are discussed. Prognostic factors for recovery of language are also presented. This chapter concludes with a discussion of issues for future research on efficacy studies of language therapy for individuals with aphasia.

Leora C. Swartzman, Margaret C. Gibson, and Tamara L. Armstrong

Through their conceptual framework of stroke as a biopsychosocial—as opposed to biomedical—event, the authors examine the literature on how the common neurobehavioral sequelae of stroke can compromise the rehabilitation process and affect long-term adjustment. This chapter updates information on current treatments and provides information on instruments for screening and tracking the neurobehavioral consequences of stroke. In addition, the importance of social supports are presented.

Ashok Devasenapathy and Vladimir C. Hachinski

Strokes may cause, contribute to, or coexist with impaired cognition and memory problems. This chapter outlines the current knowledge of the epidemiology, pathophysiology, pathology, diagnosis, and treatment of vascular cognitive impairment. Discussion of the use of the term *vascular dementia* and the distinction between preventable dementia and dementia of unknown cause are included.

Colleen Churchill

The significant effect of stroke on the immediate family of a stroke victim is often not appreciated. The acute care phase of stroke patients is often emphasized over more long-term sequelae such as psychosocial problems. This article draws attention to those social consequences of stroke that often do not receive sufficient attention, including the caregiver's involvement and adjustment and the patient's quality of life issues, such as driving and vocational issues.

Robert W. Teasell and Marc McRae

Stroke is relatively uncommon in persons younger than 50 years, and the rehabilitation of younger and older stroke patients is similar. However, there are some unique differences between older and younger stroke patients, as this chapter demonstrates. Topics covered include etiology of stroke in younger patients, recovery and prognosis in the young stroke patient, rehabilitation including return to work issues, and future needs of young stroke patients.

Stephen D. Bagg

It is becoming increasingly important to identify which patients benefit from what specific rehabilitation interventions, in what setting, at what intensity, and for how long. In addition, the cost-effectiveness of these services must be determined. This article reviews the evidence regarding the effectiveness of stroke rehabilitation and discusses factors and tools that have been found useful in predicting outcome.

1996 ISSUES

The Autonomic Nervous System
Robert W. Teasell, MD, Editor
London, Ontario, Canada

Sympathetic Pain Syndromes:
Reflex Sympathetic Dystrophy and Causalgia
C. David Tollison, PhD, and
John R. Satterthwaite, MD, Editors
Greenville, South Carolina

Physiatric Anatomic Principles
Kamala Shankar, MD, Editor
Stanford, California

1997 ISSUES

Advances in Rehabilitation Technology
Trilok N. Monga, MD, and Kuno P. Zimmermann, DO, PhD, Editors
Houston, Texas

Outcome Measurement
Richard M. Smith, PhD, Editor
Wheaton, Illinois

Functional Biomechanics and Rehabilitation of Sports Injuries
Joseph D. Fortin, DO, Frank J. E. Falco, MD, and
Hilaire A. C. Jacob, PhD, Editors
Fort Wayne, Indiana; Philadelphia, Pennsylvania; and Zurich, Switzerland

1998 ISSUES

Motor Vehicle Accidents
Ted A. Lennard, MD, and D. Wayne Brooks, MD, Editors
Springfield, Missouri, and Fayetteville, Arkansas

Injuries and Rehabilitation of the Upper Extremity
V. Jane Derebery, MD, and Morton Kasdan, MD, Editors
Austin, Texas, and Louisville, Kentucky

Stroke Rehabilitation
Robert W. Teasell, BSc, MD, Editor
London, Ontario, Canada

Subscriptions for full year and single issues available from the publisher—
Hanley & Belfus, Inc., 210 South 13th Street, Philadelphia, PA 19107.
Telephone (215) 546-7293; (800) 962-1892. Fax (215) 790-9330.

CONTRIBUTORS

Tamara L. Armstrong, MA
Department of Psychology, University of Western Ontario, London, Ontario, Canada

Stephen D. Bagg, MD, MSc, FRCPC
Assistant Professor, Department of Rehabilitation Medicine, Queen's University; Director, Stroke Rehabilitation Program, St. Mary's of the Lake Hospital, Kingston, Ontario, Canada

Michael John Borrie, BSc, MBChB, FRCPC
Associate Professor, Division of Geriatric Medicine, Department of Medicine, University of Western Ontario; Medical Director, Continence Clinic and Continence Outreach Program, Regional Geriatric Program, Parkwood Hospital, London, Ontario, Canada

James T. Butler, MBChB, FCP(Neurol) S.A.
Clinical Fellow in Epilepsy, Department of Clinical Neurological Sciences, University of Western Ontario; Fellow, Epilepsy Unit, London Health Sciences Center, London, Ontario, Canada

Colleen Churchill, BSW, MSW
Social Worker, Rehabilitation Unit, London Health Sciences Center, London, Ontario, Canada

Ashok Devasenapathy, MD
Clinical Fellow in Cerebrovascular Disease, Department of Clinical Neurological Sciences, University of Western Ontario; London Health Sciences Center, London, Ontario, Canada

Hillel M. Finestone, MD, FRCPC
Associate Professor, Department of Physical Medicine and Rehabilitation, University of Western Ontario; Staff Physiatrist, Department of Physical Medicine and Rehabilitation, London Health Sciences Center, London, Ontario, Canada

S. Jayne Garland, PhD, PT
Associate Professor, Departments of Physical Therapy and Physiology, University of Western Ontario, London, Ontario, Canada

Margaret Christine Gibson, PhD, CPsych
Adjunct Professor, Department of Psychology, University of Western Ontario; Psychologist, Veterans Care Program, Parkwood Hospital, St. Joseph's Health Center, London, Ontario, Canada

Linda S. Greene-Finestone, BSc, MSc, RD
Research Associate, Department of Physical Medicine and Rehabilitation, London Health Sciences Center; PhD candidate, Department of Epidemiology and Biostatistics, University of Western Ontario, London, Ontario, Canada

Vladimir C. Hachinski, MD, MSc, DSc (Med), FRCPC
Richard and Beryl Ivey Professor and Chairman, Department of Clinical Neurological Sciences, University of Western Ontario; Chief, Department of Clinical Neurological Sciences, London Health Sciences Center, London, Ontario, Canada

John D. Heitzner, BSc, MD, FRCPC
Fellow, Department of Physical Medicine and Rehabilitation, London Health Sciences Center, London, Ontario, Canada

Andrew Kertesz, MD, FRCPC
Professor, Department of Clinical Neurological Sciences, University of Western Ontario; St. Joseph's Health Center, London, Ontario, Canada

Gail F. Koshland, PhD, PT
Assistant Professor, Department of Physiology, University of Arizona, Tucson, Arizona

Nancy E. Mayo, BSc, MS, PhD
Associate Professor, Department of Epidemiology, School of Physical and Occupational Therapy, McGill University; Health Services and Outcomes Research Group, Division of Clinical Epidemiology, Royal Victoria Hospital, Montreal, Quebec, Canada

Marc P. McRae, BSc, MSc
Research Assistant, Department of Physical Medicine and Rehabilitation, University of Western Ontario, London, Ontario, Canada

Kimberly J. Miller, BSc, PT, MSc
Instructor, Department of Physical Therapy, University of Western Ontario, London, Ontario, Canada

J. B. Orange, PhD
Associate Professor, School of Communication Sciences and Disorders, University of Western Ontario, London, Ontario, Canada

Leora C. Swartzman, PhD, CPsych
Associate Professor, Department of Psychology, University of Western Ontario, London, Ontario, Canada

Robert W. Teasell, BSc, MD, FRCPC
Associate Professor and Acting Chair, Department of Physical Medicine and Rehabilitation, University of Western Ontario; Chief, Department of Physical Medicine and Rehabilitation, London Health Sciences Center, London, Ontario, Canada

Samuel Wiebe, MD, MSc, FRCPC
Assistant Professor of Neurology and Epilepsy, Department of Clinical Neurological Sciences, University of Western Ontario; Neurologist, Epilepsy Unit, London Health Sciences Center, London, Ontario, Canada

PREFACE

According to the Heart and Stroke Foundation of Ontario[1] an estimated 50,000 new cases of stroke occur in Canada each year. For every death, an estimated three stroke victims survive, with varying degrees of disability. Moreover, the impact of stroke is again gaining strength as the number of deaths attributable to stroke is beginning to rise after decades of decline. This trend will only accelerate as our population ages. The socioeconomic and health effects are and will continue to be substantial because the burden of disability associated with stroke remains high. Rehabilitation offers the opportunity to reduce this burden of disability; however, scientific evidence of the efficacy of a variety of rehabilitation interventions is "incomplete."[2]

This text was written as a follow-up to a previous *Physical Medicine and Rehabilitation: State of the Art Reviews* volume entitled "Long-Term Consequences of Stroke" written some $5\frac{1}{2}$ years ago. Many of the chapters have been replaced, while others have been significantly updated to try to capture the current key issues in stroke rehabilitation. We hope that this text will serve as an important resource and will be seen as another step in our quest to provide optimal care for our stroke rehabilitation patients.

Robert W. Teasell, BSc, MD FRCPC
GUEST EDITOR

REFERENCES
1. Heart and Stroke Foundation of Ontario press release. 1997.
2. Stason WB: Can clinical practice guidelines increase the effectiveness and cost-effectiveness of post-stroke rehabilitation? Topics Stroke Rehabil 4(3):1–16, 1997.

ACKNOWLEDGMENT

I would like to acknowledge Mrs. Debbi Harley, who assisted in the organization and preparation of the text.

PUBLISHED ISSUES 1987–1995

(available from the publisher)

NANCY E. MAYO, PhD

EPIDEMIOLOGY AND RECOVERY OF STROKE

From the Division of Clinical
 Epidemiology
Royal Victoria Hospital
Montreal, Quebec
Canada

Reprint requests to:
Nancy E. Mayo, PhD
Health Services and Outcomes
 Research Group
Division of Clinical Epidemiology
Royal Victoria Hospital
Ross Pavilion, 4th floor
687 Pine Avenue West
Montreal, Quebec H3A 1A1
Canada

It is well established that stroke is a major contributor to mortality and morbidity worldwide.[1-6] In Canada and other developed nations, the mortality due to stroke has been declining,[2,3,6-10] though this may be changing. Currently, Canada enjoys one of the lowest rates of death due to stroke;[1-4] however, morbidity and associated hospitalization remain unacceptably high.[3]

In Canada, death due to stroke has declined approximately 50% over the past 20 years to a current level of 50 per 100,000 Canadians, which represents 7% of all-cause mortality.[1,4] The decline in stroke-related mortality has been attributed both to improved survival following stroke[11,12] and to decreased incidence.[13-15] Both risk factor management and health promotion have played a role in the declining incidence. Population-based public health strategies targeted toward smoking cessation, diet, exercise, and weight control have contributed substantially as has medical management of hypertension, hyperlipidemia, diabetes, and cardiovascular disease.[16,17] This combined effort has increased the public's awareness of the risk factors for cardiovascular and cerebrovascular disease.

Despite this positive portrait, there is evidence that the rate of decline in incidence of stroke has reached a plateau,[11,18-21] and mortality is now no longer declining. Reasons for this are still hypothetical.[19] It is possible that more strokes are being diagnosed because of advances in diagnostic procedures. Some authors have hypothesized that current advances in the treatment of cardiovascular disease have resulted in improved survival but have placed a greater proportion of the population at risk to develop cerebrovascular disease.[19]

In addition to being an important contributor to mortality, stroke is the most disabling chronic disease affecting not only the individual, but also the family and society at large.[22] Considerable advances have been made in stroke prevention and management, but much work remains to be done because stroke continues to be an extremely prevalent and burdensome condition, particularly among the elderly.

RATES OF STROKE

A recent study of patients hospitalized for stroke in Canada has suggested that brain infarctions have declined slightly over the 10-year period ending in 1992 but that brain hemorrhages have increased.[3] By 1991–1992, the rate of cerebral infarction was approximately 170 per 100,000 men and 160 per 100,000 women. Cerebral hemorrhage is a much rarer occurrence with a rate of approximately 17 per 100,000 men and 15 per 100,000 women. These rates place Canada at about the midpoint for worldwide rates of stroke.[23] The rate of stroke is greatly determined by age, increasing from about 20 per 100,000 persons between the ages of 15 and 54 years to over 1500 per 100,000 persons between the ages of 75 and 84 years.

Finally, some authors suspect that the strokes are becoming, if not less frequent, less devastating.[24–26] Unfortunately, there is no systemic way in Canada for this important information to be documented. However, indirect evidence of this effect over time does exist in that more and more persons have been able to return home after a stroke.[3] The impact of this trend is that more persons in the community are living with the sequelae of stroke and are at risk for diminished activity level, social isolation, and recurrent stroke. Services targeted at tertiary prevention are, therefore, essential if the outcome of stroke is to improve. Tertiary prevention, or preventing the sequelae of stroke, includes access to rehabilitation services and availability of recreational, social, and educational opportunities. Currently, in Canada, access to these services is threatened as provinces look for ways to cut costs.

RECOVERY FOLLOWING STROKE

Rehabilitation and Recovery Poststroke

A growing body of evidence supports the benefits of poststroke rehabilitation in enhancing recovery. A recent synthesis by Kwakkel of eight randomized trials and one nonrandomized experiment showed that "more is better."[27]

Currently, basic science research in physical rehabilitation of stroke is focusing on biological mechanisms of gait, balance, and movement of the upper extremity.[28–34] Efforts are also being made to develop and evaluate rehabilitation interventions that target these biological mechanisms to increase function and safety of individuals with stroke.[35–38] The evaluation of effectiveness of interventions and modes of health service delivery is greatly needed in Canada so that the greatest number of patients can benefit from the best health care at the lowest cost.

Impairment, Activities, and Participation Poststroke

For the past 2 decades, the World Health Organization's *International Classification of Impairment, Disability, and Handicap* has served as a framework for considering the outcome of stroke. This organization has recently replaced the words *disability* and *handicap* with *activities* and *participation*.[39] These more positive words reflect the desired outcome of care: increased activity and participation in community life.

Tracking Recovery

Tracking the recovery following stroke is not easy because it demands the systematic follow-up of an inception cohort over time. Fortunately, there are several examples of this type of study, and they provide the most accurate portrait of recovery of stroke.

The Copenhagen Stroke Study recruited 1,197 patients with acute stroke over a 25-month period starting in 1991.[40-44] Subjects were assessed weekly until death or until the end of rehabilitation (average 37 days); initial mortality (21%) reduced the population to 947 survivors who were followed to 6 months. Table 1 summarizes the key features of this study and the main results according to initial stroke severity.

The results presented in Table 1 indicate that neurologic, functional, and walking recovery takes place very early and reaches a maximum at about 13 weeks poststroke; very little functional recovery is observed after discharge from rehabilitation. A similar pattern of recovery was also seen for the upper extremity.[41] Among a preliminary sample of 636 subjects from the Copenhagen Study, 214 (34%) had upper extremity paresis on admission, and almost half of these persons died (46%) during their hospital stay, suggesting that these persons had severe to very severe stroke. Severe paresis persisted for more than half of survivors (56%); 30% had partial recovery, and 14% achieved full recovery, as far as strength and range of motion of the arm and hand were concerned. The authors distinguished functional recovery from motor recovery and observed that the degree of functional recovery depended on the degree of motor recovery. Among persons with motor recovery, 57% gained independence in grooming and feeding, and only 6% remained unable to do these two tasks. In contrast, among persons with motor recovery, only 16% gained independence while 41% remained de-

TABLE 1. Pattern of Recovery following Stroke According to Initial Stroke Severity: Key Results from the Copenhagen Stroke Study

		Initial Stroke Severity[a]				
		Mild (41%)	Moderate (26%)	Severe (14%)	Very Severe (19%)	All (n = 1,197)
Mortality		3%	12%	33%	62%	21%
Resolution of deficits[b]		96%	81%	39%	20%	78%
Restoration of function[c]		68%	36%	26%	4%	46%
Restoration of walking[d]		89%	61%	55%	24%	n.r.
Improvement in BI from discharge to 6 months (points/100)		0.6	2.2	3.8	2.6	1.5
Time to reach best recovery (weeks)						
Neurologic[e]	80th percentile	2.5	5.5	9	10	4.5
	95th percentile	6.5	10.5	15	13	11
Functional[f]	80th percentile	3	7	11.5	11.5	6
	95th percentile	8.5	13	17	20	12.5
Walking[d]	80th percentile	3	3	5	1	5
	95th percentile	9	9	11	11	11

n. r. = not reported.

[a] Classified using the Scandinavian Neurological Stroke Scale (SSS); 80th percentile is the time when 80% of population reached maximum.

[b] Percent classified as "mild" among 947 survivors at the end of rehabilitation after an average of 37 days.

[c] Percent with no disability at discharge as indicated by a score of 100 on the Barthel Index (BI).

[d] Percent able to walk 50 m with or without assistance.

[e] Among 626 of the 873 survivors (71%) to 6 months.

[f] Based on Barthel Index; 80th percentile is the time when 80% of population reached maximum.

TABLE 2.   Evolution of Selected Indices of Impairment and Disability during First 3 Months Poststroke

Construct	Initial Evaluation Mean (SD)	1 Month Mean (SD)	3 Months Mean (SD)
Upper extremity function			
Box and Block[47] (0 to 150)[a]	25 (21)	36 (23)	42 (21)
Motor recovery			
STREAM[52] (0 to 100)[b]	75 (27)	86 (20)	89 (17)
Balance			
Balance Scale[53] (0 to 44)	37 (18)	47 (11)	49 (8)
Basic ADLs (0 to 100)			
Barthel Index[49] (0 to 100)	72 (28)	86 (20)	92 (14)
Physical mobility			
Timed Up and Go[54] (sec)[c]	73 (87)	34 (49)	21 (26)
Comfortable gait speed[28] (m/sec)[d]	0.55 (0.4)	0.82 (0.4)	0.85 (0.4)

SD = standard deviation; ADLs = activities of daily living.
[a] The maximum number of blocks, 2.54 cm in size, moved one by one from one compartment to another in one minute.
[b] Stroke Rehabilitation Assessment of Movement
[c] Time to rise up from a chair, walk 3 m, turn, and sit down.
[d] 5-m course.

pendent. Persistent upper extremity paresis was associated with a lower probability of being discharged to home (17% vs. 63% for persons with recovery).

The recovery of upper extremity function was also evaluated by Duncan in a cohort of acute stroke patients assembled in 1988.[45] Data available on 95 patients indicated that the most important recovery was made in the first 30 days and that the extent of recovery depended on the initial severity of motor impairment. Although the sample size was small, the recovery of the upper extremity did not differ appreciably from the recovery of the lower extremity. This finding was confirmed in a study by Higgins as part of the Montreal Stroke Study (Table 2).[46] In a consecutive series of 55 stroke patients, the average performance on a test of upper extremity function at approximately 8 days poststroke was 34% of age- and gender-predicted values, and this rose to 51% by 5 weeks poststroke.[47] The corresponding values for gait speed, used as a measure of lower extremity function, were 44% and 66%, at 8 days and 5 weeks, respectively. Therefore, both the upper and lower extremity experienced a 50% increase in functional ability over this 4-week period.

Another cohort study, conducted in Helsinki from 1993–1995, involved 649 persons between the ages of 55 and 85 years with acute ischemic stroke.[48] At 3 months, 425 persons were assessed on a battery of functional and neuropsychological tests. The results indicated persisting functional dependence (mean Barthel Index[49] 69; standard deviation 19), high prevalence of poststroke dementia (20%) and depression (17%), and an 8% prevalence of aphasia. With the exception of aphasia and depression, older patients had poorer outcomes than younger patients and were more often institutionalized at 3 months (21% vs. 12%).

A British study conducted in 1988–1990 recruited a cohort of persons younger than 75 years with acute stroke.[50] Subjects were assessed at 3 months and followed for up to 5 years. The estimated 5-year survival was 46%. The outcome of this group reflects a survivor phenomenon; almost all were community dwelling, and on average functional status was good (estimated Barthel Index of 84). However, 13% were considered severely disabled, 16% were considered moderately disabled, 37% had mild disability, and 54% were classified as independent according to the Barthel Index.[49]

One major limitation of the Copenhagen Stroke Study was the relatively crude outcome measures. Walking and upper extremity function were evaluated using items from the Barthel Index: the ability to walk 50 m with or without assistance and the ability to groom and eat independently.[49] These measures may not be sensitive enough to capture changes in higher level walking ability and manual dexterity, particularly in persons with mild or moderate stroke, which make up the majority of stroke survivors.

Preliminary data from an ongoing stroke cohort study in Montreal provides information about short-term recovery on physical performance and about longer term recovery, reintegration, and health-related quality of life (Tables 2 and 3).[51] Table 2 illustrates the rapid recovery of motor ability poststroke, particularly in the first 5 weeks. However, even with this steep increase over time, by 3 months a sizable proportion of patients have not met age-appropriate norms for these activities. For the upper limb,[47] only 7% reached peer values, and on basic activities of daily living (ADLs),[49] 60% reached full independence. The corresponding value for recovery of motor function using the Stroke Rehabilitation Assessment of Movement (STREAM)[52] was 33%; for balance,[53] 30%; for mobility[54] using the Timed "Up and Go" (TUG) test, 38%; and for gait speed,[28] 21%.

Table 3 compares persons approximately 1 year after stroke (range 9–15 months) with an age- and gender-matched peer group. The stroke group represents community-based survivors, and this is manifested by a high score on the Barthel Index.[49] A score of 2 on the Reintegration to Normal Living (RNL) Index[55] indicates that, on average, the stroke group had some difficulty with at least two everyday community activities; in comparison, the score on the RNL for peer controls was 1. The EuroQol thermometer rating scale (EQ-5D)[56] was used to evaluate overall health status of both groups and indicated that persons with stroke rate their health, on average, 8 points lower than peer controls. The health dimensions most strongly affected by stroke were mobility, self-care, everyday activities, and anxiety or depression.

Table 3 highlights the impact that stroke has beyond the ability to perform basic ADLs, but it is important to underline that some stroke survivors still do have difficulty even with basic ADLs. In the Montreal study survivors at 9–15 months poststroke had an overall Barthel Index of 97, and 60% had reached full independence in all ten areas of basic function. More than 90% were independent in transfers and bowel management, and more than 80% regained independence in the remaining activities except bathing, for which 76% were independent. The two activities with the highest proportion of persons with disability were stairs (18%) and bathing (24%). This is consistent with the portrait presented by Wilkinson.[50]

For higher level activities such as those captured by measures of instrumental ADLs, only 50% had reached full independence. The activities that were most problematic (requiring assistance) were housework (42%), shopping (33%), meal preparation (27%), and using transportation (25%). Less than 10% of the community-dwelling stroke population had difficulty with using the telephone and handling medications or finances. Measures of participation capture another set of activities: those dealing with role performance. On the RNL Index,[55] 43% were independent in all eleven activities. The most problematic activities were travel, social activities, establishing an important activity to fill the day, recreational activities, and moving around the community, for which 21–36% reported some difficulty.

TABLE 3. Comparison of Persons 1 Year Poststroke and Age-Matched Controls on Selected Indices of Disability, Handicap, and Health-related Quality of Life

Construct	Stroke Group (n = 136)		Controls (n = 358)	
	Mean	SD	Mean	SD
Basic ADL (0 to 100)[a]	96.9	7.0	99.6	2.4
Community integration (22 to 0)[b]	2.5	3.3	0.8	1.8
Health status (EQ-5D)[c]	69.1	18.5	77.7	14.4
Mobility problem (%)	38%		12%	
Self-care problem (%)	15%		2%	
Usual activity restriction (%)	21%		8%	
Pain or discomfort (%)	39%[g]		34%[g]	
Anxiety or depression (%)	26%		19%	
SF-36: Physical health (0–50)[d]	47.4	9.1	52.1	7.6
SF-36: Mental health (0–50)[e]	49.1	9.9	51.6	8.8
SF-36 Subscales[f]				
Physical functioning	71.6	24.4	89.1	15.3
Role—physical	68.7	41.2	87.0	31.4
Bodily pain	76.3[g]	29.2	74.9[g]	30.6
General health	73.8	18.4	82.5	16.0
Vitality	53.1	21.6	64.1	20.5
Social functioning	86.8[g]	20.7	89.6[g]	18.6
Role—emotional	72.1	43.0	87.6	32.2
Mental health	71.7	76.4	76.4	18.2

SD = standard deviation; ADL = activity of daily living.
Data have been obtained from a cohort of individuals participating in a follow-up study on the long-term outcome of stroke. Selection criteria excluded persons with a second stroke, but proxy consent was obtained for persons with cognitive and language impairments. Proxy responses were not used for physical or mental health-related quality of life. Neighborhood controls were age and gender matched, selected through telephone listings.
[a] Barthel Index.
[b] Reintegration to Normal Living (RNL) Index.
[c] Thermometer Rating Scale of the EuroQol (EQ-5D) and % indicating problem on five dimensions of the EQ-5D.
[d] Physical health component of the Measuring Outcomes Study Short Form-36 (MOS SF-36); this is standardized to have a mean of 50 and a standard deviation of 10.
[e] Mental health component (PCS) of the SF-36, with a mean of 50 and a standard deviation of 10.
[f] Subscales of the SF-36 scored out of 100.
[g] No significant difference

Health-related Quality of Life Poststroke

In contrast to the study of recovery of impairment, activities, and participation poststroke, research on health-related quality of life poststroke is less abundant but is growing as the importance of this outcome emerges. The various definitions that are currently used for quality of life and stroke-related disability have been outlined,[51] but Guyatt stated it most simply as: "all those things that one might want to measure about the health of an individual beyond death and physiologic measures of disease activity."[57]

The number of studies on health-related quality of life involving an adequate number of persons with stroke and a nonstroke population for comparative purposes is still relatively few. In 1995, de Haan and colleagues used the Sickness Impact Profile (SIP)[59] to evaluate the quality of life of 441 persons at 6 months poststroke.[58] This group represented 86% of all 6-month survivors; 14% could not be interviewed because of refusal or communication problems. A population sample of 132 elderly persons served as the reference group. The stroke group reported more serious problems than the reference group, and this was consistent across the domains captured by the SIP. In particular, persons with stroke had high levels of dysfunction in self-care, communication, eating, ambulation, and home management. Quality of life was not affected by the side of the lesion, except where communication was concerned. However, persons with supratentorial strokes reported poorer quality of life than persons with infratentorial strokes, most likely because of cognitive disturbances. This study distinguished three subgroups of stroke patients. The largest subgroup (60%) had only mildly diminished quality of life; however, 33% of these were classified as severely impaired in both the physical and psychosocial life domains. In the second, and smallest, subgroup (7%) reported problems mainly in the psychosocial domain. The third and most severely impaired group comprised older women with subcortical infarction, more than one comorbid disease, and impaired consciousness at stroke onset.

In a study done in Norway, persons (n = 165) at 1 year poststroke were approximately 20 times more likely to report poor well-being than control subjects, and upper extremity function was the strongest predictor of well-being.[60]

Anderson et al., in validating for stroke the well-known Measuring Outcomes Study Short Form 36 (SF-36),[62,63] profiled the health-related quality of life of 90 1-year survivors of stroke in southern Australia.[61] Low scores were noted for physical functioning such as vigorous activities (mean 48/100), general health (mean 64/100), and vitality (mean 56/100).

As indicated by the Copenhagen Stroke Study and other authors, most persons who survive a stroke have minimal to moderate neurologic deficits.[42,44,64] Basic functional activities can be accomplished independently, but higher level activities are often problematic. Duncan and colleagues interviewed 304 persons with prior stroke (average 2 years), 184 persons with transient ischemic attack (TIA), and 654 asymptomatic persons.[64] Of the persons with stroke, 67% had no stroke-related symptoms or their symptoms did not interfere with usual activities, 66% achieved a perfect score on the Barthel Index (100), and the average of all persons with stroke was 94 (SD = 12). Despite this positive portrait of a high level of physical function, persons with stroke, even mild stroke, reported significantly lower levels of health-related quality of life than persons with TIA or persons who were asymptomatic for cerebrovascular disease. Health-related quality of life was measured using the SF-36, and all subscales except bodily pain were affected by mild stroke. As with Anderson, the greatest impact was observed for physical function (mean 72/100), general health (mean 59/100), and vitality (57/100). Physical role (mean 65/100), which covers accomplishment of tasks, was also lower than for persons with stroke.

Early results from the Montreal Stroke Study (see Table 3) concur that persons with stroke report significantly poorer health-related quality of life at 1 year poststroke than their age and gender peers. Six of the eight subscales of the SF-36 were impacted by stroke, and only two—pain and social functioning—were equivalent between persons with stroke and controls.

Cognition, Depression, and Anxiety: The Neglected Outcomes of Stroke

Cognitive decline is a common feature of both stroke and aging. In Finland, Pohjasvaara et al. reported that 62% of persons at 3 months poststroke demonstrated impaired cognitive functioning.[65] Tatemichi et al. reported that 35% of persons, 3 months poststroke, exhibited cognitive deficits, a rate 10 times that of age peers.[66] This group of investigators also reported that improvement in cognitive status is possible over time in one third of persons with stroke.[67] In Holland, Kwa et al. found that 25% of stroke patients at 2 years poststroke had measurable cognitive deficits,[68] a finding compatible to the data reported by Tatemichi et al. and Desmond et al.[66,67]

Another study, from Italy, reported that about 25% of persons had dementia at 3 months poststroke.[69] This figure agrees very well with data for the same time period from a New York study[70] and by researchers from Finland.[48,65] Diminished cognitive status is a major problem poststroke because it affects ability to return to regular activities,[71,72] and it is also a factor identified by caregivers as affecting the quality of their relationship with the patient.[72,73] With cognitive problems affecting one fourth to one third of persons with stroke, a priority for stroke research should be directed toward improving this outcome.

Depression is another prevalent consequence of stroke, and it has been reported to be present in about 22–55% of persons 3 months poststroke.[74] Depression more often affects women than men and impacts functional outcome and participation in community activities.[75–77] Depression and anxiety often go together poststroke, and untangling them is difficult.[77,78] Schultz found that the prevalence of generalized anxiety disorder ranged from 19% just after stroke to 25% at 6 months poststroke, and persons with anxiety had higher levels of depression than persons without anxiety.[77] Interestingly, it was depression, more so than anxiety, that influenced functional outcome. Astrom found a prevalence of generalized anxiety disorder poststroke of 28%, which did not change appreciably over a 3-year follow-up period, and anxiety impacted on functional recovery.[78] While these outcomes are prevalent, most of the research in this area remains descriptive and correlational in nature.

CONCLUSION

The key points related to the recovery of stroke (Table 4) emphasize that stroke has a profound impact even on persons who, neurologically, appear to have made good recovery. Activities, participation, and health-related quality of life are the more important outcomes of stroke because the impact of stroke is felt most strongly in these areas.

Major difficulties remain in evaluating the outcome and recovery of stroke. Inception cohorts of sufficient size are rare; follow-up periods are not consistent; and outcomes vary. Basic information on mortality, institutionalization, and stroke severity is often missing, making comparisons problematic. In addition, the inclusion criteria differ as to age and type of stroke, limiting comparability and generalizability. Uniform reporting of stroke cohort studies is needed in order to assess differences and changes in outcome across health care systems and over time.

Despite these methodologic challenges, at least three aspects of the study of stroke recovery have changed from the previous review[23] that covered up to 1992 in comparison to this review, which covers the period 1993–1998.

1. More precise measurement of the timing of stroke recovery has been made possible by several large cohort studies, and these indicate the importance of early recovery (first 5 weeks). The plateau in recovery seen after this time could indicate the window of natural recovery or that not enough is being done to target recovery in the postacute phase.

2. The evaluation of recovery should target measures of a wider range of stroke outcomes and should be based on the World Health Organization's *International*

TABLE 4. Summary of Key Points Related to the Recovery of Stroke

- More rehabilitation is better than less.
- Two thirds of strokes are mild or moderate in severity, and, while neurologic deficits resolve, one third remain with limitations in basic functional activities.
- Eighty percent of neurologic and functional recovery takes place in the first 5 weeks and reaches a maximum at about 13 weeks poststroke.
- By 3 months poststroke, a sizable proportion of persons does not meet age-appropriate norms: 93% for upper extremity function, 79% for gait speed, and 40% for basic ADLs.
- Severe paresis of the upper extremity persists for more than half of survivors (56%); 30% show partial recovery, and paresis resolves for 14%.
- The most important recovery of upper extremity is made in the first 30 days.
- Poor upper extremity function is associated with a low probability of discharge home and poor rating of well-being.
- Most persons with stroke (60%) have only mildly diminished quality of life; however, 33% have severely limited quality of life.
- Even persons with mild stroke have lower than expected levels of health-related quality of life.

Classification of Impairment, Disability (Activities), and Handicap (Participation), which is gaining increasing acceptance. Research targeting recovery of upper extremity function and gait speed has demonstrated that these outcomes are profoundly affected, even for persons who are considered "independent" based on ability to perform basic ADLs. This development shows that stroke affects more than just basic ADLs and that recovery is not as complete as previously documented. This development has been more revealing for persons with mild stroke, who usually have been considered to have complete recovery.

   3. The inclusion of measures of health-related quality of life in stroke outcomes research is probably the most striking change that has occurred over the past 5 years.

REFERENCES

1. Kalache A: Stroke: The Global Burden. New York, Oxford University Press, 1995.
2. Gordon M: Monograph series on aging-related diseases: III. Stroke (cerebrovascular disease). Chron Dis Can 14:64–89, 1993.
3. Mayo NE: Hospitalization and case-fatality rates for stroke in Canada from 1982 through 1991. The Canadian collaborative study group of stroke hospitalizations. Stroke 27:1215–1220, 1996.
4. Petrasovits A, Nair C: Epidemiology of stroke in Canada. Health Rep 6:39–44, 1994.
5. Asplund K, Bonita R, Kuulasmaa K, et al: Multinational comparisons of stroke epidemiology. Evaluation of case ascertainment in the WHO MONICA Stroke Study. World Health Organization Monitoring Trends and Determinants in Cardiovascular Disease [published erratum appears in Stroke 26(8):1504, 1995]. Stroke 26:355–360, 1995.
6. Thorvaldsen P, Asplund K, Kuulasmaa K, et al: Stroke incidence, case fatality, and mortality in the WHO MONICA project. World Health Organization Monitoring Trends and Determinants in Cardiovascular Disease [published erratum appears in Stroke 26(8):1504, 1995]. Stroke 26:361–367, 1995.
7. Whisnant JP: The decline of stroke. Stroke 15:160–168, 1984.
8. Brown RD: Stroke incidence, prevalence, and survival. Secular trends in Rochester, Minnesota, through 1989. Stroke 27:373–380, 1996.
9. Modan B, Wagener DK: Some epidemiological aspects of stroke: Mortality/morbidity trends, age, sex, race, socioeconomic status. Stroke 23:1230–1236, 1992.
10. Wolf PA, D'Agostino RB, O'Neal MA, et al: Secular trends in stroke incidence and mortality. The Framingham Study [see comments]. Stroke 23:1551–1555, 1992.
11. Gillum RF: Cerebrovascular disease morbidity in the United States, 1970–1983. Age, sex, region, and vascular surgery. Stroke 17:656–661, 1986.
12. Bonita R, Beaglehole R: Monitoring stroke. An international challenge [editorial]. Stroke 26:541–542, 1995.

13. Garraway WM, Whisnant JP: The changing pattern of hypertension and the declining incidence of stroke. JAMA 258:214–217, 1987.

14. Gillum RF, Gomez-Marin O, Kottke TE, et al: Acute stroke in a metropolitan area, 1970 and 1980. The Minnesota Heart Survey. J Chronic Dis 38:891–898, 1985.

15. Kotila M: Declining incidence and mortality of stroke? Stroke 15:255–259, 1984.

16. Folsom AR, Luepker RV, Gillum RF, et al: Improvement in hypertension detection and control from 1973–1974 to 1980–1981. The Minnesota Heart Survey experience. JAMA 250:916–921, 1983.

17. Garraway WM, Whisnant JP, Furlan AJ, et al: The declining incidence of stroke. N Engl J Med 300:449–452, 1979.

18. Broderick JP, Phillips SJ, Whisnant JP, et al: Incidence rates of stroke in the eighties: The end of the decline in stroke? Stroke 20:577–582, 1989.

19. Kuller LH: Incidence rates of stroke in the eighties: The end of the decline in stroke? [editorial]. Stroke 20:841–843, 1989.

20. Mayo NE, Goldberg MS, Levy AR, et al: Changing rates of stroke in the province of Quebec, Canada: 1981–1988. Stroke 22:590–595, 1991.

21. Terent A: Increasing incidence of stroke among Swedish women. Stroke 19:598–603, 1988.

22. Lyons RA, Lo SV, Littlepage BN: Comparative health status of patients with 11 common illnesses in Wales. J Epidemiol Community Health 48:388–390, 1994.

23. Mayo NE: Epidemiology and recovery. Phys Med Rehabil State Art Rev 7:1–25, 1993.

24. Barker WH, Mullooly JP: Stroke in a defined elderly population, 1967–1985: A less lethal and disabling but no less common disease. Stroke 28:284–290, 1997.

25. Shahar E, McGovern PG, Sprafka JM, et al: Improved survival of stroke patients during the 1980s. The Minnesota Stroke Survey. Stroke 26:1–6, 1995.

26. Stegmayr B, Asplund K, Wester PO: Trends in incidence, case-fatality rate, and severity of stroke in northern Sweden, 1985–1991. Stroke 25:1738–1745, 1994.

27. Kwakkel G, Wagenaar RC, Koelman TW, et al: Effects of intensity of rehabilitation after stroke. A research synthesis. Stroke 28:1550–1556, 1997.

28. Richards CL, Malouin F, Dumas F, Tardif D: Gait velocity as an outcome measure of locomotor recovery after stroke. In Craik RL, Oatis C (eds): Analysis: Theory and Application. St. Louis, Mosby, 1995, pp 355–364.

29. Richards CL, Malouin F, Dumas F, Wood-Dauphinee S: The relationship of gait speed to clinical measures of function and muscle activations during recovery post-stroke. In Proceedings of the 2nd North American Congress on Biomechanics, Chicago, August 1992, pp 299–307.

30. Olney SJ, Griffin MP, McBride ID: Temporal, kinematic, and kinetic variables related to gait speed in subjects with hemiplegia: A regression approach. Phys Ther 74:872–885, 1994.

31. Olney SJ, Richards C: Hemiparetic gait following stroke. Part I: Characteristics. Gait Posture 4:136–148, 1996.

32. Nadeau S, Gravel D, Aresnault AB, et al: Dynamometric assessment of the plantarflexors in hemiparetic subjects: Relations between muscular, gait and clinical parameters. Scand J Rehabil Med 29:137–146, 1997.

33. Hughes MA, Duncan PW, Rose DK, et al: The relationship of postural sway to sensorimotor function, functional performance, and disability in the elderly. Arch Phys Med Rehabil 77:567–572, 1996.

34. Winstein CJ, Pohl PS: Effects of unilateral brain damage on the control of goal-directed hand movements. Exp Brain Res 105:163–174, 1995.

35. Dean CM, Shepherd RB: Task-related training improves performance of seated reaching tasks after stroke. A randomized controlled trial. Stroke 28:722–728, 1997.

36. Richards CL, Malouin F, Wood-Dauphinee S, et al: Task-specific physical therapy for optimization of gait recovery in acute stroke patients. Arch Phys Med Rehabil 74:612–620, 1993.

37. Chandler JM, Duncan PW, Kochersberger G, Studenski S: Is lower extremity strength gain associated with improvement in physical performance and disability in frail, community-dwelling elders? Arch Phys Med Rehabil 79:24–30, 1998.

38. Winstein CJ, Pohl PS, Cardinale C, et al: Learning a partial-weight-bearing skill: Effectiveness of two forms of feedback [published erratum appears in Phys Ther 77(3):328, 1997]. Phys Ther 76:985–993, 1996.

39. World Health Organization: International Classification of Impairments, Activities, and Participation: A Manual of Dimensions of Disablement and Functioning. Geneva, WHO, 1997.

40. Jorgensen HS, Nakayama H, Raaschou HO, Olsen TS: Recovery of walking function in stroke patients: The Copenhagen Stroke Study. Arch Phys Med Rehabil 76:27–32, 1995.

41. Nakayama H, Jorgensen HS, Raaschou HO, Olsen TS: Compensation in recovery of upper extremity function after stroke: The Copenhagen Stroke Study. Arch Phys Med Rehabil 75:852–857, 1994.

42. Jorgensen HS, Nakayama H, Raaschou HO, et al: Outcome and time course of recovery in stroke. Part II: Time course of recovery. The Copenhagen Stroke Study. Arch Phys Med Rehabil 76:406–412, 1995.
43. Nakayama H, Jorgensen HS, Raaschou HO, Olsen TS: The influence of age on stroke outcome. The Copenhagen Stroke Study. Stroke 25:808–813, 1994.
44. Jorgensen HS, Nakayama H, Raaschou HO, et al: Outcome and time course of recovery in stroke. Part I: Outcome. The Copenhagen Stroke Study. Arch Phys Med Rehabil 76:399–405, 1995.
45. Duncan PW, Goldstein LB, Horner RD, et al: Similar motor recovery of upper and lower extremities after stroke. Stroke 25:1181–1188, 1994.
46. Higgins J: Correlates of recovery of upper extremity function in the acute phase post-stroke [dissertation]. Montreal, McGill University, 1998.
47. Desrosiers J, Bravo G, Hebert R, et al: Validation of the Box and Block Test as a measure of dexterity of elderly people: Reliability, validity, and norms studies. Arch Phys Med Rehabil 75:751–755, 1994.
48. Pohjasvaara T, Erkinjuntti T, Vataja R, Kaste M: Comparison of stroke features and disability in daily life in patients with ischemic stroke aged 55 to 70 and 71 to 85 years. Stroke 28:729–735, 1997.
49. Granger CV, Dewis LS, Peters NC, et al: Stroke rehabilitation: Analysis of repeated Barthel Index measures. Arch Phys Med Rehabil 60:14–17, 1979.
50. Wilkinson PR, Wolfe CD, Warburton FG, et al: A long-term follow-up of stroke patients. Stroke 28:507–512, 1997.
51. Mayo NE, Wood-Dauphinee S, Ahmed S, et al: Disablement following stroke. Int J Disabil Rehabil [in press].
52. Daley K, Mayo N, Wood-Dauphinee S, et al: Verification of the stroke rehabilitation assessment of movement (STREAM). Physiother Can 49:269–278, 1997.
53. Berg K, Wood-Dauphinee S, Williams JI: The Balance Scale: Reliability assessment with elderly residents and patients with an acute stroke. Scand J Rehabil Med 27:27–36, 1995.
54. Podsiadlo D, Richardson S: The timed "Up & Go": A test of basic functional mobility for frail elderly persons. J Am Geriatr Soc 39:142–148, 1991.
55. Wood-Dauphinee S, Williams JI: Reintegration to Normal Living as a proxy to quality of life. J Chronic Dis 40:491–502, 1987.
56. Kind P: The EuroQol Instrument: An Index of Health-Related Quality of Life. In Spilker B (ed): Quality of Life and Pharmacoeconomics in Clinical Trials. 2nd ed. Philadelphia, Lippincott-Raven, 1995, pp 191–201.
57. Guyatt G, Feeny D, Patrick D: Issues in quality-of-life measurement in clinical trials. Controlled Clin Trials 12:81–90, 1991.
58. de Haan RJ, Limburg M, Van der Meulen JH, et al: Quality of life after stroke. Impact of stroke type and lesion location. Stroke 26:402–408, 1995.
59. Bergner M, Bobbitt RA, Carter WB, Gilson BS: The Sickness Impact Profile: Development and final revision of a health status measure. Med Care 19:787–805, 1981.
60. Wyller TB, Sveen U, Sodring KM, et al: Subjective well-being one year after stroke. Clin Rehabil 11:139–145, 1997.
61. Anderson C, Laubscher S, Burns R: Validation of the Short Form 36 (SF-36) health survey questionnaire among stroke patients. Stroke 27:1812–1816, 1996.
62. Ware JEJ, Kosinski M, Gandec B: SF-36 Health Survey: Manual and Interpretation Guide. 1993.
63. Ware JEJ, Kosinski M, Keller SD: SF-36 Physical and Mental Health Summary Scales: A User's Manual. 1994.
64. Duncan PW, Samsa GP, Weinberger M, et al: Health status of individuals with mild stroke. Stroke 28:740–745, 1997.
65. Pohjasvaara T, Erkinjuntti T, Vataja R, Kaste M: Dementia three months after stroke. Baseline frequency and effect of different definitions of dementia in the Helsinki Stroke Aging Memory Study (SAM) cohort. Stroke 28:785–792, 1997.
66. Tatemichi TK, Desmond DW, Stern Y, et al: Cognitive impairment after stroke: Frequency, patterns, and relationship to functional abilities. J Neurol Neurosurg Psychiatry 57:202–207, 1994.
67. Desmond DW, Moroney JT, Sano M, Stern Y: Recovery of cognitive function after stroke. Stroke 27:1798–1803, 1996.
68. Kwa VI, Limburg M, de Haan RJ: The role of cognitive impairment in the quality of life after ischaemic stroke. J Neurol 243:599–604, 1996.
69. Censori B, Manara O, Agostinis C, et al: Dementia after first stroke. Stroke 27:1205–1210, 1996.
70. Tatemichi TK, Desmond DW, Mayeux R, et al: Dementia after stroke: Baseline frequency, risks, and clinical features in a hospitalized cohort. Neurology 42:1185–1193, 1992.
71. Kalra L, Crome P: The role of prognostic scores in targeting stroke rehabilitation in elderly patients. J Am Geriatr Soc 41:396–400, 1993.

72. Galski T, Bruno RL, Zorowitz R, Walker J: Predicting length of stay, functional outcome, and after-care in the rehabilitation of stroke patients. The dominant role of higher order cognition. Stroke 24:1794–1800, 1993.

73. Browning JS, Schwirian PM: Spousal caregivers' burden: Impact of care recipient health problems and mental status. J Gerontol Nurs 20:17–22, 1994.

74. Herrmann N, Black SE, Lawrence J, et al: The Sunnybrook Stroke Study: A prospective study of depressive symptoms and functional outcome. Stroke 29:618–624, 1998.

75. Beckett LA, Brock DB, Lemke JH, et al: Analysis of change in self-reported physical function among older persons in four population studies. Am J Epidemiol 143:766–778, 1996.

76. Angeleri F, Angeleri VA, Foschi N, et al: The influence of depression, social activity, and family stress on functional outcome after stroke. Stroke 24:1478–1483, 1993.

77. Schultz CL: Predictors of anxiety in family caregivers. Aust Occup Ther J 41:153–161, 1994.

78. Astrom M: Generalized anxiety disorder in stroke patients. A 3-year longitudinal study. Stroke 27:270–275, 1996.

ASHOK DEVASENAPATHY, MD
VLADIMIR C. HACHINSKI, MD,
MSc, DSc (Med), FRCP(C)

RECENT ADVANCES IN STROKE PREVENTION AND TREATMENT

From the Department of Clinical
  Neurological Sciences
University of Western Ontario
London, Ontario
Canada

Reprint requests to:
Ashok Devasenapathy, MD
Department of Clinical Neurological
  Sciences
London Health Sciences Center
339 Windermere Road
London, Ontario N6A 5A5
Canada

Stroke remains the third leading cause of death in the United States and a major cause of disability and cognitive impairment, particularly in the elderly.[29] The atherosclerosis that affects the cerebral vasculature should be considered as one component of a systemic disorder. Patients with symptomatic or even asymptomatic cerebrovascular disease have a high morbidity from coronary artery disease and peripheral vascular disease.[2] Although great strides have been made in the last three decades in the prevention, diagnosis, and treatment of strokes and coronary artery disease, the effective prevention of strokes is still not yet possible. Unlike coronary artery disease, stroke is heterogeneous in etiology. Furthermore, the significance of risk factors that contribute to the development of the different kinds of strokes is even less clear, thereby hindering the widespread application of preventive measures.[54]

In the western world, arteriosclerosis in the carotid arteries with resultant artery-to-artery embolism from unstable plaques remains a major cause of ischemic strokes (Table 1). Cardiac emboli, as a direct manifestation of symptomatic or occult coronary artery disease, are the next most common cause of ischemic stroke. The treatment of coronary artery disease and cerebrovascular disease with the modification of vascular risk factors and the initiation of antiplatelet therapy has been effective in reducing the morbidity associated with both of these disorders.[110]

Strokes should be viewed as a preventable and potentially treatable neurologic emergency.

TABLE 1. Etiology of Transient Ischemic Attacks and Strokes

Arterial disease (thrombosis/embolism/low flow	75–80%
Extracranial large-artery (carotid, vertebrobasilar) atherothromboembolism	40%
Intracranial large-artery (e.g., middle cerebral atery) atherothromboembolism	10%
Intracranial small-artery thrombosis complicating lipohylinosis and microathenoma (lacunar strokes)	25%
Nonarteromatous arterial disease	< 5%
Cardiac disease	20%
Hematologic disease	< 5%

Adapted from Sandercock PA, Warlow CP, Jones LN, Starkey JR: Predisposing factors for cerebral infarction: The Oxfordshire Community Stroke Project. BMJ 298:75–80, 1989.

Clinical trials show that symptomatic patients with carotid stenosis have a reduction in their risk of stroke from the modification of vascular risk factors, antiplatelet therapy, and, in some instances, carotid endarterectomy. Anticoagulation has been shown to effectively prevent cardiac embolism, which causes up to 25–30% of all ischemic strokes.[40] Similarly, selected patients with acute ischemic stroke have improved neurologic recovery from intravenous thrombolytic therapy.

Although technologic advances have made it possible to identify a cause for most strokes, up to 40% of all ischemic strokes elude extensive testing and are often labeled *cryptogenic*.[110] Current and future clinical, biomedical, and epidemiologic research may help identify potentially treatable risk factors that account for many of these strokes. Such recently identified risk factors include high levels of the amino acid homocystine, which is believed to cause premature arteriosclerosis, and patent foramen ovale (PFO) as a source of cardioembolic strokes. Advances in hematology have identified lupus anticoagulant/antiphospholipid antibody as a risk factor for myocardial infarctions and ischemic strokes, especially in younger individuals.

Stroke units and acute stroke interventions may potentially reduce the morbidity and mortality associated with ischemic strokes, prompting clinicians to take an aggressive approach toward the treatment and rehabilitation of individuals with stroke.[56]

This chapter provides an overview of the recent advances in the treatment and prevention of acute strokes from diverse causes.

RISK FACTORS AND ATHEROTHROMBOTIC STROKES

The primary prevention of stroke involves the early identification and aggressive treatment of vascular risk factors (Tables 2 and 3).[60]

Over the last three decades, the mortality associated with all types of strokes has substantially decreased. Strokes remain an age-associated disease, with the incidence increasing ninefold between ages 55–64 and 85, bringing into light the limitations of primary preventive measures in cerebrovascular disease.[16]

An increased understanding of the natural history of stenotic cerebral blood vessels has contributed to the development of effective medical and surgical interventions that can prevent ischemic strokes. Additionally, the widespread availability of treatments for the vascular risk factors has contributed to an annual decrease in the incidence of ischemic strokes. Yet, strokes continue to affect 500,000 individuals annually in the United States.[15] Unfortunately, many of these strokes are the result of long-standing vascular risk factors (both known and still unidentified) compounded by racial predilection and genetic susceptibility, which provoke the development of arteriosclerosis in the cerebral vasculature. Established risk factors are described below.

Hypertension

Other than age, hypertension remains the most important independent risk factor due to its frequency and strong relationship with ischemic and hemorrhagic strokes. The overall decline in the incidence of stroke has been attributed to the judicious diagnosis and prompt treatment of high blood pressure.[68]

Ischemic Heart Disease

Ischemic heart disease remains a major cause of death—up to 30% in some series—among stroke survivors.[107] Additionally, it forms an important concurrent co-morbid condition in individuals with cerebrovascular disease.[107] Coronary artery disease

TABLE 2. TOAST Classification of High- and Medium-Risk Sources of Cardioembolism

High-Risk Sources	Medium-Risk Sources
Mechanical prosthetic valve	Mitral valve prolapse
Mitral stenosis with atrial fibrillation	Mitral anulus calcification
Atrial fibrillation (other than loan atrial fibrillation)	Mitral stenosis without atrial fibrillation
Left atrial/atrial appendage thrombus	Left atrial turbulence (smoke)
Sick sinus syndrome	Atrial septal aneurysm
Recent myocardial infarction (< 4 weeks)	Patent foramen ovale
Left ventricular thrombus	Atrial flutter
Dilated cardiomyopathy	Lone atrial fibrillation
Akinetic left ventricular segment	Bioprosthetic cardiac valve
Atrial myxoma	Nonbacterial thrombotic endocarditis
Infective endocarditis	Congestive heart failure
	Hypokinetic left ventricular segment
	Myocardial infarction (> 4 wk, < 6 mo)

TOAST = Trial of ORG 10172 in Acute Stroke Treatment

TABLE 3. Stroke Risk Factors

	Treatment Specifically Effective	Treatment of Associated Factors Effective	Treatment of Factors in Combination	Treatment Not Possible
Established Factors	Hypertension Cardiac disease Transient ischemic attacks Cigarette smoking Alcohol abuse Illicit drug abuse Elevated lipids	Age Gender Heredo-familial Race Prior strokes Diabetes mellitus	Elevated hematocrit Elevated fibrinogen Sickle cell disease Lupus anticoagulant Asymptomatic structural lesions (bruits)	
Probable Risk Factors	Homocystine			
Factors Not Well Established	Oral contraceptives Sedentary lifestyle Obesity Hyperuricemia Infection	Migraine and migraine equivalents		Geographic location Season and climate Socioeconomic factors Personality type

Adapted from Dyken ML: Stroke risk factors. In Norris JW, Hachinski VC (eds): Prevention of Stroke. New York, Springer-Verlag, 1991, pp 83–101.

contributes directly (from myocardial infarctions with resultant hypokinetic/akinetic segments, mural thrombi, or low cardiac output states, which contribute to 25% or more of cardioembolic strokes) or indirectly (nonvalvular atrial fibrillation and other cardiac rhythms that predispose to cerebral embolism and account for 45% of all identified cardioembolic strokes) to cerebrovascular disease.[20,59] All patients with cerebrovascular disease should have a basic noninvasive cardiac work-up to identify occult ischemic heart disease, which otherwise could be missed.[45]

Carotid Bruits and Asymptomatic Carotid Stenosis

Bruits heard on auscultation of the carotid arteries have sensitivity of only about 50% in predicting underlying carotid stenosis.[57] With established carotid artery stenosis, bruits carry a high positive predictive value and specificity as predictors of carotid luminal narrowing; therefore, the clinical value of auscultation of carotid arteries in asymptomatic patients remains unclear.[57]

The several prospective population-based studies that have followed hundreds of patients with asymptomatic carotid stenosis show that the risk of stroke is related to the severity and progression of carotid stenosis with a hierarchy of risk associated with increasing stenosis.[76] Published results show that the annual risk of stroke is about 3% per year in individuals with all grades of asymptomatic carotid artery stenosis; the currently accepted surgical morbidity from carotid endarterectomy is up to 3.9% for the first year after surgery.[7]

Transient Ischemic Attacks

Although transient ischemic attacks (TIAs) are major risk factors for strokes, only about 10–25% of all strokes are preceded by TIAs. About one of every three TIAs results in stroke.[106] In the Cooperative Study of Transient Ischemic Attacks, the median duration of carotid distribution TIAs was 14 minutes and that of vertebrobasilar TIAs 8 minutes.[30] TIAs may herald strokes of all types, but their frequency varies depending on their etiology. TIAs are most common in patients with large-artery atherothrombotic disease.[30,106] Recent stroke series show that TIAs occur in 25–50% of atherothrombotic infarcts, but only in 11–30% of cardioembolic strokes and 11–14% of lacunar strokes.[106]

People who have TIAs are at high risk for stroke. The overall risk of stroke after a TIA is 24–29% in the next 5 years.[30] The risk is 4–8% in the first month and 12–13% in the first year.[30] The risk of stroke increases 13- to 16-fold in the first year and about sevenfold over the next 5 years.[30] Patients with TIAs from carotid stenosis that is in excess of 70% and symptoms referable to the cerebral hemispheres have a 40% risk of stroke in 2 years.[30] Isolated monocular TIAs, such as amaurosis fugax, transient monocular blindness, and transient scotomas, and vertebrobasilar TIAs have a better prognosis.[30] Younger patients with TIAs are at lower risk for stroke than older individuals.[30]

Since TIAs serve as ominous warnings for strokes, they should be considered a neurologic emergency. The diagnostic work-up to determine the cause of the TIA should be performed in a timely manner. Unless there is extremely high suspicion that the TIA is cardiac in origin, all patients should be started on antiplatelet drugs pending diagnostic tests.[30]

Smoking

Smoking has been clearly established as a risk factor for strokes independent of age and hypertension, as shown by the 26-year follow-up from the Framingham study and the results of a meta-analysis of 32 other studies.[90] Most studies show a relative risk value of 1.5–2.[109] Heavy cigarette use further escalates the risk of stroke.

The Framingham study, the Nurses Health Study, and the Honolulu Heart Program have shown that the cessation of smoking can reduce the risk of stroke within 5 years to that of nonsmokers.[25]

Alcohol and Drug Abuse

Excessive and prolonged alcohol abuse either in isolation or compounded with illicit drug use is associated with an increased risk of ischemic and hemorrhagic strokes.[43] In contrast, consumption of 2–4 ounces of alcohol per day can increase the high-density lipoprotein cholesterol level and may lower the risk of coronary artery disease.[58]

Diabetes

Several trials have shown diabetes to be an independent risk factor for ischemic stroke.[1] The risks of stroke are particularly higher when other vascular risk factors and coronary artery disease compound diabetes.[1] The prevention of frequent or prolonged hyperglycemia and the treatment of concurrent vascular risk factors remain an effective primary prevention measure.[10] Diabetic patients are also at higher risk for complications from carotid endarterectomy and cerebral angiography.[18]

Elevated Lipid Levels

The role of elevated low-density lipoprotein (LDL) cholesterol in the development of atherothrombotic strokes is still poorly established,[47] which could reflect the heterogeneous nature of stroke and the results of studies performed prior to the availability of computed tomography.[47] These studies had methodologic flaws and had little means of excluding hemorrhagic strokes and probable cardioembolic strokes. Because LDL cholesterol is the most important independent risk factor for ischemic coronary artery disease and is easily treatable, all patients with cerebrovascular disease and elevated LDL cholesterol should be treated with pharmacologic agents.[62]

Homocystine

Elevated serum homocystine may be a treatable risk factor for strokes.[22] Hyperhomocysteinemia occurs in about 20% of the population and may account for 30–40% of all premature arteriosclerosis.[14] Additionally, homocystine may enhance coagulation-producing hypercoagulability.[44] The underlying mechanism seems to be secondary to free radical activation and endothelial damage with impaired nitric oxide function.[92] The high prevalence of hyperhomocysteinemia has been attributed to the following factors: deficiency of folic acid, vitamin B_{12}, and pyridoxine (B_6) and/or inherited abnormality of any one or more of three enzymes that are involved in the metabolism of homocystine for which the above vitamins act as cofactors.[14] Daily high-dose vitamin therapy has been shown to reduce levels of this amino acid and may reduce the risks of heart attack and stroke.[44] A major clinical trial is underway to assess the effectiveness of high-dose vitamin therapy in the reduction of vascular events among patients with nondisabling strokes and elevated homocystine levels.[92]

Antiphospholipid Antibodies and Cerebral Ischemia

Antiphospholipid antibodies are immunoglobulins of the IgG, IgM, and IgA classes with specificity for anionic and neutral phospholipids and include anticardiolipin antibody and lupus anticoagulant.[99] These antibodies can occur in isolation or with systemic lupus erythematosus, other autoimmune disorders, and systemic malignancy.[99] Antiphospholipid antibodies are associated with systemic thromboembolic events, myocardial infarction, and ischemic strokes, particularly in younger individuals with no other risk factors.[99] Some of these patients may develop recurrent strokes and vascular cognitive impairment. Prevention of systemic thromboembolic events and ischemic strokes involves anticoagulation with warfarin.[99]

Patent Foramen Ovale and Atrial Septal Aneurysm

PFO has been linked to stroke in multiple case-control studies involving young individuals.[26] The proposed mechanism for stroke from PFO involves paradoxical embolism.[26] Echocardiography with the intravenous injection of saline bubbles demonstrates some degree of intra-arterial shunting, particularly with Valsalva-provoking activities such as coughing and during cardiac systole, in 10–22% of normal control subjects.[86] Transesophageal echocardiography (TEE) is more sensitive than precordial echocardiography in the detection of small shunts.[86]

Case-control studies typically show that PFOs have an increased prevalence among younger individuals with TIA or ischemic stroke (32–48%), particularly in cryptogenic strokes (49–61%).[105]

About 25% of young patients with PFO-associated strokes have atrial septal aneurysms, which have been associated with a considerably higher stroke risk than either abnormality alone.[11]

Atrial septal aneurysms are detected by TEE in about 0.2–4% of patients undergoing echocardiography and in 1–21% of patients with TIAs and ischemic strokes.[11] Atrial septal aneurysms are often associated with PFO, atrial septal defects, and mitral valve prolapse.[28] Potential mechanisms for embolism include paradoxical embolism, intra-aneurysm thrombi formation, and coexistent myxomatous degeneration of the mitral valve.[28]

SURGICAL PREVENTION OF STROKE

Symptomatic Carotid Stenosis

Carotid endarterectomy has become an accepted surgical procedure for selected symptomatic patients with angiographic stenosis in excess of 70%.[77]

Despite the negative results of the carotid endarterectomy trial in 1970, the number of surgical procedures for symptomatic carotid artery stenosis continued to increase.[35] However, in the first 15 years following this study the surgical morbidity was variable.[66] Published results from different case series had shown both benefit (low morbidity) and unacceptably high complication rates (above 10%).[12]

In the late 1980s, the European Carotid Surgery Trial (ECST) and North American Carotid Endarterectomy Trial (NASCET) started to assess the presumed benefit of carotid endarterectomy as a preventive measure for strokes, for different grades of carotid stenosis, compared to best available medical management.[33,77] The NASCET results for high-grade carotid artery stenosis (70–99%) were available within 4 years after the beginning of the trial. NASCET had shown carotid endarterectomy to be clearly more beneficial than medical management in the prevention of strokes for patients with 70–99% carotid stenosis, on the ipsilateral side of either a TIA or nondisabling stroke within 120 days of the vascular event.[77] A 17% absolute risk reduction and a 65% relative risk reduction from carotid endarterectomy illustrated the benefit of surgery.[77] A declining benefit from carotid endarterectomy was observed with decreasing stenosis from 99–70%.[77] The ECST had shown similar results although the mode of estimation of carotid stenosis was different.[33]

Preliminary results for the NASCET moderate stenosis group (40–69%) show an overall benefit from carotid endarterectomy for 50–69% stenosis. There is incremental benefit from surgery with higher degrees of moderate stenosis.

Symptomatic patients with low moderate stenosis (50–60%) require careful presurgical assessment based on concurrent medical problems. As a group, patients with moderate stenosis and ocular events derive no benefit from surgery. The interval between the ischemic event and surgery is also important; for the group of patients with 40–69% stenosis, the overall benefit from surgery equals that of medical management in 2 years. Women and diabetics with symptomatic moderate stenosis receive no benefit from surgery.

Carotid endarterectomy is an effective preventive measure for stroke only when associated with acceptable morbidity and mortality rates (NASCET 5.8%, ECST 7.5%). Perioperative morbidity or mortality rates that approach 10% annul any observed benefit from this procedure.[71a]

Asymptomatic Carotid Stenosis

Five prospective randomized clinical trials have assessed the benefit of prophylactic carotid endarterectomy in asymptomatic carotid stenosis for the primary prevention of stroke: the Carotid Artery Surgery Asymptomatic Operation Versus Aspirin trial, Mayo Asymptomatic Carotid Endarterectomy trial, the Veterans Administration Cooperative Asymptomatic Stenosis Study, the Asymptomatic Carotid Surgery Trial, and the Asymptomatic Carotid Atherosclerosis Study. The results of all but the latter trial were either inconclusive or showed no benefit of carotid endarterectomy versus medical management.[8]

The Asymptomatic Carotid Atherosclerosis Study failed to show any benefit from carotid endarterectomy in preventing disabling strokes; however, there was an overall benefit from surgery (for stenosis $\geq$ 60%). The benefits of surgery versus medical treatment were observed only after 3–5 years or more, depending on the surgical morbidity and mortality.[8] Furthermore, women did not benefit from carotid endarterectomy. This study was not able to determine a possible benefit of prophylactic carotid endarterectomy for higher grades of asymptomatic carotid stenosis, where the risks of stroke may be higher.[8]

Current recommendations for the management of patients with asymptomatic carotid artery stenosis include the aggressive modification of all identified vascular risk factors and empiric aspirin therapy for the primary prevention of related coronary morbidity or mortality and possibly TIAs and strokes. Patients should not have carotid endarterectomy for asymptomatic carotid stenosis except under exceptional circumstances.[8,17a]

Carotid plaque morphology may be another important factor contributing to the instability of arteriosclerotic plaques.[31] The European trial, Asymptomatic Carotid Stenosis at Risk Study, plans to assess the relationship between carotid plaque morphology on ultrasound and cerebrovascular events.[74] Although carotid plaque ulcers and interplaque hemorrhage have been implicated in escalating the risk of stroke in symptomatic patients, the significance of these phenomena in asymptomatic carotid artery stenosis is unclear.[31]

MEDICAL PREVENTION OF STROKE

Antithrombotic Therapy in Stroke Prevention

PRIMARY PREVENTION WITH ASPIRIN

Aspirin continues to be the most widely used antiplatelet agent for the primary prevention of ischemic strokes and cardiovascular disease.[74] European and North

American studies show that aspirin can significantly reduce the incidence of nonfatal myocardial infarction (MI) in individuals older than 50.[9,94] The same studies show a less dramatic reduction in the incidence of ischemic stroke (25% relative risk reduction) with the same dose of aspirin (80–325 mg/day).[9,94]

In the 1993 meta-analysis of 145 randomized trials testing antiplatelet agents, the Antiplatelet Trialists Collaboration Group (ATCG) concluded that "antiplatelet treatment might reduce vascular events (nonfatal MI, stroke or vascular death) by about 25%."[5] Therefore, current data suggest that asymptomatic individuals older than 50 who are at risk for coronary artery disease and ischemic strokes can benefit by consuming 100–325 mg of aspirin daily for the primary prevention of vascular disease.[5]

SECONDARY PREVENTION WITH ASPIRIN, TICLOPIDINE, CLOPIDOGREL, AND DIPYRIDAMOLE

Aspirin.   Aspirin remains a safe and effective medication for the long-term secondary prevention of strokes and coronary artery disease.[5] The ATCG meta-analysis of 17 trials among people with a past history of stroke or TIA reported aspirin to demonstrate a 22% odds reduction for nonfatal stroke, nonfatal MI, or vascular death.[5] The 2-year risk was 18% for patients treated with antiplatelet drugs and 22% for control groups. Although this meta-analysis had shown a similar risk reduction in men and women, young and elderly, hypertensive and nonhypertensive patients, and diabetic and nondiabetic patients, some of the individual aspirin studies failed to show any benefits of aspirin for women.[5]

The optimal dose of aspirin that is needed for the secondary prevention of stroke remains unsettled.[39] The Food and Drug Administration recommends an aspirin dose of 1300 mg/day for the secondary prevention of stroke. In Europe 30–80 mg of aspirin per day continues to be in favor.[100,101] Data for the efficacy of lower doses of aspirin are available only from trials involving minor strokes and TIAs.[51]

The ATCG retrospectively compared the incidence of major vascular events, including strokes, in three trials that had used an aspirin dosage of 300–325 mg/day and 15 other trials that had used 900–1500 mg/day.[5] The patients on lower doses of aspirin had more strokes than the patients taking higher doses.[5] Therefore, the authors concluded that 975 mg or more of aspirin might be necessary for the optimal prevention of strokes even though gastrointestinal hemorrhage and other toxic manifestations were less common in individuals taking lower doses of aspirin.[5]

Ticlopidine.   Ticlopidine is biochemically, structurally, and pharmacologically different than aspirin. Ticlopidine acts on the platelet adenosine phosphate system. In the Canadian American Ticlopidine Study (CATS) ticlopidine was compared to placebo in noncardioembolic strokes in 1053 patients.[42] Ticlopidine had produced a 23% risk reduction in an intention-to-treat analysis and a 30% risk reduction in the efficacy analysis.[42] The risk reduction for nonfatal or fatal recurrent stroke was 33%.[42] In the Ticlopidine Aspirin Stroke Study (TASS), ticlopidine was compared to aspirin (1300 mg/day) among 3069 patients who had a TIA or minor stroke.[52] There was an overall 12% reduction in stroke or death at 3 years but a dramatic 47% risk reduction in fatal or nonfatal stroke in the first year for individuals treated with ticlopidine versus aspirin.[52]

Therefore, the two major studies of ticlopidine—CATS and TASS—had shown ticlopidine to be more beneficial than aspirin in the secondary prevention of TIAs and stroke, particularly in the first year of treatment, with an added benefit for women and vertebrobasilar circulation symptoms; however, the 1993 meta-analysis by ATCG determined that ticlopidine added only an approximated 10% increment to the benefit of aspirin,[5] which did not appear to be statistically significant.[5] Additionally, treatment with ticlopidine is associated with a significant increase in diarrhea (6.4%) and rash (3.4%) relative to placebo (1.7% and 0.9%, respectively).[42,52] Ticlopidine also can cause neutropenia in 1% of patients and, rarely, thrombotic thrombocytopenic purpura.[38]

Clopidogrel. The recently completed trial, Clopidogrel Versus Aspirin in Patients at Risk for Ischemic Events (CAPRIE), had assessed the efficacy of clopidogrel 75 mg/day over aspirin 325 mg/day in reducing the incidence of ischemic strokes, MI, and vascular deaths in patients with recent ischemic stroke, recent MI, and symptomatic peripheral vascular disease.[19] Data were collected on 2144 patients who were randomized to one of the two treatments modalities, with a mean follow-up of 1.91 years.[19]

The primary analysis of CAPRIE using the outcomes of ischemic stroke, MI, or vascular death showed that 939 patients randomized to clopidogrel and 1021 to aspirin experienced one of these events. The intention-to-treat analysis showed a relative risk reduction of 8.7% in favor of clopidogrel over aspirin (absolute risk reduction is less impressive—about one third of 1% a year).[19] A subgroup analysis showed a relative risk reduction over aspirin of 7.3% for stroke and MI, with 23.8% for peripheral vascular disease.[19]

The pharmacologic actions of clopidogrel are similar to those of ticlopidine, and the incidence of side effects, particularly diarrhea, rash, and neutropenia, is lower.[19]

Dipyridamole. Dipyridamole was shown to add no benefit to aspirin in the French AICLA trial. However, the results of the European Stroke Prevention Study 2 suggested that 200 mg twice a day of time-release dipyridimole was more effective than aspirin (25 mg/day) in the prevention of stroke, MI, and vascular disease after TIAs or minor strokes.[27] The relative risk reduction for stroke was 19% for aspirin, 16% for dipyridamole, and 37% for the combination of both. The relative risk reduction for stroke or death was 13% for aspirin, 15% for dipyridamole, and 24% for the combination.[27] The quality of the monitoring in this trial was shown to be suboptimal, thereby bringing into question the reliability of the results.[32]

ACUTE STROKE

No published data exist on the differences in vascular outcomes associated with the use of aspirin, ticlopidine, or clopidogrel in acute strokes even though all of these drugs have an established role in the secondary prevention of strokes.[13] Although the optimal dose of aspirin that is necessary for the secondary prevention of TIAs and strokes is unknown, data suggest that the cardiac dose of aspirin (80 mg) may not be enough.[84] Current recommendations are that patients should start taking aspirin at a dose of 1300 mg/day. Individuals who experience gastrointestinal toxicity with higher doses of aspirin may reduce the dose to a minimum of 325 mg/day.[5,9,39,74,94] Patients who are on optimal dose of aspirin at the time of a stroke may require the use of an alternate antiplatelet agent, but little research exists to support this statement.

Anticoagulation with standard heparin or with the low–molecular-weight heparinoids has not shown any added benefit in improving functional outcome from atheroembolic strokes.[48] Additionally, heparin and heparin-like compounds may provoke hemorrhagic transformation of ischemic strokes. The indication for heparin in progressing strokes, crescendo TIAs, and vertebrobasilar thrombosis remains unproven.[91] Anticoagulation is clearly beneficial in the secondary prevention of cardioembolic strokes, as discussed below.

Treatment for Elevated Lipids

In 1987, the introduction of HMG CoA (3-hydroxy-3-methylglutaryl coenzyme A) synthetase inhibitors had revolutionized antilipid therapy. The Asymptomatic Carotid Artery Progression Study had shown lovastatin (20–40 mg/day) was effective in reducing the maximal intimal-medial thickness in the extracranial arteries of asymptomatic individuals with moderate arteriosclerosis and elevated LDL cholesterol.[41]

In the Scandinavian Simvastatin Survival Study, 4444 patients with MI and total serum cholesterol of 5.5–8.0 mmol/L were randomized to receive simvastatin or placebo.[87] Rates of nonfatal cerebrovascular events were 2.7% (n = 14) and 4.3% (n = 12) in the simvastatin and placebo groups, respectively.[87] There was no difference in the incidence of fatal strokes in the placebo or treatment groups.[87] A post hoc analysis of all cerebrovascular events, fatal and nonfatal, had shown a reduction in the incidence of TIAs, nonembolic strokes, and intervention-related strokes (70 events in the simvastatin group and 98 events in the placebo group, resulting in a relative risk of 0.70, 95% confidence interval 0.52–0.96, p = 0.024).[3] Such results have led researchers to postulate a potential plaque-stabilizing effect from the HMG-CoA synthase inhibitors such as simvastatin.[98]

Postmenopausal Estrogen Therapy

Postmenopausal hormone replacement has a well-established role in the prevention of coronary artery disease and ischemic strokes.[69] In the 10-year follow-up of 50,000 women in the Nurses Health Study, postmenopausal estrogen use was associated with a reduction in the incidence of coronary morbidity and mortality, but no such effect was seen with ischemic stroke.[93] An analysis of follow-up data from the National Health and Nutrition Examination Survey revealed that postmenopausal hormone replacement therapy in caucasian women was associated with a 31% decrease in the incidence of stroke and a 63% reduction of mortality from strokes.[37]

CARDIAC EMBOLISM AND ISCHEMIC STROKE

Epidemiology

Embolic events from the heart cause 25–30% of all identified ischemic strokes (see Table 1).[40] Newer technologic advances such as TEE and magnetic resonance imaging of the heart have facilitated the identification of an increased number of cardiac anomalies that may account for cardioembolic strokes (see Table 2). Some case series show that up to 45% of all cryptogenic ischemic strokes have a probable cardioembolic etiology.[85]

Diagnosis and Management

Although the identification of cardiac disease that may cause TIAs or strokes is desirable, in many instances the neurologic history, mode of presentation of the symptoms, and relevant cardiac/neuroradiologic tests may be the only means of assessing the likelihood that an embolic event is cardiac in etiology rather than from the carotid vessels, because the prevention of embolism from the heart is different than that of carotid artery-to-artery embolism.

About 15–40% of ischemic strokes have no identifiable cause. TEE has made it possible to define a greater variety of cardiac structural abnormalities that may potentially contribute to cerebral embolism.[55,85] Examples of such recent findings include PFO, spontaneous echo contrast in the left atrium, left atrial size in excess of 2.5 cm, and aortic arch arteriosclerotic plaques.[55,61,85] Conventional transthoracic echocardiograms have a low yield in identifying such pathology.[89] Holter and prolonged electrocardiographic monitoring also have a low yield in the diagnosis of paroxysmal cardiac arrhythmias such as atrial fibrillation and sick sinus syndrome. Using a combination of these modalities, these paroxysmal arrhythmias are diagnosed in only 4% of patients.[65,89]

The issue of early versus delayed anticoagulation for a potential cardioembolic stroke remains unclear; the TOAST (Trial of ORG 10172 in Acute Stroke Treatment) study showed the risks of a recurrence as about 3% per day in the first 2 weeks.[67] The early initiation of anticoagulation for cardioembolic strokes should be weighed against the possibility of hemorrhagic conversion of the acute stroke. Although petechial hemorrhage forms the normal pathologic change observed in all ischemic strokes, cardioembolic strokes have a propensity for spontaneous hemorrhagic conversion.[50] The time limit for hemorrhagic transformation has not been well studied but is felt to occur 2–4 days after the stroke.[78] Potential predictors of hemorrhagic change include large strokes, older patients, and persistent uncontrolled hypertension after the stroke.[4]

Atrial Fibrillation

Atrial fibrillation remains a common cardiac arrhythmia, particularly in individuals older than 60.[108] It occurs in 5% of persons older than 60 and escalates to affect 13% of individuals older than 82.[108] Nonvalvular atrial fibrillation is associated with a fivefold increase in the risk of stroke and accounts for 45% of all cardioembolic strokes.[108] The overall stroke risk in patients with chronic atrial fibrillation is about 5% per year.[108]

Randomized clinical trials have shown that warfarin anticoagulation is beneficial in reducing the stroke risk in asymptomatic patients with nonvalvular atrial fibrillation.[6] The relative risk reduction for stroke ranges from 42–86%, and the major hemorrhagic rates for warfarin range from 0.8–2.1%.[6] These studies also show that there is a modest risk reduction for stroke with aspirin.[6] The Stroke Prevention in Atrial Fibrillation III trial among high-risk individuals with nonvalvular atrial fibrillation demonstrated that warfarin therapy with an INR (international normalized ratio) of 2–3 was superior to aspirin and low-dose warfarin (INR < 1.5) in the prevention of stroke.[6,95]

The recommendations of the Fourth American College of Chest Physicians Consensus Conference on Antithrombotic Therapy are for long-term warfarin therapy (INR 2–3) for nonvalvular atrial fibrillation (individuals should have no contraindications for anticoagulation), except in patients younger than 60 without any associated cardiovascular disease where aspirin therapy is enough.[63]

Prosthetic Cardiac Valves

Warfarin is beneficial in preventing strokes among patients with prosthetic cardiac valves. Although patients with mechanical heart valves require life-long anticoagulation, individuals with bioprosthetic valves require only temporary anticoagulation with warfarin before maintenance therapy with antiplatelet agents.[24] The combination of low-dose aspirin and warfarin is more effective than warfarin alone in reducing mortality and major embolic events in patients with prosthetic cardiac valves and associated atrial fibrillation.[102]

Myocardial Infarction and Cardiac Hypokinetic Segments

Anticoagulation for possible embolism from acute anterior MI or ventricular aneurysm (with or without mural thrombi) remains controversial.[34] The Warfarin in Reinfarction study had shown that warfarin is superior to aspirin in reducing the incidence of recurrent MI, strokes, and death in individuals younger than 75 with acute MI.[34,104]

The current recommendation for an individual with acute MI and associated thrombi includes heparin therapy that is subsequently followed by warfarin.[103] Patients with only hypokinetic segment(s) from an acute anterior MI are less at risk for stroke and warrant oral warfarin therapy at least temporarily (3–6 months) to minimize the risk of systemic and cerebral thromboembolism.[103]

STROKE PREVENTION IN CARDIAC SURGERY

Coronary artery bypass grafting (CABG) surgery is associated with overt clinical strokes in 1–5% of patients.[72] There may be up to a 66% incidence of cognitive impairment for 12 months or more after such surgery, most likely from the effect of perioperative cerebral ischemia compounded by cerebral embolism from particulate arteriosclerotic debris.[72,97] Risk factors that may account for at least some of these strokes include aortic arteriosclerosis with embolization of plaque at the time of aortic clamping; hemodynamic cerebral ischemia from asymptomatic carotid stenosis and intraoperative hypotension/hypovolemia; mechanical ventilation; postoperative atrial fibrillation in up to 35% of patients; and acute myocardial ischemia/infarctions related to surgery.[49]

Carotid Stenosis

PREOPERATIVE RISK

Most studies fail to show a relationship among carotid bruits, asymptomatic carotid stenosis, and CABG-related perioperative strokes, even in patients with severe carotid stenosis.[82] Data pertaining to the risk of perioperative stroke in symptomatic high-grade carotid stenosis and hemodynamically significant carotid artery stenosis are limited or inconclusive.[21,82]

PERIOPERATIVE AND INTRAOPERATIVE RISK

Although current recommendations are to delay CABG surgery up to 3 months in individuals with TIAs and nondebilitating strokes, the necessity for emergent surgical intervention often arises, such as with medically refractory unstable angina.[83] The risk of perioperative stroke may be assessed and possibly reduced by the application of preoperative transcranial Doppler (TCD) blood flow measurements, which is still an experimental technique, to assess the cerebrovascular reserve prior to surgery.[73] Assessment of cerebral perfusion with intraoperative TCD blood flow studies may be useful in identifying an acute compromise of cerebral perfusion and may aid in determining the necessity for pharmacologic intervention to improve cerebral blood flow.[73]

More than 2 hours of extracorporeal pump time during CABG surgery may be an independent risk factor for strokes and cognitive impairment.[96] Cerebral perfusion pressure below 60 mm Hg has been implicated as a risk factor for stroke, especially in high-risk patients, such as those with long-standing hypertension, history of strokes or recent TIAs, hemodynamically significant carotid stenosis, older individuals with autonomic insufficiency, and generalized arteriosclerosis.

Surgical expertise with the modification of technique may aid in reducing the shower of emboli to the brain with intraoperative TCD microemboli detection aiding in assessment of the extent of cerebral embolization.[80]

POSTOPERATIVE RISK

Atrial fibrillation after CABG surgery occurs in about 30–40% of patients. Although there may be a higher incidence of stroke in such patients, the relative risk of stroke from CABG associated atrial fibrillation is unclear.[79]

Postoperative encephalopathy may occur in 4–12% of all patients who undergo CABG. Subtle neuropsychological evidence of cognitive deficits has been described in 65–85% of CABG patients, even after 1 year; up to 35% of these patients develop frank cognitive impairment of different degrees.[23]

Acute Stroke Interventions

THROMBOLYSIS

Intravenous thrombolysis with tissue plasminogen activator (TPA) has been approved by the Food and Drug Administration for thrombolysis in acute ischemic stroke and should be administered within 3 hours after the onset of symptoms using the criteria of the National Institutes of Health's TPA Stroke Study (NIH-TPA).[81] The NIH-TPA trials have demonstrated a consistent and persuasive improvement in the 3-month outcomes based on three different outcome assessment scales: Barthel Index, Rankin Scale, and Glasgow Outcome Scale.[75] The guidelines for the safe use of this drug are similar to those found in the NIH-TPA stroke study protocol. The use of TPA is associated with an approximated tenfold increase in intracerebral hemorrhage (6% for TPA and 0.6% in placebo).[75] The risk of intracerebral hemorrhage is relatively higher in patients with larger strokes, cardioembolic strokes, and uncontrolled hypertension at the time of the acute stroke.[75]

Patients older than 79 were not included in the study. It remains unclear whether age is an independent risk factor for intracerebral hemorrhage from TPA at the dose used for thrombolysis in strokes.[64]

All forms of intra-arterial thrombolysis for occluded cerebral vessels remain research techniques until proven otherwise. The efficacy of intra-arterial infusions of pro-urokinase by the superselective catheterization of the middle cerebral artery is under study by the Prolysis in Acute Cerebral Thrombo-Embolism Trial (PROACT). The application of urokinase for intra-arterial thrombolysis for basilar artery thrombosis is under investigation by the Australian Urokinase Stroke Trial Collaborators.[17]

Several neuroprotective agents are under investigation in phase 2 and 3 clinical trials, but none of them are currently available for widespread clinical use.

Prevention of Subarachnoid Hemorrhage

NATURAL HISTORY

About 60% of subarachnoid bleeds are due to ruptured aneurysms.[71] The immediate mortality rate from aneurysmal subarachnoid hemorrhage is high; about 30% of patients die before admission to hospital.[71] There is a further 65% mortality over the first 3 months after aneurysmal bleeds.[71] Much of the morbidity and mortality from aneurysmal bleeds occurs within 2 weeks after the initial hemorrhage, with the risks of rebleeding being greatest in the first 24 hours. Rebleeding accounts for up to 60% of all mortality from aneurysm ruptures.[71]

DIAGNOSIS

Up to 70% of patients have symptoms such as focal headaches, eye pain, facial pain, and dizziness that may herald a major bleed.[88] These nonspecific symptoms are often taken lightly by physicians and patients, at a time when diagnosis and interventions are desirable.[88] Efforts should be made to identify patients with these nonspecific symptoms, especially when a family history of subarachnoid bleeding exists.

Although computed tomography has 90% sensitivity in identifying subarachnoid hemorrhages, sentinel bleeds are often missed. High-resolution magnetic resonance imaging/MR-angiography of the brain may be useful in identifying both minor sentinel bleeds and moderate-size aneurysms (> 4 mm), but cerebral angiography remains the gold standard test to diagnose, localize, and estimate the size of aneurysms.[53] It is most desirable to diagnose cerebral aneurysms prior to hemorrhage, when interventions are relatively safer.

Routine screening of patients at high risk for cerebral aneurysms may be useful. Such high-risk groups include a family history of aneurysms, Marfan's disease, polycystic kidney disease, fibromuscular dysplasia, and coarctation of the aorta.[36,53,88]

PREVENTION OF REBLEEDING

The rate of rebleeding peaks between day 1–14, with the risks being highest in the first 24 hours.[88] Up to 20% of patients who do not have surgical intervention have another hemorrhage in the first 2 weeks, 50% have another hemorrhage within the first 6 months, and the rate thereafter is 3% per year.[88] The mortality associated with rebleeding is higher than with the initial bleed. Early surgical intervention is therefore a logical way of reducing mortality in all patients, except in those who appear to be in stupor or coma.[88] Patients who are poor surgical candidates or have aneurysms that are surgically inaccessible or surgically technically difficult may be candidates for endovascular treatment.[53,88] Endovascular treatment, consisting of platinum coiling of aneurysms to induce thrombosis, is generally reserved for unruptured aneurysms and is limited to specialized centers because of the technical expertise that is necessary to perform it.[53,88]

Preoperative patients with ruptured aneurysms ideally should be managed in a neurologic intensive care unit where the mean arterial pressures are carefully regulated pharmacologically to minimize tension on the aneurysm wall and reduce the risk of rebleeding. Patients also may require careful regulation of cerebral perfusion pressures and intracranial pressures, in the face of a dysfunctional cerebral autoregulatory mechanism.[53,88]

Seizures may occur in 10–25% of patients and can precipitate rehemorrhage.[88] Hydrocephalus is another common complication that may occur during the acute (0–24 hours), subacute (24 hours–7 days), or delayed (> 10 days after hemorrhage) phases.[88] Subacute hydrocephalus is often difficult to differentiate from vasospasm.[88] Cardiopulmonary complications also may occur. Neurogenic pulmonary edema and cardiac rhythm disturbances including supraventricular and ventricular arrhythmias are present in up to 90% of patients.[88]

Vasospasm remains a leading cause of disability following subarachnoid bleeds. Angiographic evidence of vasospasm occurs in up to 60–75% of patients.[88] Clinically delayed cerebral ischemia within the first 2 weeks from vasospasm occurs in 14–40% of patients. Aneurysmal rehemorrhage, subacute hydrocephalus, and metabolic disturbances should be ruled out prior to diagnosing vasospasm.[88] Typical clinical manifestations of vasospasm include worsening of headache, personality change, and agitation.[88] Additionally, hemiparesis, aphasia, and hemisensory deficit may occur if the middle cerebral artery is involved with the vasospasm. Anterior cerebral artery involvement typically produces an abulic state.[88] Vasospasm involving the posterior circulation is less common and may produce decreased level of consciousness, dysconjugate eye movements, abnormal breathing patterns, and autonomic derangement.[88]

Prevention of vasospasm involves empiric prophylactic treatment with the calcium channel blocker nimodipine for 21 days.[88] Confirmation of vasospasm and its treatment involves cerebral angiography and angioplasty of amenable lesions.[88] Hypervolemic hydration or induced hypertensive therapy with phenylephrine and dopamine have been proven to counteract vasospasm.[88]

CONCLUSION

Strokes remain the most common neurologic emergency. Acute strokes should be conceived as "brain attacks," warranting the same sense of urgency as heart attacks. There is no longer a place for therapeutic nihilism in the treatment of strokes, because acute ischemic strokes are responsive both to primary and secondary prevention and to acute therapeutic interventions.

The "decade of the brain" has witnessed a tremendous explosion of knowledge not only in basic neurobiology but also in the application of knowledge attained from clinical trials. Clinical trials have clearly shown antithrombotic therapy to be an effective treatment modality for the primary and secondary prevention of strokes and anticoagulation for the primary prevention of cardioembolic strokes. Additionally, the NASCET had established clinical criteria for carotid endarterectomy in symptomatic patients. An understanding of the relative importance of vascular risk factors involved in the development of strokes and cardiovascular disease has led to the development of effective pharmacologic agents for the treatment of these risk factors.

Technologic advances in noninvasive imaging modalities such as magnetic resonance imaging have made it possible to visualize acute strokes using magnetic resonance imaging-diffusion techniques. Color and power Doppler technology have made it feasible to noninvasively screen for and estimate carotid stenosis. Interventional radiology has witnessed the development of angioplasty and stenting procedures for extracranial and intracranial blood vessels. Endovascular therapy has facilitated the treatment of vascular malformations in the brain and cerebral aneurysms through the use of synthetic compounds and metallic coils.

Although intravenous TPA is currently the only approved treatment option for selected patients with acute ischemic stroke, TPA should be considered as a prototype for the many other acute stroke treatments in development.

REFERENCES

1. Abott RD, Donahue RP, MacMahon SW, et al: Diabetes and the risk of stroke: The Honolulu Heart Program. JAMA 257:949–952, 1987.
2. Adams H, Brott T, Crowell R, et al: Guidelines for management of patients with acute ischemic stroke: A statement for healthcare professionals from a special writing group of the Stroke Council, American Heart Association. Stroke 25:1901–1914, 1994.
3. Adams HP Jr, Byington RP, Byington RP, et al: Effect of cholesterol lowering medication on progression of mild arteriosclerotic lesions and on the risk of stroke. Cerebrovasc Dis 5:171–177, 1995.
4. Anderson JL, Kargonounis L, Allen A, et al: Older age and elevated blood pressure are risk factors for intracerebral hemorrhage after thrombolysis. Am J Cardiol 68:166–170, 1991.
5. Antiplatelet Trialists' Collaboration: Collaborative overview of randomized trials of antiplatelet treatment: Part 1. Prevention of death, myocardial infarction, and stroke by prolonged antiplatelet treatment in various categories of patients. BMJ 308:81–106, 1994.

6. Atrial Fibrillation Investigators: Risk factors for stroke and efficacy of antithrombotic therapy in atrial fibrillation: Analysis of pooled data from 5 randomized clinical trials. Arch Intern Med 154:1449–1457, 1994.

7. Barnett HJM, Haines HJ: Carotid endarterectomy for asymptomatic carotid stenosis. N Engl J Med 328:276–279, 1993.

8. Barnett HJM, Meldrum HE, Eliaziw M: The dilemma of surgical treatment for patients with asymptomatic carotid disease. Ann Intern Med 123:723–725, 1995.

9. Barnett HJM, Meldrum HE, Eliaziw M: Drugs and surgery in the prevention of ischemic stroke. N Engl J Med 332:238–248, 1995.

10. Barrett-Connor E, Khaw KT: Diabetes mellitus: An independent risk factor for stroke? Am J Epidemiol 128:116–123, 1988.

11. Belkin RN, Hurwitz BJ, Kisslo J: Atrial septal aneurysm: Association with cerebrovascular and peripheral embolic events. Stroke 18:856–862, 1988.

12. Bernstein EF, Humber PB, Collins GM, et al: Life expectancy and late stroke following carotid endarterectomy. Ann Surg 198:80–86, 1983.

13. Biller J: Medical management of acute cerebral ischemia. Neurol Clin 10:63–85, 1992.

14. Boers GHJ, Trijbels FMJ, Fowler B, et al: Heterozygosity for homocystinuria in premature peripheral and cerebral occlusive vascular disease. N Engl J Med 313:709–714, 1985.

15. Bonita R, Stewart A, Beaglehole R: International trends in stroke mortality. Stroke 21:989–992, 1990.

16. Broderick JP, Phillips SJ, Whisnant JP, et al: Incidence rates of stroke in the eighties: The end of the decline in stroke? Stroke 20:577–582, 1989.

17. Brott TG: Reopening occluded cerebral arteries. In Bogousslavsky J (ed): Acute Stroke Management. St. Louis, Mosby, 1997, pp 109–148.

17a. Brott T, Toole J: Medical compared with surgical treatment of asymptomatic carotid artery stenosis. Ann Intern Med 123:720–722, 1995.

18. Burgos LG, Ebert TL, Asiddo C, et al: Increased intraoperative cardiovascular morbidity in diabetics with autonomic neuropathy. Anesthesiology 70:591–597, 1989.

19. CAPRIE Steering Committee: A randomized clinical trial of clopidogrel versus aspirin in patients at risk for ischemic events (CAPRIE). Lancet 348:1329–1339, 1996.

20. Cerebral Embolism Task Force: Cardiogenic brain embolism. The second report of the Cerebral Embolism Task Force. Arch Neurol 46:727–743, 1989.

21. Chimowitz MI, Furlan AJ: Preventing cerebral complications of cardiac surgery. In Norris JW, Hachinski VC (eds): Prevention of Stroke. New York, Springer-Verlag, 1991, pp 219–227.

22. Clark R, Dally L, Robinson K, et al: Homocysteinemia: An independent risk factor for vascular disease. N Engl J Med 324:1149–1155, 1991.

23. CNS dysfunction after cardiac surgery: Defining the problem. Ann Thorac Surg 59:1287–1362, 1995.

24. Cohn LH, Allred EN, Disesa VJ, et al: Early and late risk of aortic valve replacement: A 12-year concomitant comparison of porcine bioprosthetic and tilting disk prosthetic aortic valves. J Thorac Cardiovasc Surg 88:695–705, 1984.

25. Colditz GA, Bonita R, Stampfer MJ, et al: Cigarette smoking and the risk of stroke in middle-aged women. N Engl J Med 318:937–941, 1988.

26. Cujec B, Polasek P, Voll C, et al: Transesophageal echocardiography in the detection of potential cardiac source of embolism in stroke patients. Stroke 22:727–733, 1991.

27. Diener HC, Cumha L, Forbes C, et al: European Stroke Prevention Study 2: Dypiradamole and aspirin in the secondary prevention of stroke. J Neurol Sci 143:1–13, 1992.

28. Di Pasquale G, Andreoli A, Grazi P, et al: Cardioembolic strokes from atrial septal aneurysm. Stroke 19:640–643, 1988.

29. Dyken ML: Stroke risk factors. In Norris JW, Hachinski VC (eds): Prevention of Stroke. New York, Springer-Verlag, 1991, pp 83–103.

30. Dyken ML, Conneally M, Haerer AF, et al: Cooperative study of the hospital frequency and character of transient ischemic attacks. 1: Background, organization and clinical survey. JAMA 237:882–886, 1997.

31. Eliasziw M, Streifler J, Fox AJ, et al: Significance of plaque ulceration in symptomatic patients with high grade carotid stenosis. Stroke 25:304–308, 1994.

32. Ensinerk M: Fraud and ethics charges hit stroke drug trial. Science 274:2004–2005, 1996.

33. European Carotid Surgery Trialists' Collaborative Group: MRC European Carotid Surgery Trial: Interim results for symptomatic patients with severe (70–99%) or with mild (0–29%) carotid stenosis. Lancet 337:1235–1243, 1991.

34. Ezekowitz MD, Azrin MA: Should patients with large anterior myocardial infarctions have echocardiography to identify left ventricular thrombus in myocardial infarction: A rationale in support of masterly inactivity. J Am Coll Cardiol 14:903–911, 1989.

35. Fields WS, Maselinkov V, Meyer JS, et al: Joint study of extracranial artery occlusion: V. Progress report of prognosis following surgery of nonsurgical treatment of transient ischemic attacks and carotid artery lesions. JAMA 211:1993–2003, 1970.
36. Findlay JM, Weir BKA: Prevention of aneurysmal subarachnoid hemorrhage. In Norris JW, Hachinski VC (eds): Prevention of Stroke. New York, Springer-Verlag, 1991, pp 247–260.
37. Finucane FF, Madans JH, Bush TL, et al: Decreased risk of stroke among post menopausal hormone users: Results from a national cohort. Arch Intern Med 153:73–79, 1994.
38. Fisher MC: Medical therapy for ischemic stroke. In Fisher M, Bougousslavsky J (eds): Current Review of Cerebrovascular Disease. Philadelphia, Current Medicine, 1993, pp 18–20.
39. Fishman WH, Dollery CT, Cruckshank JM (eds): Current Cardiovascular Drugs. Philadelphia, Current Medicine, 1994.
40. Foulkes MA, Wolf PA, Price TR, et al: The stroke data bank design, methods and baseline characteristics. Stroke 19:547–554, 1988.
41. Furberg CD, Adams HP Jr, Applegate WB, et al: Effect of lovastatin on early carotid atherosclerosis and cardiovascular events. Circulation 90:1679–1687, 1994.
42. Gent M, Blakely J, Easton JD, et al: The Canadian American Ticlopidine Study (CATS) in thromboembolic stroke. Lancet 1:1215–1220, 1989.
43. Gorelick PB: The status of alcohol as a risk factor for stroke. Stroke 20:1607–1610, 1989.
44. Grahm IM, Daly L, Refsum H, et al: Plasma homocystine as a risk factor for vascular disease. JAMA 277:1175–1181, 1997.
45. Guidelines for the management of transient ischemic attacks: From the Ad Hoc Committee on Guidelines for the Management of Transient Ischemic Attacks of the Stroke Council of the American Heart Association. Stroke 25:1320–1335, 1994.
46. [Reference deleted.]
47. Hachinski VC, Graffanino C, Beaudry M, et al: Lipids and stroke: A paradox resolved. Arch Neurol 53:303–308, 1996.
48. Haley EC, Kassell NF, Torner JC: Failure of heparin to prevent progression in progressing ischemic infarction. Stroke 19:10–14, 1988.
49. Hammon JW, Stump DA, Hines M, et al: Prevention of embolic events during coronary artery bypass graft surgery. Perfusion 9:412–413, 1994.
50. Hart RG, Easton JD: Hemorrhagic infarcts. Stroke 17:586–589, 1986.
51. Hart RG, Harrison MJG: Aspirin wars: The optimal dose of aspirin to prevent stroke. Stroke 27:585–587, 1996.
52. Hass WK, Easton JD, Adams HP Jr, et al: A randomized trial comparing ticlopidine hydrochloride with aspirin for the prevention of stroke in high-risk patients. N Engl J Med 321:501–507, 1989.
53. Heiseman JE, Bird RC: Cerebral aneurysms. Neuroimaging Clin North Am 4:799–819, 1994.
54. Horowitz DR, Tuhrim S, Weinberger JM, et al: Mechanisms in lacunar infarction. Stroke 23:325–327, 1992.
55. Humphrey RD, Harrison MJ: How often can an embolic stroke be diagnosed clinically? A clinicopathological correlation. Postgrad Med J 61:1039–1042, 1985.
56. Indredavik B, Bakke F, Solberg R, et al: Benefits of a stroke unit: A randomized controlled trial. Stroke 22:1026–1031, 1991.
57. Ingall TJ, Homer D, Whisnant JP, et al: Predictive value of carotid bruit for carotid arteriosclerosis. Arch Neurol 46:418–422, 1989.
58. Kazararevic D, Mc Gee D, Vojovodic N, et al: Frequency of alcohol consumption and morbidity and mortality: The Yugoslavian Cardiovascular Disease Study. Lancet 1:613–616, 1980.
59. Kittner SJ, Sharkness CM, Price TR, et al: Infarcts with a cardiac source of embolism in the NINCDC Stroke Data Bank: Historical features. Neurology 40:281–284, 1990.
60. Klag MJ, Whelton PK: The decline in stroke mortality: An epidemiological perspective. Ann Epidemiol 3:571–575, 1993.
61. Labovitz AJ, Camp A, Castello R, et al: Usefulness of transesophageal echocardiography in unexplained cerebral ischemia. Am J Cardiol 72:1448–1452, 1993.
62. La Rosa JC, Hunninghake D, Bush D, et al: The cholesterol facts: A summary of the evidence relating dietary fats, serum cholesterol, and coronary artery disease. A joint statement by the American Heart Association and the National Lung and Blood Institute: The task force on Cholesterol Issues, American Heart Association. Circulation 81:1721–1733, 1990.
63. Laupacis A, Albers G, Dunn M, Feinberg W: Antithrombotic therapy in atrial fibrillation. Chest 102(suppl):426–433, 1992.
64. Levy DE, Brott TG, Hailey C, et al: Factors related to intracranial hematoma formation in patients receiving tissue-type plasminogen activator for ischemic stroke. Stroke 25:291–297, 1994.

65. Lindgren A, Rogers A, Norrving B, et al: Carotid artery and heart disease in subtypes of cerebral infarction. Stroke 25:2365–2362, 1994.

66. Lord RS: Late survival after carotid endarterectomy for transient ischemic attacks. J Vascular Surg 1:512–519, 1984.

67. Low molecular weight heparinoid, ORG 10172 (danaprinoid), and outcome after acute ischemic stroke: A randomized controlled trial. The Publications Committee for the Trial of ORG 10172 in Acute Stroke Treatment (TOAST) Investigators. JAMA 279:1265–1272, 1998.

68. MacMahon S, Cutler JA, Stamler J: Antihypertensive drug treatment: Potential, expected and observed effect on stroke and coronary artery disease. Hypertension 13:145–150, 1989.

69. Manson JE, Tostenson H, Ridker PM, et al: The primary prevention of myocardial infarction. N Engl J Med 326:1406–1416, 1992.

70. [Reference deleted.]

71. Miller J, Diringer M: Management of aneurysmal subarachnoid hemorrhage. Neurol Clin 13:451–478, 1995.

71a. Moore WS, Barnett HJ, Beebe HG, et al: Guidelines for carotid endarterectomy: A multidisciplinary consensus statement from the Ad Hoc Committee, American Heart Association. Circulation 91:566–579, 1995.

72. Murkin JM: The role of CPB management in neurobehavioral outcomes after cardiac surgery. Ann Thorac Surg 59:1308–1311, 1995.

73. Newman ME, Croughwell NV, Blumenthal JA, et al: Predictors of cognitive decline after cardiac operation. Ann Thorac Surg 59:1326–1330, 1995.

74. Nicolaides AN: Asymptomatic carotid stenosis and risk of stroke. Identification of a high-risk group (ACSRS). A natural history study. Int Angiol 14:21–23, 1995.

75. NINDS rt-PA Stroke Study Group: Tissue plasminogen activator for acute ischemic stroke. N Engl J Med 333:1581–1587, 1995.

76. Norris JW, Zhu CZ, Bornstein NM, Chambers BR: Vascular risks of asymptomatic carotid stenosis. Stroke 22:1485–1490, 1991.

77. North American Symptomatic Carotid Endarterectomy Trial Collaborators: Beneficial effect of carotid endarterectomy for high-grade carotid stenosis. N Engl J Med 325:445–453, 1991.

78. Okada Y, Yamaguchi T, Minematsu K, et al: Hemorrhagic transformation in cerebral embolism. Stroke 20:598–603, 1989.

79. O'Neill BJ III, Furlan AJ, Hobbs RD: Risk of stroke in patients with transient postoperative atrial fibrillation/flutter. Stroke 14:133, 1983.

80. Protection of the brain during cardiopulmonary bypass: Diagnosis, etiology and therapeutics. J Cardiothor Vasc Anesth 10:1–138, 1996.

81. Quality Standards Subcommittee of the American Academy of Neurology: Practice advisory: Thrombolytic therapy for acute ischemic-summary statement. Neurology 47:835–839, 1996.

82. Reed GL III, Singer DE, Picard EH, et al: Stroke following coronary artery bypass surgery: A case control estimate of the risk from carotid bruits. N Engl J Med 319:1246–1250, 1988.

83. Rorick M, Furlan AJ: Risk of cardiac surgery in patients with prior stroke. Neurology 40:835–837, 1990.

84. Rothrock JF, Hart RG: Antithrombotic therapy in cerebrovascular disease. Ann Intern Med 115:885–895, 1991.

85. Sacco RF, Ellenberg JH, Mohr JP, et al: Infarcts of undetermined cause: The NINDS stroke data bank. Ann Neurol 25:382–390, 1989.

86. Sardesi SH, Marshall RJ, Mourant AJ, et al: Paradoxical and systemic embolism through a patent foramen ovale. Lancet 1:732–733, 1989.

87. Scandinavian Simvastatin Study Survival Group: Randomised trial of cholesterol lowering in 4444 patients with coronary heart disease: The Scandinavian Simvastatin Survival Study (4S). Lancet 344:1383–1389, 1994.

88. Sekhar L, Heros R: Origin, growth and rupture of saccular aneurysms: A review. Neurosurgery 8:248–260, 1981.

89. Sherman DG: Prevention of cardioembolic stroke. In Norris JW, Hachinski VC (eds): Prevention of Stroke. New York, Springer-Verlag, 1991, pp 149–159.

90. Shinton R, Beevers G: Meta-analysis of the relation between cigarette smoking and stroke. BMJ 298:789–794, 1989.

91. Slivka A, Levy D: Natural history of progressive ischemic stroke in a population treated with heparin. Stroke 21:1657–1666, 1990.

92. Spence JD: New approaches to atherosclerosis based on endothelial function. In Fisher M, Bogousslavsky J (eds): Current Review of Cerebrovascular Disease. Philadelphia, Current Medicine, 1998.

93. Stampfer MJ, Colditz GA, Willett WC, et al: Post menopausal estrogen replacement and cardiovascular disease: 10 year follow-up from the Nurses Health Study. N Engl J Med 325:756–762, 1991.
94. Steering Committee on the Physicians' Health Study Research Group: Final report on the aspirin component of the ongoing physicians' health study. N Engl J Med 321:129–135, 1989.
95. Stroke Prevention in Atrial Fibrillation Investigators: Adjusted-dose warfarin versus low intensity, fixed dose warfarin plus aspirin for high risk patients with atrial fibrillation: Stroke Prevention in Atrial Fibrillation III randomized clinical trial. Lancet 348:633–638, 1996.
96. Stump DA, Wallenhaupt SL, Newman SP, et al: Cardiopulmonary bypass time and neuropsychological deficits after cardiac surgery. Perfusion 8:249, 1993.
97. Stump DA: Selection and clinical significance of neuropsychologic tests. Ann Thorac Surg 59:1331–1335, 1995.
98. Tell GS, Crouse JR, Furberg CD: Relationship between blood lipids, lipoproteins and cerebrovascular arteriosclerosis. A review. Stroke 19:423–430, 1988.
99. The Antiphospholipid Antibodies in Stroke Study Group: Clinical and laboratory findings in patients with antiphospholipid antibodies and cerebral ischemia. Stroke 21:1268–1273, 1990.
100. The Dutch TIA Trial Study Group: A comparison of two doses of aspirin (30 mg vs 283 mg a day) in patients after a transient ischemic attack or minor ischemic stroke. N Engl J Med 325:1261–1266, 1991.
101. The SALT Collaborative Group: Swedish Aspirin Low-dose Aspirin Trial of 75 mg. Aspirin for the secondary prophylaxis of cerebrovascular events. Lancet 338:1345–1349, 1991.
102. Turpie AG, Gent M, Laupacis A, et al: A comparison of aspirin with placebo in patients treated with warfarin after heart valve replacement. N Engl J Med 329:524–529, 1993.
103. Vitkus PT, Barnathan ES: Embolic potential, prevention and management of mural thrombus following anterior myocardial infarction: A meta-analysis. J Am Coll Cardiol 22:1004–1009, 1993.
104. WARRS, APASS, PICSS, and HAS study groups: The feasibility of a collaborative double-blind study using an anticoagulant: The Warfarin-Aspirin Recurrent Stroke Study (WARSS), the Antiphospholipid Antibodies and Stroke Study (APASS), the Patent Foramen Ovale in Cryptogenic stroke (PICSS), and the Hemostatic System Activation Study (HAS). Cerebrovasc Dis 7:100–112, 1997.
105. Webster MMI, Chancelor AM, Smith HJ, et al: Patent foramen ovale in young stroke patients. Lancet 19:640–643, 1988.
106. Weldin L, Juhler M: The course of transient ischemic attacks. Neurology 38:677–680, 1988.
107. Wolf PA, Kannel WB, Sorlie P, et al: Asymptomatic carotid bruit and the risk of stroke. The Framingham study. JAMA 245:1442–1445, 1981.
108. Wolf PA, Abbott RD, Kannel WB, et al: Atrial fibrillation: A major contributor to stroke in the elderly. Arch Intern Med 147:1561–1564, 1987.
109. Wolf PA, D'Agostino RB, Kannel WB, et al: Cigarette smoking as a risk factor for stroke: The Framingham study. JAMA 259:1025–1029, 1988.
110. Wolf PA, D'Agostino RB, Belanger AJ, et al: Secular trends in stroke incidence and mortality. The Framingham study. Stroke 22:312–318, 1991.

JOHN D. HEITZNER, MD, FRCPC
ROBERT W. TEASELL, MD, FRCPC

CLINICAL CONSEQUENCES OF STROKE

From the Department of Physical
  Medicine and Rehabilitation
University of Western Ontario
London, Ontario
Canada

Reprint requests to:
John D. Heitzner, MD, FRCPC
London Health Sciences Center
University Campus
339 Windermere Road
London, Ontario N6A 5A5
Canada

Cerebrovascular disorders represent the third leading cause of mortality and the second major cause of long-term disability in North America.[10] The impairments associated with a stroke exhibit a wide diversity of clinical signs and symptoms. Disability, which is multifactorial in its determination, varies according to the degree of neurologic recovery, the site of the lesion, the patient's premorbid status, and the environmental support systems.

One of the first tasks in the neurologic diagnosis of stroke is localization of the lesion. Certain types of strokes tend to occur in specific areas; for instance, lacunar infarcts and intracerebral hemorrhages occur most often in subcortical regions. The most common presentation of a stroke patient requiring rehabilitation is contralateral hemiparesis or hemiplegia. Other neurologic manifestations vary depending on the side of the stroke lesion and whether the stroke occurs in the cerebral hemispheres or the brain stem. The arterial territory that is affected will determine the clinical manifestations; hence, localization of a stroke is often described in such terms.

The clinical consequences of stroke are best classified based on the anatomic regions of the brain that are affected. This is best understood by dividing the brain according to the left and right hemispheres (carotid/anterior circulation) and the brain stem (vertebral-basilar/posterior circulation) (Fig. 1). A large degree of specialization exists within the brain. Different neurologic functions are divided among the two hemispheres and the brain stem. The clinical picture of a stroke

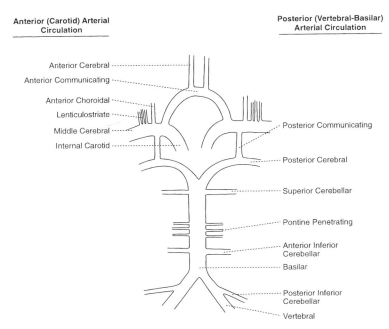

Anterior (Carotid) Arterial Circulation

Anterior Cerebral
Anterior Communicating
Anterior Choroidal
Lenticulostriate
Middle Cerebral
Internal Carotid

Posterior (Vertebral-Basilar) Arterial Circulation

Posterior Communicating
Posterior Cerebral
Superior Cerebellar
Pontine Penetrating
Anterior Inferior Cerebellar
Basilar
Posterior Inferior Cerebellar
Vertebral

FIGURE 1.   Arterial blood supply to the brain can be divided into the carotid/anterior circulation and the posterior/vertebral-basilar circulation.

depends on which specialized centers have been damaged with subsequent loss of the specialized neurologic function they control. However, this schematic view of the brain is in many ways too simplistic. Brain functioning generally occurs in a more integrated fashion. Even a simple activity such as bending to pick up an object requires the integrated function of the entire central nervous system (CNS). When damage occurs in one region of the brain, not only are the specialized centers associated with the impaired region that is affected, but the entire brain also suffers from loss of input from the injured part.

CEREBRAL HEMISPHERES

A stroke in this vascular distribution often results in contralateral paralysis or weakness (hemiparesis/hemiplegia), sensory loss, and visual field loss (homonymous hemianopsia). Middle cerebral artery (MCA) involvement is common, but anterior cerebral artery (ACA) strokes are uncommon.

Anterior Cerebral Artery

The ACA supplies the anterior two thirds of the medial surface of the cerebral hemisphere. This vascular territory includes the medial aspect of the frontal and parietal lobes, the anterior half of the internal capsule, the anterior inferior head of the caudate, the anterior four fifths of the corpus callosum, and the supplementary motor area and the primary motor and sensory areas for the contralateral lower extremity (Fig. 2).

Infarction involving the ACA territory accounts for only 3% of all strokes. The circle of Willis generally compensates for lesions proximal to the anterior

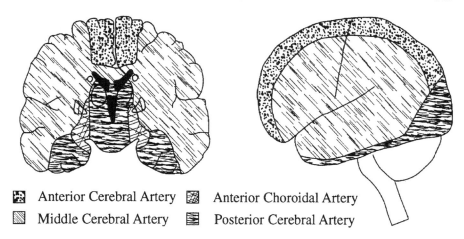

🔲 Anterior Cerebral Artery   🔲 Anterior Choroidal Artery
🔲 Middle Cerebral Artery   🔲 Posterior Cerebral Artery

FIGURE 2.   Vascular territories of anterior, middle, and posterior cerebral arteries.

communicating arteries. However, with distal occlusions there is weakness of the opposite leg and a contralateral cortical sensory deficit, which is most marked in the leg. Bilateral lesions often present with incontinence, abulia or slow mentation, and the appearance of primitive reflexes. Proximal occlusion of the ACA results in all of the above signs plus facial and proximal arm weakness and frontal apraxia. Apraxia occurs as a consequence of the interruption of commissural fibers between the two frontal lobes. Patients typically present with right motor paresis and left apraxia, the latter being prominent when the patients attempt to follow commands.

Middle Cerebral Artery

Cortical branches of the MCA supply two thirds of the lateral surface of the hemispheres as well as the temporal pole. Important areas of neurologic specialization within the MCA territory include the primary motor and sensory areas for the face and upper extremity as well as Broca's and Wernicke's language areas in the dominant hemisphere (Figs. 3 and 4). An infarction in the MCA territory is the most common site of cerebral ischemia. In North America, this infarction is generally embolic rather than atherothrombotic. However, an atherothrombotic infarction

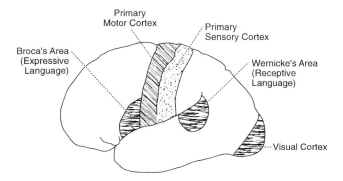

FIGURE 3.   Areas of the cerebral cortex associated with specific functions.

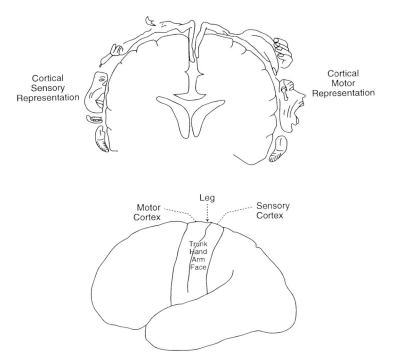

FIGURE 4. Representation of the body on the primary motor and sensory cortex. This explains greater arm involvement in a middle cerebral artery occlusion and greater leg involvement in an anterior cerebral artery occlusion.

of the internal carotid artery invariably presents with symptoms predominantly in the MCA territory. The clinical consequences are similar to those with involvement of the anterior/carotid circulation (see above). Unlike strokes involving the ACA, there is greater facial and upper extremity involvement. Additional clinical signs and symptoms occur depending on whether the right or left hemisphere is involved.

Right Versus Left Hemispheric Lesions

Each hemisphere is responsible for initiating motor activity and receiving sensory information from the opposite side of the body. However, each hemisphere has a large degree of specialization. Despite this specialization, normal thinking and performance of activities requires the integrated function of both hemispheres, neither of which is truly dominant over the other. Many stroke patients have diffuse cerebrovascular disease and other conditions resulting in impaired cerebral circulation. While there may be one major area of infarction, there may be other areas of ischemic damage located throughout the hemispheres that may complicate the clinical presentation.

THE RIGHT HEMISPHERE

The right hemisphere is effective in mediating learned behaviors that require voluntary initiation, planning, and spatial-perceptual judgment. Clinical signs and symptoms include visuospatial perceptual deficits, emotional disorders, and subtle communication problems.

Visuospatial Perceptual Disorders. The right hemisphere is dominant for visuospatial orientation, constructional praxis, and judgment in more than 90% of the population.[10] Therefore, in a right hemispheric middle cerebral infarct, visuospatial perceptual disorders include left-sided neglect, right-left confusion, astereognosis, figure-ground disorientation, and constructional apraxia. Stone et al. noted that visuospatial neglect was equally common in patients with right hemisphere and left hemisphere strokes 3 days after the stroke (72% vs 62%).[40] However, the severity of the neglect was greater in right hemispheric stroke patients and was more likely to be a permanent deficit than in patients with a left hemispheric stroke.[40] Anosognosia has been associated with right hemisphere strokes. Such patients may perceive that they have no deficit and may disregard the existence of the affected half of their bodies.[10] Frequently, an associated left homonymous hemianopsia exists that may further compound these deficits.

A strong relationship has been established between visual, spatial, perceptual, and motor dysfunction and the performance of activities of daily living (ADLs) by right hemispheric stroke victims.[8] Such perceptual impairments have been shown to adversely influence the rate of achieving independent sitting and stair climbing.[33]

Delaney and Potter note: "As the extent of perceptual, motor and sensory deficits and left-sided neglect increases, a summation effect often occurs in regard to the disability seen. Such difficulties together restrict safety in locomotion and many specific daily tasks such as cooking. However, when only isolated lesions are present such as sensory deficit without neglect, homonymous hemianopsia without neglect, or perceptual problems, patients can often learn to accommodate to the discrete deficits."[10]

Emotional Disorders. Because patients with right hemispheric lesions may speak well, their actual abilities are often overestimated. These patients tend to have a lack of insight into their own deficits. Difficulties generally labeled as emotionally related include indifference reaction or flat affect, impulsivity (often leading to multiple accidents), and emotional lability.

Communication Problems. Although aphasia is common with left hemispheric strokes, it rarely occurs in right hemispheric strokes. Annett demonstrated that aphasia occurred after right hemispheric strokes in 30% of left-handers and 5% of right-handers.[1] Moreover, patients with nondominant hemispheric lesions often have associated communication difficulties, whereby they have difficulty using intact language skills effectively. The patient may not observe turn-taking rules of conversation, may have difficulty telling jokes (frequently missing the punchline), and may have fewer tendencies to appropriately initiate conversation. This tends to result in social dysfunction that may negatively affect family and social support systems.[10]

LEFT HEMISPHERE

The left hemisphere is more effective in learning and using language symbols. Clinical signs and symptoms include aphasia, apraxia, and, arguably, emotional disorders.

Aphasia. About 93% of the population is right-handed, with the left hemisphere being dominant for language in 99% of right-handed individuals.[10] In left-handed individuals, 70% have language control in the left hemisphere, 15% in the right hemisphere, and 15% in both hemispheres.[35] Therefore, language control is primarily in the left hemisphere in 96.9% of the population. The exception is the

TABLE 1. Characteristic Features of Aphasia

Type	Fluency	Comprehension	Repetition
Broca's aphasia	Nonfluent	Good	Poor
Transcortical motor	Nonfluent	Good	Good
Wernicke's aphasia	Fluent	Poor	Poor
Transcortical sensory	Fluent	Poor	Good
Global	Nonfluent	Poor	Poor
Conduction	Fluent	Good	Poor

35% of left-handers (3% of population) who use the right hemisphere for language function. A disorder of language is called aphasia, and expressive (Broca's) aphasia is the language disorder most commonly seen with left hemispheric MCA strokes. Table 1 describes characteristic features of the aphasias.

Apraxia. Apraxia is a disorder of voluntary movement wherein one cannot execute willed, purposeful activity despite the presence of adequate mobility, strength, sensation, coordination, and comprehension. Left hemispheric stroke patients often demonstrate apraxias. General apraxias are known as the motor or ideational apraxias, and specific apraxias include constructional apraxias, apraxias of speech, dressing apraxias, and apraxias of gait[43] (Table 2).

Emotional Disorders. Major poststroke depression develops in up to 75% of patients with left frontal lobe lesions. Rage and frustration reactions occasionally are seen, especially in nonfluent or receptive aphasics (see chapter entitled "Psychosocial Considerations in Adjustment to Stroke").

BRAIN STEM

A stroke in this vertebral-basilar/posterior vascular distribution can produce diverse manifestations because the vertebral-basilar artery system provides the vascular supply to the occipital lobes, brain stem, and cerebellum (Table 3). In contrast to the major cognitive or language disorders seen with hemispheric strokes, brain stem strokes in isolation spare cognitive and language functions. Intact cognitive abilities are important later in regaining functional abilities that are lost as a consequence of the stroke.[17]

TABLE 2. Types of Apraxias

Type	Site of Lesion	Manifestation
Motor or ideomotor	Often left hemisphere	Can automatically perform a movement but cannot repeat it on command
Ideational	Often bilateral parietal	Can perform separate movements but cannot coordinate all steps into an integrated sequence
Constructional	Either parietal lobe but right more often than left	Unable to synthesize individual spatial elements into a whole (e.g., cannot draw a picture)
Verbal	Commonly associated with Broca's aphasia	Sparse verbal output, poor articulation, abnormal phrase length and melody
Dressing	Either hemisphere, right more often than left	Inability to dress oneself despite adequate motor ability
Gait	Frontal lobes	Difficulty initiating and maintaining a normal walking pattern when sensory and motor functions seem otherwise unimpaired

TABLE 3.   Clinical Signs and Symptoms of Vertebral-basilar Artery Disorders

System	Signs and Symptoms
Cranial nerves	Bilateral visual and cranial nerve disturbances
	Vertigo
	Dysarthria/dysphagia
	Diplopia
	Facial numbness or paresthesia
	Ataxia
Motor	Hemiparesis or quadriparesis
Sensory	Hemi- or bilateral sensory loss
Other	Drop attacks

Brain stem strokes are categorized into a variety of well-defined syndromes (Table 4) depending on the vascular territory involved (Fig. 5). Specific impairments resulting from brain stem syndromes include the involvement of ipsilateral cranial nerves (dysarthria and dysphagia), pyramidal tracts (hemiparesis), sensory tracts

TABLE 4.   Classic Brain Stem Syndromes

Syndrome	Location of Lesion	Clinical Picture
Wallenburg's	Lateral medulla (posterior inferior cerebellar artery and/or vertebral artery)	Vertigo Nausea and vomiting Sensory loss of ipsilateral face of contralateral limbs Ipsilateral ataxia Rotatory or horizontal gaze nystagmus Hoarseness and dysphonia Dysphagia and dysarthria Ipsilateral Horner's syndrome
	Medial medulla	Contralateral limb paralysis (facial sparing) Contralateral decrease in position and vibration sense Ipsilateral tongue paralysis
Jackson's	Medulla	Hoarseness and dysphonia Weakness of trapezius and sternocleidomastoid muscles
Millard-Gubler	Lower pons	Alternating or crossed hemiparesis Unilateral upper motor neuron facial palsy Contralateral limb paralysis with no contralateral facial palsy
Fouille's	Lower pons	Crossed (alternating hemiparesis) Ipsilateral lateral gaze palsy
Raymond's	Lower pons	Abducens nerve palsy Contralateral hemiparesis
Parinaud's	Superior colliculus	Paralysis of upward conjugate convergence and frequently of downward gaze
Cerebellum	Cerebellum	Unilateral ataxia Vertigo Headache Occasionally patient may become comatose
Weber's	Midbrain	Contralateral hemiparesis Ipsilateral oculomotor paralysis with dilated pupil, lateral gaze only, ptosis
Benedict's or Claude's	Midbrain	Contralateral hemiparesis Tremor in paretic limbs on voluntary movement Frequently contralateral sensory loss Ipsilateral oculomotor paralysis

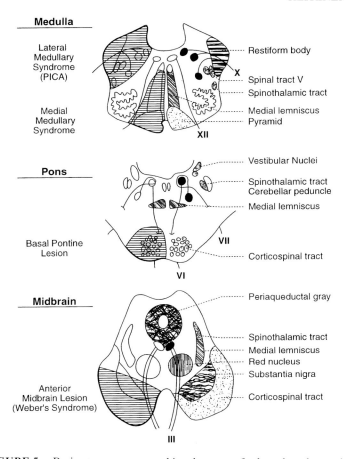

FIGURE 5.   Brain stem anatomy and involvement of selected stroke syndromes.

(hemisensory deficits), and cerebellar tracts (ipsilateral ataxia and incoordination). Dysarthria is characterized by unclear speech of various types, including slurred, scanning, spastic, monotonous, lisping, nasal, or expulsive speech.[37] Dysphagia is simply defined as difficulty with swallowing. The management of brain stem strokes with dysphagia often requires the use of prolonged feeding by an alternate route.

Posterior Inferior Cerebellar Artery

The posterior inferior cerebellar arteries (PICAs) originate from the vertebral arteries about 1 cm below the junction of the two vertebral arteries where they form the basilar artery. Each PICA courses around the lateral surface of the medulla and then loops back to supply portions of the cerebellum. It supplies a wedge of the lateral medulla and the inferior aspect of the cerebellum (see Fig. 5). Occlusion of the PICA results in a lateral medullary or Wallenburg's syndrome (see Table 4).

Basilar Artery

The basilar artery is formed at the junction of the medulla with the pons by the merger of the two vertebral arteries. There are three major branches of the basilar

TABLE 5. Signs and Symptoms Resulting from Stenosis of Basilar Artery Branches

System	Signs and Symptoms
Sensorium	Alterations in consciousness
Cranial nerves	Pupil abnormalities
	III, IV and VI with dysconjugate gaze
	Horner's syndrome
	V with ipsilateral facial hypoalgesia
	Nystagmus
	VII with unilateral lower motor neuron facial paralysis
	Caloric and oculocephalic reflexes
	Vertigo
	IX and X with dysphagia, dysarthria
Motor	Quadriplegia or contralateral hemiplegia
Sensory	Contralateral limb hypoalgesia
Cerebellum	Ipsilateral or bilateral cerebellar abnormalities
Respiratory	Respiratory irregularities
Cardiac	Cardiac arrhythmias and erratic blood pressure

artery: the anterior inferior cerebellar artery, the superior cerebellar artery, and the internal auditory or labyrinthine artery. These are known as the long circumferential arteries. There are also short circumferential arteries and small penetrating arteries that supply the pons and paramedian regions. Occlusion of these vessels may result in a variety of signs and symptoms (Table 5).

Posterior Cerebral Artery

Although the posterior cerebral arteries (PCAs) primarily supply the occipital cerebral hemispheres, they usually arise from the posterior circulation. The posterior cerebral arteries arise as terminal branches of the basilar artery in 70% of individuals, from one basilar and the opposite carotid in 20–25%, and directly from the carotid circulation in 5–10%. Both PCAs receive a posterior communicating vessel from the internal carotid artery and then arch posteriorly around the cerebral peduncles to the tentorial surface of the cerebrum. They supply the inferolateral and medial surfaces of the temporal lobe, the lateral and medial surfaces of the occipital lobe, and the upper brain stem. Included in this area is the midbrain, visual cortex, cerebral peduncles, thalamus, and splenium of the corpus callosum (see Fig. 2). Occlusion of the PCA or any of its branches may produce a wide variety of syndromes (Table 6).

LACUNAR INFARCTS

Short penetrating arteries that are end arteries with no anastomotic connections supply the medial and basal portions of the brain and brain stem. These small arteries arise directly from large arteries, causing the gradation between arterial and capillary pressure to occur over a relatively short distance and exposing these small arteries to high arterial pressures. Occlusion of small penetrating arteries (50–100 μ in diameter) may lead to small cerebral infarcts (usually < 10–12 mm) in the deep subcortical regions of the brain. They are associated with hypertension. Marked hypertrophy of the subintimal hyaline (lipohyalinosis) occurs with eventual obliteration of the vascular lumen. On healing after infarction, a small cavity, or "lacune," forms.

TABLE 6.   Syndromes of Posterior Cerebral Artery Occlusions

Thalamoperforate Branch Occlusion	Thalamogeniculate Branch Occlusion (Thalamic Syndrome)	Cortical Branch Occlusion	Bilateral Posterior Cerebral Artery Occlusions
Involuntary movement disorders	Contralateral sensory loss	Contralateral homonymous hemianopsia	Visual agnosia or cortical blindness (intact pupillary reflexes)
Hemiataxia	Transient contralateral hemiparesis	Dominant hemisphere— alexia, memory impairment or anomia, especially for naming colors	Severe memory loss (Korsakoff's amnesia)
Intention tremor	Contralateral mild involuntary movements		
Ipsilateral oculomotor palsy with contralateral hemiplegia (Weber's syndrome)	Intense, persistent, burning pain	Nondominant hemisphere—topographic disorientation prosopagnosia (failure to recognize faces)	
Ipsilateral oculomotor palsy with contralateral cerebellar ataxia (Claude's or Benedict's syndrome)			

Most lacunar infarcts occur within the deep gray nuclei, and some may involve multiple sites (Table 7). The onset of a focal deficit may occur suddenly or progress over several hours. Similarly, both the time frame and extent of recovery is variable. Lacunar infarcts are often mistaken for a thromboembolic transient ischemic attack. Computed tomography may show a small, deep infarct; however, many are too small to be seen without magnetic resonance imaging. Smaller lacunar infarcts may be asymptomatic. Fischer has described 21 lacunar syndromes.[20] The four most common lacunar syndromes are described in Table 8.

RECOVERY

Course of Recovery Poststroke

Most spontaneous or intrinsic recovery occurs within the first 3 months poststroke. Recovery may continue at a slower pace for at least 6 months; in up to 5% of patients recovery may continue for up to 1 year, especially in the patients who were most severely disabled at the time of initial examination.[4,12,18,27,44,45] Progress toward recovery may be arrested or may plateau at any stage of recovery, and only about 10% of patients with moderate or severe stroke achieve full recovery. The return of motor power is not synonymous with recovery of function; function may be hampered by the inability to perform skilled coordinated movements, apraxias, sensory

TABLE 7.   Sites of Lacunar Infarcts

Localization	Percentage (%)
Lenticular nuclei (especially putamen)	65
Pons	39
Thalamus	32
Internal capsule (posterior limb) and corona radiata	27
Caudate	24
Frontal white matter	17

Adapted from Dombovy ML: Stroke: Clinical course and neurophysiologic mechanisms of recovery. Crit Rev Phys Rehabil Med 2:171–188, 1991.

TABLE 8. Common Lacunar Syndromes

Syndrome Manifestation	Site of Lesion	Clinical
Pure motor hemiparesis	Posterior limb of internal capsule Lower pons (basis pontis)	Weakness of face, arm, and leg No sensory involvement
Pure sensory stroke	Sensory nucleus of the thalamus	Sensory signs and/or symptoms involving half of the body
Dysarthria—clumsy hand	Upper pons (basis pontis)	Dysarthria and dysphagia Weakness of one side of the face and tongue Clumsiness and mild weakness of the hand
Ataxic hemiparesis	Upper pons (basis pontis)	Hemiplegia and cerebellar type of ataxia on the same side

deficits, communication disorders, and cognitive impairment. Functional improvements may occur in the absence of motor recovery.[14,34]

Type of Recovery

Recovery following a stroke is generally one of two types: (1) spontaneous or intrinsic neurologic recovery and (2) functional or adaptive recovery.

As a rule, the severity of the initial deficit is inversely proportional to the prognosis for recovery. Most spontaneous recovery occurs during the first 3–6 months after the onset of the stroke. This type of recovery has until recently been regarded as largely inaccessible to medical intervention or manipulation.

Functional recovery refers to improvement of independence in such areas as self-care and mobility. It depends on the patient's motivation, ability to learn, and family supports as well as the quality and intensity of therapy. This type of recovery is accessible to intervention/manipulation and is influenced by, but may occur independently of, neurologic recovery.

Processes Involved in Recovery

Various processes have been identified as playing a role in neurologic recovery after a stroke (Table 9). The role that these factors play in intrinsic or spontaneous recovery is not completely understood. Recovery from stroke is often attributed to resolution of edema and return of circulation to the ischemic penumbra.[11] However, these mechanisms do not account for recovery that occurs after 4–6 weeks poststroke.[7] Factors that contribute to recovery can be grouped into three categories: (1)

TABLE 9. Mechanisms of Recovery from Stroke

Mechanism	Time Frame of Occurrence
Local Processes	
Resolution of edema	Weeks to 2 months
Resolution of ischemic penumbra	Hours to weeks
Resolution of remote functional depression (diaschisis)	Days to months
Central Nervous System Reorganization	
Neurotransmitter alterations	Immediate to a few months
Unmasking (release from inhibition) of ipsilateral and alternate pathways	Weeks to months
Synaptogenesis	Weeks to years

Adapted from Dombovy ML: Stroke: Clinical course and neurophysiologic mechanisms of recovery. Crit Rev Phys Rehabil Med 2:171–188, 1991.

local CNS processes (early recovery), (2) CNS reorganization (later recovery), and (3) secondary peripheral factors.

LOCAL CNS PROCESSES

The following processes leading to initial clinical improvement occur independently of behavior or stimuli:

Local Edema. Poststroke edema surrounding the lesion may disrupt nearby neuronal functioning. As the edema subsides, the neurons may regain function. Much of the early recovery is probably due to resolution of edema surrounding the infarcted area.[32] This process may continue for up to 8 weeks but is generally completed much earlier.[23] Cerebral hemorrhages tend to have more edema, which would then take longer to subside.

Diaschisis. This is a state of low reactivity or depressed function as a result of a sudden interruption of a major input to a part of the brain remote from the site of brain damage. With brain injury to one area of the brain, other areas of normal brain tissue are suddenly deprived of a major source of stimulation. One example of this is thought to be "spinal shock."[32] The term *diaschisis* was coined by von Monakow to describe the distant effects of brain lesions that appeared to be reversible.[6,42] Neuronal function may return with resolution of diaschisis. This is particularly true of noncortical structures after cortical injury.[6]

Reperfusion of the Ischemic Penumbra. A focal ischemic injury consists of a core of low blood flow that eventually infarcts, surrounded by a region of moderate blood flow—the ischemic penumbra—that is at risk of infarction but still salvageable. Reperfusion of this area causes affected and previously nonfunctioning neurons to resume functioning with subsequent clinical improvement.

CNS REORGANIZATION

Dombovy notes that some of the basic mechanisms thought to underlie the later return of function are "the bilaterality of the brain, dendritic sprouting and synaptogenesis, unmasking of alternative pathways, and development of cortical inhibition. Additionally, numerous alterations in neurotransmitters and cerebral metabolism occur following brain injury. These contribute to the observed deficits via interactions, both at the site of injury and in remote areas of the brain (diaschisis)."[11]

Importance of Brain Plasticity. The potential for significant plasticity of the human CNS is now widely accepted. Recovery of function can continue for months or years. Neurology traditionally has emphasized the correlation between the localization of the lesion and the deficit in functioning. This suggests that certain areas of the brain control certain functions and, once that area is destroyed, the function is lost. While this approach is essential to an understanding of neurologic symptoms and syndromes, it frequently has led to a therapeutic nihilism. Greater emphasis is being placed on the plasticity of the brain and increased efforts are being made to obtain maximum recovery and reorganization of function of the damaged nervous system.

There is increasing evidence that much of the recovery after CNS insult depends on adaptive restructuring of the residual functioning brain tissue. In large strokes the deficit is greater and recovery more limited because there is less residual brain tissue. Kertesz and McCabe found that the prognosis for anomic, conduction, and Broca's aphasia was far better than that of global aphasia, where the lesion was more extensive.[28] Hier et al. found that after right hemispheric lesions, recovery from unilateral neglect and anosognosia was the most rapid.[22] Recovery from constructional and dressing apraxias was intermediate, and recovery was slowest for hemiparesis, hemianopsia, and extinction.

One explanation for these varying rates of recovery states that the rate of recovery depends on the functional role of the damaged structures. Recovery is delayed after injury to structures that control elementary functions requiring immediate execution. These functions, including movement, sensation, and vision, involve precise neural networks, and injury results in slower recovery and long-lasting dysfunction. In contrast, the structures mediating higher cortical functions are diffuse and extensive. As a result they are capable of adaptive restructuring with quicker and more complete return of the lost function (aphasia, apraxia, neglect). If there is a large lesion and the entire network responsible for the higher cortical function is destroyed, there may be little, if any, recovery, i.e., global aphasia.

The concept of a tight relationship between brain structure and a given cognitive or behavioral function has led to the belief that loss of a specific area of the brain results in irrevocable loss of function by that brain tissue. Laboratory and clinical findings do not necessarily support strict localization, which provides support for recovery.[31] For example, results in animals show that brain damage created in two temporally separated surgeries often produces much less behavioral dysfunction than when the same tissue is removed in one surgery.[19] In addition, slowly evolving tumors often produce much less behavioral dysfunction than rapidly evolving strokes affecting the same region.[6] The structure-determines-function concept does not account for spontaneous recovery in the absence of lost tissue.[6] This process of CNS reorganization or adaptation is not felt to be spontaneous but results from responses to stimuli or learning. The younger the individual, the greater the ease with which adaptations can occur. There is evidence that a stimulating environment, in contrast to a nonstimulating environment, promotes intrinsic recovery in brain-damaged animals. Optimal recovery would then seem to be dependent to a large degree on patient motivation, ability to learn, and the guidance of trained rehabilitation staff.

Redundancy/Unmasking of Pathways. Some redundancy is built into the CNS pathways. An activity may be controlled through multiple pathways.[32] However, many of the pathways are selectively inhibited in favor of the more efficient dominant pathway. If the predominant pathway is destroyed by the stroke, the subordinate pathway may be "unmasked," strengthened, and may achieve a high degree of efficiency[2]; however, this alternative pathway is never as efficient as the previously dominant pathway. This may explain why some stroke patients initially have great difficulty producing a movement but require less effort as recovery progresses.

Substitution. Multiple centers within the CNS often control a given function. A stroke damages one or more of these centers, upsetting the balance between the remaining centers. Lost function can sometimes be partially restored by the remaining intact ipsilateral centers. Homologous centers in the contralateral hemisphere may partially take over the lost function. For example, children whose left cerebral hemisphere language area has been damaged early in life can regain language functioning in the right hemisphere. Such complete substitutions are unlikely to occur in adults, but more limited contralateral substitution is felt to play a major role in neurologic recovery.[32]

Regeneration. Regeneration, which also has been referred to as "sprouting" or "synaptogenesis," refers to the new growth of axonal branches following neuronal loss. Regenerative sprouting refers to severed or injured axons issuing side sprouts, which form new synapses on other nearby neurons. Axonal sprouting has been observed in the peripheral nervous system of humans and in the CNS of animals.[15,38]

However, the relevance of regenerative sprouting to recovery from CNS damage is likely minimal.[30] Collateral sprouting refers to denervated but intact neurons attracting side sprouts from nearby uninjured axons after some or all of their normal input has been destroyed.[30] Studies have demonstrated collateral sprouting in the human CNS.[30] Regeneration may play some role in functional recovery in human beings. Bach-y-Rita notes that sprouting, also known as reactive synaptogenesis, also may be maladaptive in nature.[2] Different types of axons converging on cells bring in different types of input. If one type of neuron is lost after a stroke and surrounding neurons make up the loss, the input may be different and the resulting function abnormal. Boyeson et al. have noted that although structural modifications of the brain in the form of collateral sprouting is generally accepted, there is a lack of research that links these modifications with beneficial functional recovery following brain injury.[6] Evidence of this type of compensation is more often associated with the appearance of behaviors that may be maladaptive, such as spasticity.[5]

Neurotransmitter Changes.   Dombovy[11] notes: "Multiple changes in neurotransmitters take place over varying time frames, and some may be directly responsible for, or associated with, observed decreases in brain metabolism and function."[16] Evidence from multiple animal studies and, increasingly, human research suggests that pharmacologic intervention can influence recovery. This is currently the subject of intense research.

SECONDARY PERIPHERAL CONSEQUENCES

The general deconditioning and muscle weakness that accompanies any period of prolonged bed rest can add to the already apparent neurologic deficits. Relative immobility after a stroke can lead to a variety of reversible problems (Table 10).

TABLE 10.   Potential Complications of Immobilization

System	Effect
Musculoskeletal	Atrophy and contracture of muscle Osteoporosis
Respiratory	Decreased overall ventilation Regional changes in ventilation and perfusion Atelectasis Pulmonary embolism Difficulty coughing
Endocrine and renal	Decreased basal metabolism Increased diuresis, natriuresis, and extracellular fluid shift Negative nitrogen balance Glucose intolerance Hypercalcemia and calcium loss Renal stones
Gastrointestinal	Anorexia Constipation
Skin	Pressure sores
Vascular	Deep venous thrombosis
Central nervous system	Altered sensation Decreased motor activity Autonomic instability Emotional and behavioral disturbances Intellectual deficit Poor coordination

	TABLE 11.	Outline of Recovery for Stroke	
Disease	Impairment	Disability	Handicap
Infarct Hemorrhage	Site of lesion Type of lesion	Activities of daily living	Based on: Impairment and/or disability Attitude of society
	For example: Motor Sensory Visual Dysarthria Dysphagia Attention Memory	For example: Bowel Bladder Dressing Self-care Communication Locomotor	For example: Physical dependence Mobility Orientation Occupation Economic self- sufficiency

These complications can account for much of the functional loss and are generally reversible. Hence, a discussion of recovery would not be complete without taking these secondary complications into account.

Recovery and Functional Outcome

In 1980 the World Health Organization published *The International Classification of Impairments, Disabilities and Handicaps.*[46] This conceptual model suggests that disease may give rise to impairment, which in turn may lead to the development of disability. Handicap may result from an impairment or disability. This recovery from stroke (Table 11) is simplistic but can be used as a basic foundation to discuss recovery and related issues.

Stroke recovery consists of impairments (signs and symptoms) defined by the localization of the lesion. Disability results from the neurologic deficits (impairments), and it is measured in terms of functions such as ADLs.

Jorgensen and colleagues studied 1,197 acute stroke patients in the Copenhagen Stroke Study.[25,26] This study consisted of a large unselected community-based population. Impairments were classified using the Scandinavian Neurological Stroke Scale (SNSS), and functional disability was defined according to the Barthel Index (BI). The initial impairments of stroke patients were divided into thirds: a third were severe to very severe, a third were moderate, and a third mild. Table 12 outlines the impairments and functional disability of the survivors; 21% of the stroke patients died. Typically, recovery from impairment and functional disability meant the highest recorded score in SNSS and BI, respectively, with no further improvement. Neurologic recovery occurred an average of 2 weeks earlier than functional recovery. In surviving patients, the best neurologic recovery in 80% of the patients occurred within 4.5 weeks, and the best ADL function was achieved by 6 weeks. In 95% of the patients, the best neurologic recovery was reached by 11 weeks and best ADL function within 12.5 weeks. In another study, Jorgensen et al. reported that best walking function was reached within 4 weeks for patients with mild paresis of the affected lower extremity, 6 weeks for those with moderate paresis, and 11 weeks for severe paralysis.[24] Consequently, the time course of neurologic and functional recovery was strongly related to both initial stroke severity and functional disability.

Although Jorgensen demonstrated that two thirds of all stroke survivors had mild to moderate strokes and are able to achieve independence in ADL, Duncan et al. have shown that even individuals with mild and moderate stroke exhibit limitations in higher physical functions, physical and social role functioning, and return to work.[14,24–26]

TABLE 12. Impairment and Functional Disability Outcome of the Survivors in the
Copenhagen Stroke Study

Impairment: Recovery			Functional Disability: Recovery		
Category	% of Survivors*	Weeks†	Category	% of Survivors*	Weeks†
Very severe	4	10	Very severe	14	11
Severe	7	9	Severe	6	11.5
Moderate	11	5.5	Moderate	8	6
Mild/No	78	2.5	Mild	26	2.5
			No	46	

* Percentage of the survivors after completion of rehabilitation
† Time required for best recovery reached in 80% of the patients after completion of rehabilitation
Adapted from Jorgensen HS, Nakayama H, Raaschou HO, et al: Outcome and time course of recovery in stroke. Part I. The Copenhagen Stroke Study. Arch Phys Med Rehabil 76:399–405, 1995, and Jorgensen HS, Nakayama H, Raaschou HO, et al: Outcome and time course of recovery in stroke. Part II. The Copenhagen Stroke Study. Arch Phys Med Rehabil 76:406–412, 1995.

Generally, survivors of brain stem strokes have reportedly better prognosis for recovery and long-term survival than those with hemispheric infarctions.[21,41] Chua and Kong retrospectively studied 53 consecutive patients with brain stem strokes admitted to an inpatient rehabilitation unit.[9] They found that 96% of the patients were discharged home and that patients with a lower Modified Barthel Index (MBI) score on admission had a worse functional outcome. The total MBI was the only significant factor to influence outcome. Nonsignificant factors included age, pattern of motor weakness, presence or absence of ataxia, and urinary incontinence.

Reporting on the ADL recovery of 100 stroke patients, Duncan and Lai found that the most dramatic recovery occurred in the first 30 days for individuals with mild to moderate strokes.[13] Severe strokes had a much more protracted recovery, with most recovery occurring 1–3 months poststroke. This group also had the greatest degree of variability in ADL recovery. A strong correlation was noted between motor recovery and ADL recovery, but the percentage of ADL recovery was always greater than the percentage of motor recovery. The authors felt that this suggested that stroke patients might achieve independence in basic ADLs in the presence of significant residual motor impairment.[13]

Stroke recovery is not merely the result of neurologic improvement. Roth et al. were able to objectively confirm the additional benefit of comprehensive rehabilitation of stroke patients with respect to improving function.[39] Their study consisted of 402 patients consecutively admitted to an acute stroke rehabilitation program. Significant improvements in functional performance occurred regardless of whether patients had experienced reduction in their impairments. Thus, improvements in functional outcome cannot be solely explained by the natural recovery taking place during the rehabilitation admission. The efficacy of comprehensive rehabilitation is additionally supported by the findings of two meta-analyses.[29,36]

REFERENCES

 1. Annet M: Hand preference and the laterality of cerebral speech. Cortex 11:305–328, 1975.
 2. Bach-y-Rita P: Central nervous system lesions: Sprouting and unmasking in rehabilitation. Arch Phys Med Rehabil 62:413–417, 1981.
 3. Benson DF: Aphasia, Alexia, and Agraphia. New York, Churchill Livingstone, 1979.
 4. Bonita R, Beaglehole R: Recovery of motor function after stroke. Stroke 19:1497–1500, 1988.
 5. Boyeson MG, Bach-y-Rita P: Determinants of brain plasticity. J Neurol Rehabil 3:35–57, 1989.

6. Boyeson MG, Jones JL, Harmon RL: Sparing of motor function after cortical injury. Arch Neurol 51:405–414, 1994.

7. Brodal A: Self-observations and neuroanatomical considerations after a stroke. Brain 96:675–694, 1973.

8. Campbell A, Brown A, Schildroth C, et al: The relationship between neuropsychological measures and self-care skills in patients with cerebrovascular lesion. J Natl Med Assoc 83:321–324, 1991.

9. Chua KSG, Kong K-H: Functional outcome in brain stem stroke patients after rehabilitation. Arch Phys Med Rehabil 77:194–197, 1996.

10. Delaney G, Potter P: Disability post stroke. Phys Med Rehabil State Art Rev 7:27–42, 1993.

11. Dombovy ML: Stroke: Clinical course and neurophysiologic mechanisms of recovery. Crit Rev Phys Rehabil Med 2:171–188, 1991.

12. Duncan PW, Goldstein LB, Matchar D, et al: Measurement of motor recovery after stroke: Outcome assessment and sample size requirements. Stroke 23:1084–1089, 1992.

13. Duncan PW, Lai SM: Stroke recovery. Top Stroke Rehabil 4:51–58, 1997.

14. Duncan PW, Samsa GP, Weinberger M, et al: Health status of individuals with mild stroke. Stroke 28:740–745, 1997.

15. Easter SS, Purves D, Spitzner NC: The changing view of neural specificity. Science 230:507–511, 1985.

16. Feeney DM, Sutton RL: Pharmacotherapy for recovery of function after brain injury. Crit Rev Neurobiol 3:135–197, 1987.

17. Feigenson JS, McCarthy ML, Greenberg SD, Feigenson WD: Factors influencing outcome and length of stay in a stroke rehabilitation unit. Part 2. Comparison of 318 screened and 248 unscreened patients. Stroke 8:657–662, 1977.

18. Ferrucci L, Bondinelli S, Gufalnick JM, et al: Recovery of functional status after stroke: A post rehabilitation follow-up study. Stroke 24:200–205, 1993.

19. Finger S, Stein DG: Brain Damage and Recovery: Research and Clinical Perspectives. New York, Academic Press, 1982.

20. Fischer CM: Lacunar stroke and infarcts—a review. Neurology 32:871–876, 1982.

21. Garrison SJ, Rolak LA: Rehabilitation of the stroke patient. In DeLisa JA, Gans BM (eds): Rehabilitation Medicine: Principles and Practice. Philadelphia, JB Lippincott, 1993, pp 801–824.

22. Hier DB, Mondlock J, Caplan LR: Recovery of behavioral abnormalities after right hemisphere stroke. Neurology 33:345–350, 1983.

23. Inoue Y, Takemoto K, Miyamoto T, et al: Sequential computed tomography scans in acute cerebral infarction. Radiology 135:655–662, 1980.

24. Jorgensen HS, Nakayama H, Raaschou HO, Olsen TS: Recovery of walking function in stroke patients: The Copenhagen Stroke Study. Arch Phys Med Rehabil 76:27–32, 1995.

25. Jorgensen HS, Nakayama H, Raaschou HO, et al: Outcome and time course of recovery in stroke. Part I. The Copenhagen Stroke Study. Arch Phys Med Rehabil 76:399–405, 1995.

26. Jorgensen HS, Nakayama H, Raaschou HO, et al: Outcome and time course of recovery in stroke. Part II. The Copenhagen Stroke Study. Arch Phys Med Rehabil 76:406–412, 1995.

27. Kelly-Hayes M, Wold PA, Kase CS, et al: Time course of functional recovery after stroke: The Framingham Study. J Neurol Rehabil 3:65–70, 1989.

28. Kertesz A, McCabe P: Recovery patterns and prognosis in aphasia. Brain 100:1–18, 1977.

29. Langhorne P, Williams BO, Gilchrist W, Howie K: Do stroke units save lives? Lancet 342:395–398, 1993.

30. Laurence S, Stein DG: Recovery after brain damage and concept of localization of function. In Finger S (ed): Recovery from Brain Damage. New York, Plenum Press, 1978, pp 369–407.

31. Layton BS: Optimal recovery after stroke. Presented at the 54th annual meeting of the American Academy of Physical Medicine and Rehabilitation, San Francisco, November 13–16, 1992.

32. Lo RC: Recovery and rehabilitation after stroke. Can Fam Physician 32:1851–1853, 1986.

33. Mayo NE, Korner-Bitensky NA, Becker R: Recovery time of independent function post-stroke. Am J Phys Med Rehabil 70:5–12, 1991.

34. Nakayama H, Jorgenson HS, Raaschou HO, Olsen T: Compensation in recovery of upper extremity function after stroke: The Copenhagen Stroke Study. Arch Phys Med Rehabil 75:852–857, 1994.

35. O'Brien MT, Pallet PJ: Total Care of the Stroke Patient. Boston, Little, Brown, 1978.

36. Ottenbacker KJ, Jannell S: The results of clinical trials in stroke rehabilitation research. Arch Neurol 50:37–44, 1993.

37. Pryse-Phillips W, Murray TJ: Essential Neurology. Garden City, NY, Medical Examination Publishing, 1978.

38. Raisman G, Field PM: A quantitative investigation of the development of collateral reinnervation of the septal nuclei. Brain Res 50:241–264, 1973.

39. Roth EJ, Heinemann AW, Lovell LL, et al: Impairment and disability: Their relation during stroke re-habilitation. Arch Phys Med Rehabil 79:329–335, 1998.
40. Stone SP, Wilson B, Wroot A, et al: The assessment of visuo-spatial neglect after acute stroke. J Neurol Neurosurg Psychiatry 54:345–350, 1991.
41. Turney TM, Garraway MG, Whisnant JP: The natural history of hemispheric and brainstem infarction in Rochester, Minnesota. Stroke 15:790–794, 1984.
42. Von Monakow C: Gehirpathologie. Vienna, A. Holder, 1905.
43. Wade DT, Langton-Hewer R, Skilbeck CE, David RM: Stroke: A Critical Approach to Diagnosis, Treatment and Management. Chicago, Year Book, 1985.
44. Wade DT, Langton-Hewer R: Functional abilities after stroke: Measurement, natural history, and prognosis. J Neurol Neurosurg Psychiatry 50:177–182, 1987.
45. Wade DT, Langton-Hewer R, Wood VA, et al: The hemiplegic arm after stroke: Measurement and recovery. J Neurol Neurosurg Psychiatry 46:521–524, 1983.
46. World Health Organization: The International Classification of Impairments, Disabilities and Handicaps. Geneva, WHO, 1980.

SAMUEL WIEBE, MD, MSc, FRCPC
JAMES T. BUTLER, MBCHB, FCP (NEUROL) S.A.

POSTSTROKE SEIZURES AND EPILEPSY

From the Department of Clinical
  Neurological Sciences
University of Western Ontario
London, Ontario
Canada

Reprint requests to:
Samuel Wiebe, MD
London Health Sciences Center,
  University Campus
339 Windermere Road
London, Ontario N6A 5A5
Canada

Hughlings Jackson was one of the first to record the association between stroke and seizures. In 1864 he wrote: "It is not very uncommon to find when a patient has recovered or is recovering from hemiplegia, the result of embolism of a middle cerebral artery, or some branch of this vessel, that he is attacked by convulsion beginning in some part of the paralysed region."[37] William Gowers reported on 66 patients with hemiplegia and epilepsy and introduced the term "post-hemiplegic epilepsy."[28] Since then, numerous studies have analyzed this association. This chapter summarizes current evidence pertaining to the relation between stroke and seizures or epilepsy and discusses issues of relevance to clinicians dealing with this patient population.

Vascular disease is the most common documentable cause of seizures in the elderly[1,35,46,67,68,84] (Table 1). The average age of patients with poststroke seizures (PSS) or epilepsy is 60 years across studies.[12,15,29,56,69,76] Thus, the known increased incidence of epilepsy in later life may be partly explained by stroke. For example, in the United Kingdom's National General Practice Study of Epilepsy, epilepsy was attributed to vascular causes in 15% of all patients and 49% of patients older than 60.[64]

The incidence of seizures following ischemic or hemorrhagic stroke in earlier series is highly variable, ranging from 7.7–42.8% depending on study design, patient population, diagnostic methods, and follow-up.[5,16,17,36,49,53] High-resolution imaging such as with computed tomography (CT) and magnetic resonance imaging (MRI) has

TABLE 1.   Etiology of Seizures in Older Patients

	White et al.	Ang and Utterback	Hildick-Smith	Seifer and Ignacio	Schold et al.
Age of patient (yrs)	> 50	> 40	> 60	> 40	> 69
No. of patients	107	96	50	153	50
Cardiovascular (total)	49	46	22	26	15
Hypertension	6	5	—	—	—
Hemorrhage	—	6	—	8	2
Systemic/metabolic	2	7	4	—	5
Degenerative/atrophic	5	11	7	2	0
Tumor	21	4	5	26	1
Trauma	3	5	1	4	4
Other	2	6	4	10	0
Unknown	25	17	7	85	25

From Lesser RP, Luders H, Dinner DS, et al: Epileptic seizures due to thrombotic and embolic cerebrovascular disease in older patients. Epilepsia 26:622–630, 1985; with permission.

improved the ability to identify and classify strokes, resulting in better estimates of their clinical course and consequences.

In comparison to earlier studies, recent reports reveal less variability in the risk of PSS. The average risk of seizures is 10% within 1–10 years after stroke (Table 2), and well-conducted prospective studies report a 5-year cumulative incidence of 11.5%[7] (Fig. 1). At least two studies suggest a higher incidence of PSS (15–17%) in patients in rehabilitation units.[41,57] It is not clear whether this reflects seizure ascertainment bias (e.g., seizures are less likely to be missed in closely observed patients), a true increased seizure risk in this population (e.g., more extensive cerebral injury), or both. Analyses based on neurologic services[59] and stroke registries[7] confirm that PSS are more likely to occur after severe strokes.

RISK OF POSTSTROKE SEIZURES AND EPILEPSY: THE EVIDENCE

Validity of the Evidence

As the literature on PSS proliferates, clinicians must interpret the results of numerous and often conflicting studies. To assess the validity and potential application of the evidence on PSS, clinicians can quickly apply the following five-point test to the methods section of relevant articles[44] (Table 3).

1. Does the study have a well-defined, representative sample of stroke patients assembled at a common point in the course of disease—preferably early after stroke?

TABLE 2.   Risk of Seizures following Stroke of All Types in Recent Studies

Series	Study Type/Source	No. Patients	Probability of Seizures	Follow-Up
Burn, 1997	Prospective/Stroke registry	675	11.5%	5 years
Paolucci, 1997	Prospective/Rehabilitation service	306	15%	—
So, 1996	Retrospective/Population	535	8.9%	10 years
Lancman, 1993	Retrospective/Hospital	219	10%	1 year
Kotila, 1992	Prospective/Rehabilitation service	200	17%	3 years

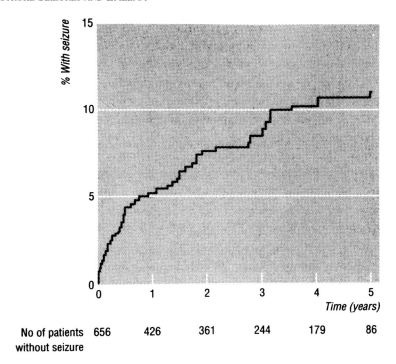

No of patients 656   426   361   244   179   86
without seizure

FIGURE 1. Cumulative risk of poststroke seizures (Kaplan-Meier estimate) after first stroke. Patients with a history of seizures were excluded, and deaths were censored. The number of patients at risk of seizures is indicated. From Burn J, Dennis M, Bamford J, et al: Epileptic seizures after a first stroke. BMJ 315:1582–1587, 1997; with permission.

Because patient populations may differ in their risk of PSS, authors should describe how and which patients were included. Because the risk of PSS is thought to change with time (higher frequency early after stroke), including patients at dissimilar points after stroke makes it difficult to interpret the results.

2. Is the endpoint of interest—seizures—systematically and explicitly assessed in all patients?

Establishing the presence of seizures is not always straightforward. Patients or inexperienced clinicians may miss certain seizure types or misdiagnose syncope, movement disorders, or other phenomena as seizures. This is particularly problematic in surveys or retrospective chart reviews. Information may be ambiguous and subject to interpretation, and corroboration by a neurologist may not be possible, resulting in spuriously inflated or deflated estimates of risk.

TABLE 3.　Assessing the Evidence for Poststroke Seizures and Epilepsy

Is the evidence valid?
1. Are patients well defined, representative, and assembled at a similar point in the course of stroke?
2. Are seizures systematically, explicitly, and equally assessed in all study patients?
3. Is follow-up sufficiently long and complete?
4. Does stroke precede seizures in all patients?
5. Is the study a prospective analysis?

TABLE 4. Appraisal of 11 Large Studies Assessing the Risk of Poststroke Seizures

Methodologic Feature	No. of Studies (%)
Patients captured at similar point	10 (91)
Patients captured early after stroke	8 (73)
Study population well defined	11 (100)
Seizures systematically and explicitly assessed	2 (18)
Adequate follow-up (complete, sufficiently long)	8 (73)
Exclusion of seizures before stroke	7 (64)
Prospective study	5 (45)

3. Was follow-up sufficiently long and complete?

Incomplete or insufficiently long follow-up may bias risk estimates because events are missed in specific patient groups. For example, loss to follow-up may select out those with worse or better outcomes.

4. Does stroke precede seizures?

Temporal association is important. Inclusion of patients with preexisting epilepsy results in inflated estimates of PSS.

5. Is the study a prospective analysis?

Prospective analyses avoid the biases common to retrospective studies, such as incomplete information, nonsystematically obtained data, and ambiguous recording of events of interest.

Table 4 summarizes the validity of the evidence for PSS derived from 11 large studies published since 1990 and containing an adequate description of the patient population.[2,7,27,39,41,42,48,57,59,73,77] Patients were seen at a similar point in the course of their illness in 10 (91%) of studies, but only eight (73%) captured patients early after stroke. Follow-up was explicit in eight (73%) of the studies, but, only one contained actuarial analysis, which is pertinent when the duration of follow-up varies among patients.[7] Incidence of PSS was generally lower in seven (64%) studies that excluded patients with seizures preceding stroke. Data were prospectively collected in five (45%) of the studies. Finally, only two studies (18%) assessed the presence of seizures in a systematic and explicit manner.[2,7] Studies with the highest score on this five-point check provide the strongest evidence.

Helpfulness of the Evidence

To determine whether the evidence is useful, clinicians can apply a three-point check to the results section of valid studies[44] (Table 5).

1. Are the patients similar to my own?

Studies should describe the patients with enough detail to allow clinicians to compare and, if possible, extrapolate to their own patients.

2. How large is the risk, and what are the prognostic factors?

A simple statement of frequency of PSS may not be sufficiently informative unless the clinician knows how it compares to a control group or to the general population.

TABLE 5. Applying the Evidence for Poststroke Seizures and Epilepsy to Patients

Is the evidence useful?

1. Are the study patients similar to my own?

2. How large is the risk for poststroke seizures, and what are the important prognostic factors?

3. How precise (certain) are the results?

For example, Burn et al. found that the risk of seizures is 35 times higher after stroke than in the general population.[7] They also compare graphically the risk of PSS in various subgroups and state that hemorrhagic stroke has a risk of PSS ten times higher than ischemic stroke.

3. How precise are the results?

Even when valid, a prognostic study provides only an estimate of the true risk. The precision of the estimate is best examined with a confidence interval (CI). The wider the CI, the less precise, and less certain, the results. Only three of the eleven studies cited above provide a useful estimate of the precision of their results.[2,7,59] The importance of this point is illustrated by considering that the cumulative risk of seizures 5 years after subarachnoid hemorrhage was 34% in one study, but the true risk (expressed as 95% CI) could be from 0–100%.[7] Therefore, when discussing risks with patients, one may prefer to use short-term but more precise estimates, e.g., the 2-year risk of seizures after subarachnoid hemorrhage is 27.8% (95% CI 5.3–50.7%).

SEIZURE TYPES IN CEREBROVASCULAR DISEASE

Seizures are the clinical expression of excessive, hypersynchronous discharge of neurons in the cerebral cortex. The area of cerebral cortex involved in a seizure determines its clinical expression. The latter often evolves as seizure activity spreads through the brain.[19]

Although most stroke-related seizures are simple partial (especially focal motor), in some series up to 50% are either primary or secondarily generalized. On the other hand, complex partial seizures are uncommon, and absence seizures do not occur as a result of stroke[7,46] (Table 6).

TIMING OF SEIZURE OCCURRENCE IN RELATION TO STROKE

As compared with earlier series, recent studies show remarkable agreement in the frequency of early PSS (Table 7).

Studies with short follow-up create the impression that virtually all PSS occur early. In Black's prospective study, 39% of patients had their PSS in the first 24 hours and 88% in the first year.[5] In contrast, the 5-year prospective Oxfordshire study demonstrates that only 43% of patients had their PSS in the first year.[7] Thereafter, an average of 1.5% new patients per year continued to develop PSS.[7] As the period of observation (the denominator) increases, the proportion of patients with early PSS diminishes in relation to the total. Studies with longer follow-up may continue to show small but long-term incremental risks of PSS.

TABLE 6. Types of Seizures in Patients with Cerebrovascular Disease

	Ang and Utterback	Louis and McDowell	Meyer et al.	Schold et al.	Cocito et al.	Franck	DeCarolis et al.	Total
Focal motor	14	34	14	27	11	13	2	115
Complex partial	—	—	—	1	2	3	—	6
Adversive	—	—	—	—	1	—	—	1
Focal with secondary generalization	15	—	—	—	4	—	16	35
Generalized only	17	26	4	22	4	1	—	74

From Lesser RP, Luders H, Dinner DS, et al: Epileptic seizures due to thrombotic and embolic cerebrovascular disease in older patients. Epilepsia 26:622–630, 1985; with permission.

TABLE 7.   Incidence of Early Poststroke Seizures in Six Large Studies

Series	Study Type	No. Patients	Incidence	Time
Burn, 1997	Prospective	675	2.0%	< 24 hours
Arboix, 1997	Retrospective	1200	2.4%	< 48 hours
Reith, 1997	Prospective	1197	4.2%	< 2 weeks
Lo, 1994	Retrospective	1200	2.5%	< 2 weeks
Giroud, 1994	Retrospective	1640	5.4%	< 2 weeks
Kilpatrick, 1990	Prospective	1000	4.4%	< 2 weeks

Epilepsy Preceding Stroke

Epilepsy may precede a clinically apparent stroke.[4] The importance of this recognition resides in the tendency for established seizure disorders to produce recurrent seizures, creating an erroneous impression of worse seizure outcome in PSS.

A prospective, case-control, British study found the prevalence of epilepsy prior to the first known stroke to be 4.5%,[70] almost eight times higher than the prevalence of epilepsy in the general population (0.6%). The prevalence rose to 9.3% in cases of recurrent stroke. The median duration of epilepsy before the first stroke was 9.5 years, and the median age of the patients was 60. Problems with this study include its retrospective nature, patient admission bias, and selection of controls, all of which could contribute to a spuriously high prevalence of prestroke seizures.

Well-conducted, prospective cohort studies report a lower frequency of prestroke seizures. For example, the prevalence of unprovoked seizures preceding stroke in the Oxfordshire project was 2% (95% CI 1–3%).[7]

One explanation for this phenomenon is that some late-onset epilepsies may be caused by clinically silent strokes, which have been demonstrated by necropsy studies[17] and by CT and MRI.[71] The development of hemiplegia in three of four patients with prior ipsilateral partial seizures in the British case-control study supports the occurrence of silent strokes.[70] Furthermore, in a subset of patients in this study, only those with prior seizures continued to have seizures during a follow-up period of 30 months.[69]

A case-control study of first seizures has shown by multiple logistic regression analysis that hypertension, a well-known stroke risk factor, also independently increases the risk of developing adult-onset seizures.[55] Therefore, a heretofore unexplained association between risk factors for stroke and seizures seems to operate.

Seizures at Onset of Stroke

Almost 10% of strokes may be accompanied at onset by focal motor epileptic seizures.[4,12,15,20,49,61] Recent series find stroke-onset seizures in 2–4% of patients (see Table 7).

The finding by DeRueck et al. that other possible causes for seizures were usually present—renal failure, severe hypertension and cerebral edema—have not been confirmed by others.[16] Interestingly, in two other large studies seizures occurred in five patients in association with transient ischemic attacks (TIAs) alone.[12,20] Distinguishing Todd's postictal paralysis from vascular paralysis may be difficult in such circumstances.

The possibility of an ischemic event should always be considered when an individual at risk for stroke presents with new-onset seizures, whether single or in status epilepticus.[46] Seizures can be causally related to stroke if they follow rather than precede stroke, if localizing focal ictal features exist, and if there is clinical or radiologic evidence of vascular disease in the corresponding area.

Early-Onset Versus Late-Onset Seizures

Gupta et al. found no difference in risk of recurrence with early- versus late-onset seizures after a follow-up of only 30 months.[29] However, Hauser et al. found the cumulative risk 6 years after stroke to be 19%.[32] The risk increased 22-fold in patients with early-onset seizures. Similarly, Burn et al. report an eightfold late seizure risk increase in patients with early seizures.[7] On the other hand, Sung et al. and Paolucci et al. find that late seizures are better predictors of the development of epilepsy.[57,77] In the latter studies, the definition of epilepsy may predetermine the results.

Most studies agree that early-onset seizures are not associated with a higher mortality or a worse functional outcome.[30,39,69,70,75]

Epilepsy after Stroke

Epilepsy can be defined as a condition characterized by a tendency for recurrent seizures that are not caused by an immediately preceding insult. This excludes childhood febrile convulsions and seizures due to an acute metabolic derangement or an acute insult to the brain.[19,31]

Retrospective studies looking at all stroke types have consistently found the prevalence of poststroke epilepsy to be below 10%.[3,20,49,51,61] Olson prospectively followed 61 patients with supratentorial stroke for 2–4 years; seven patients (9%) developed epilepsy, most within 6–12 months.[56]

The long-term risk of poststroke epilepsy has been analyzed prospectively using the life table method in a Swedish cohort of 409 stroke patients followed for 3.5–7 years.[81] The cumulative risk was 3% at 1 year and 5% at 5 years. The annual incidence was highest in the first year (3%) and thereafter decreased to 0.4% per year. More recently, using similar methodology, the Oxfordshire project found that the cumulative 5-year risk of epilepsy (recurrent seizures) was almost identical to that found in the Swedish study: 5.4% (95% CI 0.3–10.5%). The relative benign character of PSS is reflected in this study's finding that recurrent seizures occur in only 50% and frequent seizures in only 15% of patients with PSS.[7]

In a retrospective study of 206 patients hospitalized for ischemic stroke, Hauser et al. found a cumulative risk for epilepsy of 19% at 6 years, a figure that is four times higher than in the Swedish and British studies.[32] The risk increased to 56% in patients with a history of seizures prior to stroke, as has been suggested in other studies.[69] Differences in patient population, with selection of more severe cases in the Hauser study, may explain the discrepancies.

In Olsen's study, seizures were focal motor or generalized and were easily controlled with antiepileptic drugs.[56] The patients at highest risk for epilepsy had persistent hemiparesis and cortical involvement (six of seven) regardless of the nature of the stroke.

Several studies have analyzed the electroencephalographic (EEG) features of poststroke epilepsy. Focal delta or theta has been found in most series and epileptiform activity in some of the series. However, the EEG does not help to determine the risk of developing epilepsy after stroke.[20,49,51,56]

STROKE TYPES AND SEIZURES

Thrombotic Versus Embolic Stroke

Early studies support the notion that seizures are more common with embolic than with thrombic infarcts.[36,53,54,61] The main criticism of these studies is that

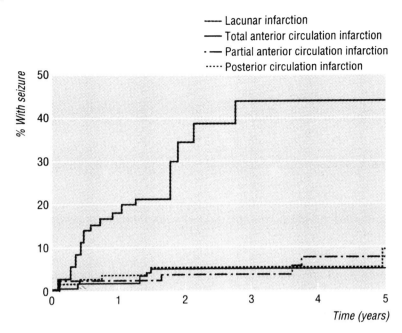

FIGURE 2. Cumulative risk of poststroke seizures (Kaplan-Meier estimate) after ischemic stroke, subdivided by clinical subtype. From Burn J, Dennis M, Bamford J, et al: Epileptic seizures after a first stroke. BMJ 315:1582–1587, 1997; with permission.

"embolic" stroke is presumed rather than documented. Several more recent studies fail to support these observations[5,39,56,69] and emphasize the difficulties in distinguishing between thrombotic and embolic stroke clinically, radiologically, and even pathologically.[37]

In the prospective study of Black et al., a potential source of cardiac embolism was found in 32 (38%) patients with seizures following stroke and in 200 (27%) patients with stroke and no seizures; the difference was not statistically significant.[5] Similarly, in a case-control study, Shinton et al. found no difference in the frequency of seizures after embolic, thrombotic, or hemorrhagic stroke.[69]

More recently, Kilpatrick et al. prospectively studied 1,000 patients with TIA or stroke of all types and locations in the brain.[39] Early seizures occurred in 44 patients (4.4%). No difference in incidence of seizures was found between presumed embolic and thrombotic stroke.

The prospective study of Olsen et al. found no difference in seizure incidence among thrombotic, embolic, or hemorrhagic stroke.[56] However, heart failure and recent myocardial infarction, both risk factors for embolic stroke, were among the many exclusion criteria.

Cortical Versus Subcortical Stroke

Earlier studies have emphasized that cortical involvement is essential for the production of PSS. Olsen et al.[56] and Kilpatrick et al.[39] found that a vascular lesion involving the cerebral cortex, irrespective of size or nature, was a prerequisite for the development of epilepsy and that purely subcortical lesions did not produce

TABLE 8. Reports on Seizures in Patients with Intracerebral Hemorrhage

Author	Year	Diagnostic Method	No. of Patients	Study Period	Patients with Seizure	Incidence of Seizure (%)
Aring and Merritt	1935	Autopsy	116	Admission	16	13.8
Richardson and Dodge	1954	Autopsy	23	Admission	1	4.3
Schaafsma	1968	Autopsy	42	Admission	1	2.0
Fentz	1971	Chart review	23	Acute stage	2	6.0
Fentz	1971	Chart review	12	Late stage	2	17.0
Mohr et al. Harrison	1978	Prospective, clinical diagnosis	115	Acute stage	7	6.0
Kase et al.	1980	CT	62	Acute stage	4	6.0
Lipton et al.	1985	CT and autopsy	24	Acute stage	3	12.5
Berger et al.	1987	CT	112	Acute stage	19	17.0
Sung and Chu	1988	CT	112	Acute stage	19	17.0
	1989	CT	1402	Acute and late stage	64	4.6

CT = computed tomography
From Sung CY, Chu NS: Epileptic seizures in intracerebral haemorrhage. J Neurol Neurosurg Psychiatry 52:1273–1276, 1989; with permission.

seizures.[39,56] This concept requires revision in light of recent evidence. At least three studies demonstrate the occurrence of seizures following basal ganglia hemorrhage or lacunar infarcts without any cortical involvement.[7,27,76] In Burn's study, 10% of all PSS patients had exclusively lacunar strokes, and a similar amount had posterior circulation and partial anterior circulation strokes[7] (Fig. 2).

Intracerebral Hemorrhage

Intracerebral hemorrhage (ICH) is the third most frequent cause of stroke after infarction and embolism. The major causes of hemorrhage are vascular malformations, hypertension, bleeding disorders, and, in the elderly, amyloid angiopathy.

Table 8 highlights the features of 11 earlier studies addressing the frequency of seizures after ICH, as summarized by Sung and Chu.[76] The risk of seizures in these studies ranged from 2–17%, due in part to study design and diagnostic method of ICH.

Although recent large series continue to show a broad range in the frequency of post-ICH seizures (4.3–15%), all demonstrate that the risk is higher after ICH than after ischemic stroke (Table 9). The highest risk applies to subarachnoid hemorrhage, followed by ICH, and lastly by ischemic stroke (Fig. 3).

TABLE 9. Risk of Poststroke Seizure by Stroke Type

Series	Hemorrhage	Infarct	Length of Follow-Up
Kilpatrick, 1990	15%	7%	≤ 2 weeks
Lo, 1994	15%	2.3%	≤ 2 weeks
Arboix, 1997	4.3%	2%	≤ 2 weeks
Reith, 1997	8%	3%	≤ 2 weeks
Giroud, 1994	15%	6%	≤ 2 weeks
Burn, 1997	26%	9.7%	5 years

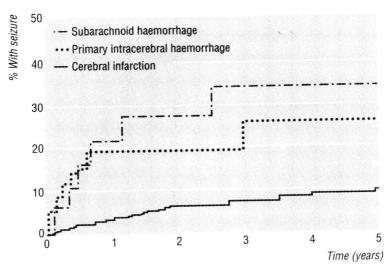

FIGURE 3. Cumulative risk of poststroke seizures (Kaplan-Meier estimate), subdivided by stroke type. From Burn J, Dennis M, Bamford J, et al: Epileptic seizures after a first stroke. BMJ 315:1582–1587, 1997; with permission.

As with ischemic stroke, cortical involvement by ICH is a stronger risk factor for seizures. Although deep-seated hemorrhages may cause seizures, the risk is 7–15 times higher when the cortex is involved.[39,48,56,76]

It has been proposed that ICH is more frequently associated with late-onset than with early-onset seizures, in distinction to other stroke types.[46] However, in a series of 1402 patients with primary ICH, Sung and Chu found that 64 patients (4.6%) had seizures whose timing was similar to that reported for other stroke entities: 19 (30%) occurred in the first 24 hours, 38 (60%) in the first 2 weeks, and 58 (90%) by the first year after ICH.[76] Seizure phenomenology was similar to that which occurred in other stroke types. Epilepsy occurred in 37 (58%) of patients with seizures. Those with late-onset seizures, defined as occurring more than 2 weeks after ICH, seemed particularly at risk.

Subarachnoid Hemorrhage

Subarachnoid hemorrhage (SAH), a spontaneous, nontraumatic, intracranial hemorrhage caused by aneurysms, accounts for about 10% of all strokes.[34,80] The frequency, time of onset, and consequences of seizures in SAH have not been systematically studied, and the available data are controversial.[21]

Several difficulties occur in the analysis of such data. For example, alteration of consciousness at onset is a prominent feature of SAH; it occurs transiently in up to 45% of patients, but 21% of patients are comatose at onset.[83] Seizures in these patients may be subtle. Likewise, intracranial pressure may acutely increase, producing episodes of decerebrate posturing that may be mistaken for seizures.[78]

Sundaram and Chow retrospectively studied 131 consecutive cases of spontaneous SAH with a highly disciplined protocol; prior epilepsy, decerebrate posturing, and vague "blackouts" were excluded, and an accurate seizure description

TABLE 10. Time of Seizures in Relation to Subarachnoid Hemorrhage

Early seizures (within the first 2 weeks)		26 (20%)
Less than 24 hours of bleeding	19	
24–48 hours	2	
48 hours–1 week	3	
1–2 weeks	2	
Delayed seizures		5 (4%)
(First seizure more than 2 weeks after hemorrhage)		

From Sundaram MBM, Chow F: Seizures associated with spontaneous subarachnoid hemorrhage. Can J Neurol Sci 13:229–231, 1986; with permission.

was sought.[75] Seizure incidence was 24%, 84% of which took place in the first 2 weeks of SAH, mostly within the first few hours or minutes of initial bleeding or rebleeding (Table 10). Late-onset (more than 2 weeks) seizures occurred in 4% of all patients and 16% of patients with seizures. More than 60% of the patients had multiple seizures, with a range of two to four seizures per patient over 2 years. As in other recent studies, there was no evidence that SAH patients with seizures have a higher mortality or rebleeding rate than patients without seizures. Half of all seizures were partial with or without secondary generalization, and half appeared to be primarily generalized although an occult focus was likely present. Importantly, partial seizure phenomenology did not correlate with location of the aneurysm.

Retrospectively analyzing 100 consecutive cases of aneurysmal SAH from two centers, Hart et al. found a similar seizure incidence of 26%.[30] More than half of all attacks happened within the first 12 hours of hemorrhage, and most occurring after 12 hours were related to acute rebleeding as documented by new blood in the cerebrospinal fluid. All seizures were easily controlled with anticonvulsants and had no relationship with mortality or short-term prognosis. Other recent studies concur that seizures are easily controlled and that long-term prophylactic anticonvulsants are probably not indicated.[2,7,59]

Seizures have been reported to occur at some point during the acute period of SAH in 3–26% of patients.[3,8,30,33,39,63,75,82,83,85] After recovery from SAH, 4–10% of patients continue to have seizures.[30,63,75,82,83,85]

Vascular Malformations and Epilepsy

ARTERIOVENOUS MALFORMATIONS

The incidence of seizures among series of patients with arteriovenous malformations (AVMs) ranges from 23–58%.[6,24,58] Crawford et al. found that seizures were more likely to occur among younger patients, in patients with large AVMs, and among patients whose AVMs involved the cerebral cortex.[14] In two studies, the risk of a subsequent bleed was 36–67% among patients presenting with hemorrhage and was 22–27% in patients presenting with seizures.[14,24] However, one other study found no difference.[6]

Crawford et al. found that an average of 10 years elapsed before an AVM was discovered as the cause of epilepsy[14]; this would likely be shortened with even greater access to neuroimaging.

One study has related seizure origin to AVM location. In addition to seizures arising from the vicinity of the AVM, Yeh and Privitera found remote foci in eight of 27 patients, all of which were ipsilateral mesial temporal in location.[87]

CAVERNOUS ANGIOMAS

The natural history of cavernous angiomas (CAs) is poorly understood. Because CAs may be asymptomatic and difficult to diagnose, epidemiologic estimates of their consequences, i.e., seizures, are difficult to obtain. However, it is possible to describe their mode of presentation. Retrospective data from pre-MRI studies have led to the widespread belief that one third of CA patients present with seizures, one third with hemorrhage, and one third with nonspecific or no symptoms.[72] However, MRI-based studies show a much higher prevalence of seizures or epilepsy and a lower incidence of symptomatic hemorrhage.[62] In one recent study, 21 of 31 (68%) patients presented with seizures.[38] Seizures are more likely to occur if CAs involve the cortex, and they are medically refractory in almost half of the patients. The EEG is abnormal in 54% of patients with seizures.[9] At least 45% of children with CA present with seizures.[23] Surgical removal of CAs in cases of medically refractory seizures leaves 60–70% of patients free of seizures.[9,13]

CEREBRAL VENOUS THROMBOSIS

Cerebral venous thrombosis (CVT) can involve the cerebral cortex or deep veins, the dural venous sinuses, or, more often, a combination of these.

The neurologic features reflect the production of increased intracranial pressure, hemorrhagic infarct, intracerebral or subarachnoid hemorrhage, or seizures.

In contrast with most cerebrovascular conditions associated with epilepsy, CVT frequently affects young adults and children with conditions such as meningitis, otitis, dehydration, systemic malignancy, hypercoagulable states, pregnancy, postpartum, and use of oral contraceptives.[25]

Seizures occur in about half of patients with CVT, particularly with cortical vein and superior sagittal sinus thrombosis. Most paroxysmal events occur at the onset; they may be focal or generalized; and repeated seizures or status epilepticus at onset are said to be characteristic. Seizures may be followed by a worsening hemiparesis.[10]

CVT is one of the few vascular diseases in which seizures may originate in a multifocal manner.[10] Most seizures respond to antiepileptic monotherapy.

STROKE IN CHILDREN

Lanska et al. studied the clinical profile of 42 children with stroke.[43] Strokes in days-old infants almost always presented as seizures; a cortically originating neurologic deficit is usually not apparent at that age. Other authors found a similar presentation at this age.[11,22,47,74,79] In contrast, infants with strokes identified later in the first year of life usually presented with an early hand preference but without a history of ictus. Strokes in older children most commonly presented as a sudden hemiparesis or hemiplegia, occasionally associated with seizures. The incidence of late seizures in childhood stroke has varied among studies from 11–49%.[43] Possible risk factors for epilepsy following childhood stroke include seizures at stroke onset, epileptiform activity in the EEG, an early age of stroke onset, cortical involvement, and residual motor deficit.

About 12–18% of AVMs in children present as seizure disorder.[26,40] Surgical excision of the AVM and associated epileptogenic regions has relieved seizures in more than 70% of patients in various series.[40,45,86]

One specific condition that involves stroke and seizures is mitochondral encephalomyopathy, lactic acidosis, and stroke-like episodes (MELAS).[50] MELAS may become clinically apparent from age 2 to young adulthood. Patients are of short stature and have partial or generalized seizures, and some children have episodic headaches with vomiting. In association with the headaches or seizures, stroke-like episodes may develop. Such episodes of cerebral infarction may lead to a progressive loss of cognitive function, alternating hemiparesis with bilateral upper motor neuron signs, cortical deafness, and visual impairment. Muscle weakness and atrophy occur in some patients. The seizure disorder may be moderately therapy-resistant because of its multifocality.

DIFFERENTIAL DIAGNOSIS OF SEIZURES WITH STROKE

In patients with cerebrovascular disease, associated neurologic conditions that resemble epileptic seizures may occur.

Syncope

Syncope is the most common neurologic condition of systemic origin that is confused with epilepsy. The common mechanism for the several types of syncope is cerebral hypoxia. Although syncope is characterized by attacks of loss of consciousness with loss of motor tone, a recent videometric and EEG analysis illustrates the plethora of syncopal motor phenomena that resemble seizures (Table 11). During syncope, tonic spasms, myoclonus, and clonic movements may occur after the fall; however, in epileptic seizures the tonic component precedes and causes the fall. Sphincter incontinence is more common with seizures but may occur with syncope. The duration of syncope is usually less than 1 minute, followed by prompt arousal without confusion. Cardiac arrhythmia and postural hypotension, spontaneous or precipitated by antihypertensive therapy, are common causes of syncope in the elderly.[18,46]

Transient Ischemic Attacks

Both TIAs and partial seizures may produce intermittent, focal neurologic deficits. TIAs usually consist of "negative" phenomena, such as paresis, visual or

TABLE 11. Videometric Analysis of Provoked Syncope in 42 Healthy Young Adults; Mean Age = 24 Years

Features	Number (Range) or Percentage
Duration	12.1 (4.5–21.7) sec
Fall backward	83%
Atonic/Tonic	48%/52%
Myoclonus	90%
Duration	6.6 (0.7–16) sec
Outlast responsiveness	22%
Multifocal	52%
Generalized	2%
Face	58%
Other motor	79%
Extensor posture	7%
Tongue biting	2%
Moan	40%

Adapted from Lempert T, Bauer M, Schmidt D: Syncope: A videometric analysis of 56 episodes of transient cerebral hypoxia. Ann Neurol 36:233–237, 1994.

sensory deficit, and aphasia, but partial seizures tend to have "positive" phenomena, such as jerking or stiffening of a limb, which may spread rapidly over seconds to engage other parts.

Todd's paralysis refers to temporary focal weakness reflecting postictal cerebral dysfunction but not resulting from a new lesion. Transient sensory, visual, auditory, and language cerebral dysfunctions also may occur after a seizure. Distinguishing such dysfunction from TIA may be difficult in the presence of cerebrovascular disease, but Todd's paralysis without a motor seizure is unusual.

Other Abnormal Movements and Posture

In comatose patients, decerebrate posturing and intermittent muscle spasms should not be mistaken for epileptic seizures. They occur in subarachnoid hemorrhage or in parenchymal hemorrhages and infarcts with severe intracranial hypertension.

Axial and multifocal myoclonus may be present in hypoxic-ischemic encephalopathy, especially after cardiac arrest, and entails a poor prognosis.

Finally, hemiballismus or flailing movements of the limbs may occur after a stroke in the contralateral subthalamic nucleus or its connections.

TREATMENT

In the absence of adequate studies assessing the impact of antiepileptic drugs (AEDs) on the quality of life or seizure frequency in stroke patients, treatment principles are based on treatment for epilepsy in general. Much of the evidence for the latter is limited to accumulated clinical experience. The principles include (1) using anticonvulsants as monotherapy where possible, (2) starting at a low dose and escalating it slowly and only where clinically indicated, such as when seizures are recurrent, and (3) monitoring for drug toxicity using clinical findings.

Starting Treatment

Any decision to start treatment should be based on evidence that the patient has a propensity to recurrent seizures and that the seizures are not related to an immediately remediable metabolic cause such as nonketotic hyperglycemia or hyponatremia. A diagnosis of epileptic seizures is frequently subject to clinical judgment, with attendant risks for diagnostic error. If doubt exists, expert opinion or EEG evidence for seizures should be obtained.

Previously discussed evidence suggests that at least 50% of patients with PSS have a single seizure.[7] The risk of recurrence appears larger after severe strokes involving entire anterior circulation territories and after hemorrhagic stroke.

In addition to considering risk of recurrence, the decision to recommend AED therapy should take into account the following:

1. Seizure severity. Infrequent, simple partial (motor, sensory, or limbic) seizures that do not interfere with consciousness or vital functions such as breathing and swallowing may be less onerous to the patient than the side effects of therapy.

2. The physical and psychological impact of seizures on the patient and caregivers and the possibility of side effects should be considered.

3. Correctable seizure-precipitating factors should be investigated before embarking on treatment. Factors include metabolic disturbances, intercurrent illnesses, and medications such as theophylline, cyclosporine, and penicillin.

In patients with recurrent PSS who seem refractory to AED, one must consider the following before deciding on changes in AEDs: (1) impaired compliance due to unwillingness or inability to follow physician's instructions and (2) progressive lesions such as enlarging AVMs or unsuspected brain tumors.

Monotherapy

Most seizure disorders are as effectively managed with single antiepileptic medications as with multiple drugs.[52,60,65,66] Many patients with vascular disease are elderly and already take several medications. They may have less-than-average comprehension of medication regimens and may have limited financial resources. Monotherapy will be associated with fewer drug interactions, and the effectiveness of an antiepileptic medication can be more accurately assessed.

Choice of Medication

No evidence exists to support the choice of one particular AED in these patients. Many AEDs have proven beneficial in improving partial and secondarily generalized seizures of various causes. However, no trials have been conducted in this patient population, and limited numbers of patients make future trials unlikely. Furthermore, no methodologically sound trials have assessed the effectiveness of AEDs in the elderly. Therefore, the choice of AED is usually based on the clinician's comfort level with a particular drug and on the drug's side effect profile.

Regardless of the AED that is chosen, it should be remembered that metabolic clearance rates peak in childhood and decline with age. Thus, the elderly usually require fewer daily dosages and lower total doses.

ACKNOWLEDGMENT

We wish to thank Mrs. Zena Pellegatta for secretarial assistance.

REFERENCES

1. Ang RT, Utterbach RA: Seizures with onset after forty years of age; role of cerebrovascular disease. South Med J 59:1404–1408, 1966.
2. Arboix A, Garcia-Eroles L, Massons JB, et al: Predictive factors of early seizures after acute cerebrovascular disease. Stroke 28:1590–1594, 1997.
3. Aring CC, Merritt HH: Differential diagnosis between cerebral hemorrhage and cerebral thrombosis; clinical and pathologic study of 245 cases. Arch Intern Med 56:435–456, 1935.
4. Barolin GS: The cerebrovascular epilepsies. Electroencephalogr Clin Neurophysiol 35:287–295, 1982.
5. Black SE, Norris JW, Hachinski VC: Post-stroke seizures. Stroke 14:134, 1983.
6. Brown RD, Wiebers DO, Forbes G, et al: The natural history of unruptured intracranial arteriovenous malformations. J Neurosurg 68:352–357, 1988.
7. Burn J, Dennis M, Bamford J, et al: Epileptic seizures after a first stroke: The Oxfordshire Community Stroke Project. BMJ 315:1582–1587, 1997.
8. Cabral RJ, King TT, Scott DF: Epilepsy after two different neurosurgical approaches to the treatment of ruptured intracranial aneurysms. J Neurol Neurosurg Psychiatry 39:1052–1056, 1976.
9. Casazza M, Broggi G, Franzini A, et al: Supratentorial cavernous angiomas and epileptic seizures: Preoperative course and postoperative outcome. Neurosurgery 39:26–32, 1996.
10. Chopra JS, Banerjee AK: Primary intracranial sinovenous occlusions in youth and pregnancy. In Vinken PJ, Bruyn GW, Klawans HL (eds): Handbook of Clinical Neurology. Vol 54. New York, Elsevier, 1989, pp 425–452.
11. Clancy R, Malin S, Laraque D, et al: Focal motor seizures heralding stroke in full-term neonates. Am J Dis Child 139:601–606, 1985.
12. Cocito L, Favale E, Reni L: Epileptic seizures in cerebral arterial occlusive disease. Stroke 13:189–195, 1982.
13. Cohen DS, Zubay GP, Goodman RR: Seizure outcome after lesionectomy for cavernous malformations. J Neurosurg 83:237–242, 1995.
14. Crawford PM, West CR, Shaw MDM, et al: Cerebral arteriovenous malformations and epilepsy: Factors in the development of epilepsy. Epilepsia 27:270–275, 1986.

15. Daniele O, Mattaliano A, Tassinari CA, et al: Epileptic seizures and cerebrovascular disease. Acta Neurol Scand 80:17–22, 1989.

16. De Rueck J, Krahel N, Sieben G, et al: Epilepsy in patients with cerebral infarcts. J Neurol 224:101–109, 1980.

17. Dodge PR, Richardson EP, Victor M: Recurrent convulsive seizures as a sequel to cerebral infarction: A clinical and pathological study. Brain 77:610–638, 1954.

18. Engel J Jr: Differential diagnosis. In Engel J Jr (ed): Seizures and Epilepsy. Philadelphia, FA Davis, 1989, pp 340–379.

19. Engel J Jr: Terminology and classifications. In Engel J Jr (ed): Seizures and Epilepsy. Philadelphia, FA Davis, 1989, pp 3–21.

20. Fentz V: Epileptic seizures in patients with cerebrovascular accidents [abstract]. Nord Medicine 86:1023–1025, 1971.

21. Ferguson GG: Intracranial arterial aneurysms: A Surgical Perspective. In Vinken PJ, Bruyn GW, Klawans HL (eds): Handbook of Clinical Neurology. Vol 55. New York, Elsevier, 1989, pp 41–88.

22. Filipek PA, Krishnamoorthy KS, Davis KR, et al: Focal cerebral infarction in the newborn: A distinct entity. Pediatr Neurol 3:141–147, 1987.

23. Fortuna A, Ferrante L, Mastronardi L, et al: Cerebral cavernous angioma in children. Childs Nerv Syst 5:201–207, 1989.

24. Fults D, Kelly DL: Natural history of arteriovenous malformations of the brain: A clinical study. Neurosurgery 15:658–662, 1984.

25. Gates PC, Barnett HJM: Venous disease: Cortical veins and sinuses. In Barnett HJM, Stein BM, Mohr JP, et al (eds): Stroke, Pathophysiology, Diagnosis and Management. New York, Churchill Livingstone, 1986, pp 731–743.

26. Gerosa MA, Cappellotto P, Licata C, et al: Cerebral arteriovenous malformations in children (56 cases). Childs Brain 8:356–371, 1981.

27. Giroud M, Gras P, Fayolle H, et al: Early seizures after acute stroke: A study of 1,640 cases. Epilepsia 35:959–964, 1994.

28. Gowers WR: Epilepsy and other chronic convulsive disorders. In Gowers WR (ed): Epilepsy and Other Chronic Convulsive Disorders. New York, Dover, 1964.

29. Gupta SR, Naheedy MH, Elias D, et al: Post infarction seizures, a clinical study. Stroke 19:1477–1481, 1988.

30. Hart RG, Byer JA, Slaughter JR, et al: Occurrence and implications of seizures in subarachnoid hemorrhage due to ruptured intracranial aneurysms. Neurosurgery 8:417–421, 1981.

31. Hauser WA, Hesdorffer DC: Incidence and prevalence. In Hauser WA, Hesdorffer DC (eds): Epilepsy: Frequency, Causes and Consequences. New York, Demos, 1990, pp 1–51.

32. Hauser WA, Ramirez-Lassepas M, Rosenstein R: Risk for seizures and epilepsy following cerebrovascular insults. Epilepsia 25:666, 1984.

33. Heidrich R: Subarachnoid hemorrhage. In Vinken PJ, Bruyn GW (eds): Handbook of Clinical Neurology. Vol 12. New York, American Elsevier, 1972, pp 68–204.

34. Heros RC, Zervas NT: Subarachnoid hemorrhage. Annu Rev Public Health 34:367–375, 1983.

35. Hildick-Smith M: Epilepsy in the elderly. Age Ageing 3:203–208, 1974.

36. Holmes GL: The electroencephalogram as a predictor of seizures following cerebral infarction. Clin Electroencephalogr 11:83–86, 1980.

37. Jackson JH: Epileptiform convulsions from cerebral disease. In Taylor J, Holmes G, Walshe FMR (eds): Selected Writings of John Hughlings Jackson on Epilepsy and Epileptiform Convulsions. London, Hodder and Stoughton Ltd., 1931, pp 330–340.

38. Kattapong VJ, Hart BL, Davis LE: Familial cerebral cavernous angiomas: Clinical and radiologic studies. Neurology 45:492–497, 1995.

39. Kilpatrick CJ, Davis SM, Tress BM, et al: Epileptic seizures in acute stroke. Arch Neurol 47:157–160, 1990.

40. Kondziolka D, Humphreys RP, Hoffman JH, et al: Arteriovenous malformations of the brain in children: A forty-year experience. Can J Neurol Sci 19:40–45, 1992.

41. Kotila M, Waltimo O: Epilepsy after stroke. Epilepsia 33:495–498, 1992.

42. Lancman ME, Golimstok A, Norscini J, et al: Risk factors for developing seizures after a stroke. Epilepsia 34:141–143, 1993.

43. Lanska MJ, Lanska DJ, Horwitz SJ, et al: Presentation, clinical course, and outcome of childhood stroke. Pediatr Neurol 7:333–341, 1991.

44. Laupacis A, Wells G, Richardson WS, et al: Users' guides to the medical literature. V. How to use an article about prognosis. Evidence-Based Medicine Working Group. JAMA 272:234–237, 1994.

45. Leblanc R, Feindel W, Ethier R: Epilepsy from cerebral arteriovenous malformations. Can J Neurol Sci 10:91–95, 1983.

46. Lesser RP, Luders H, Dinner DS, et al: Epileptic seizures due to thrombotic and embolic cerebrovascular disease in older patients. Epilepsia 26:622–630, 1985.

47. Levy SR, Abroms IF, Marshall PC, et al: Seizures and cerebral infarction in the full-term newborn. Ann Neurol 17:366–370, 1985.

48. Lo YK, Yiu CH, Hu HH, et al: Frequency and characteristics of early seizures in Chinese acute stroke. Acta Neurol Scand 90:83–85, 1994.

49. Louis S, McDowell F: Epileptic seizures in non-embolic cerebral infarction. Arch Neurol 17:414–418, 1967.

50. Maertens P, Dyken PR: Inborn errors of metabolism I. Neurologic degenerative diseases. In David RB (ed): Pediatric Neurology for the Clinician. Norwalk, CT, Appleton & Lange, 1992, pp 303–362.

51. Marquardsen J: The Natural History of Acute Cerebrovascular Disease. Copenhagen, Munksgaard, 1969.

52. Mattson RH, Cramer JA, Collins JF, et al: Comparison of carbamazepine, phenobarbital, phenytoin, and primidone in partial and secondarily generalized tonic-clonic seizures. N Engl J Med 313:145–151, 1985.

53. Meyer JS, Charney JZ, Rivera VM, et al: Cerebral embolization. Prospective clinical analysis of 42 cases. Stroke 2:541–554, 1971.

54. Mohr JP, Caplan LR, Melski JW, et al: The Harvard Cooperative Stroke Registry: A prospective registry. Neurology 28:754–762, 1978.

55. Ng SA, Hauser WA, Brust JCM, et al: Risk factors for adult onset first seizures. Ann Neurol 18:153, 1985.

56. Olsen TS, Hogenhaven H, Thage O: Epilepsy after stroke. Neurology 37:1209–1211, 1987.

57. Paolucci S, Silvestri G, Lubich S, et al: Poststroke late seizures and their role in rehabilitation of inpatients. Epilepsia 38:266–270, 1997.

58. Perret G, Nishioka H: Arteriovenous malformations: An analysis of 545 cases of cranio-cerebral arteriovenous malformations and fistulae reported to the Co-operative Study. J Neurosurg 25:467–490, 1966.

59. Reith J, Jorgensen HS, Nakayama H, et al: Seizures in acute stroke: Predictors and prognostic significance. The Copenhagen Stroke Study 28:1585–1589, 1997.

60. Reynolds EH, Shorvon SD: Monotherapy or polytherapy for epilepsy. Epilepsia 22:1–10, 1981.

61. Richardson EP, Dodge PR: Epilepsy in cerebral vascular disease. Epilepsia 3:49–74, 1954.

62. Robinson JR, Awad IA, Little JR: Natural history of the cavernous angioma. J Neurosurg 75:709–714, 1991.

63. Rose FC, Sarner M: Epilepsy after ruptured intracranial aneurysm. BMJ 1:18–21, 1965.

64. Sander JW, Hart YM, Johnson AL, et al: National General Practice Study of Epilepsy: Newly diagnosed epileptic seizures in a general population. Lancet 336:1267–1271, 1990.

65. Schmidt D: Two antiepileptic drugs for intractable epilepsy with complex-partial seizures. J Neurol Neurosurg Psychiatry 45:1119–1124, 1982.

66. Schmidt D: Reduction of two-drug therapy in intractable epilepsy. Epilepsia 24:368–376, 1983.

67. Schold C, Yaruell PR, Earnest MP: Origin of seizures in elderly patients. JAMA 238:1177–1178, 1977.

68. Seifer FP, Ignacio OJ: Seizures in patients over the age of 40: A general hospital study. J Ky Med Assoc 72:371–373, 1974.

69. Shinton RA, Gill JS, Melnick SC, et al: The frequency, characteristics and prognosis of epileptic seizures at the onset of stroke. J Neurol Neurosurg Psychiatry 51:273–276, 1988.

70. Shinton RA, Gill JS, Zezulka AV, et al: The frequency of epilepsy preceding stroke. Case-control study in 230 patients. Lancet 1:11–13, 1987.

71. Shorvon SD, Gilliat RW, Cox TCS, et al: Evidence of vascular disease from CT scanning in late onset epilepsy. J Neurol Neurosurg Psychiatry 47:225–230, 1984.

72. Simard JM, Garcia Bengochea F, Ballinger WE Jr, et al: Cavernous angioma: A review of 126 collected and 12 new clinical cases. Neurosurgery 18:162–172, 1986.

73. So EL, Annegers JF, Hauser WA, et al: Population-based study of seizure disorders after cerebral infarction. Neurology 46:350–355, 1996.

74. Sran SK, Baumann RJ: Outcome of neonatal strokes. Am J Dis Child 142:1086–1088, 1988.

75. Sundaram MBM, Chow F: Seizures associated with spontaneous subarachnoid hemorrhage. Can J Neurol Sci 13:229–231, 1986.

76. Sung CY, Chu NS: Epileptic seizures in intracerebral haemorrhage. J Neurol Neurosurg Psychiatry 52:1273–1276, 1989.

77. Sung CY, Chu NS: Epileptic seizures in thrombotic stroke. J Neurol 237:166–170, 1990.

78. Toole JF, Robinson MK, Mercuri M: Primary subarachnoid hemorrhage. In Vinken PJ, Bruyn GW, Klawans HL (eds): Handbook of Clinical Neurology. Vol 55. New York, Elsevier, 1989, pp 1–40.

79. Trauner DA, Mannino FL: Neurodevelopmental outcome after neonatal cerebrovascular accident. J Pediatr 108:459–461, 1986.

80. Uttley D: Subarachnoid hemorrhage. Br J Hosp Med 19:138–154, 1978.

81. Viitanen M, Eriksson S, Asplund K: Risk of recurrent stroke, myocardial infarction and epilepsy during long-term follow-up after stroke. Eur Neurol 28:227–231, 1988.

82. Walton JN: The electroencephalographic sequelae of spontaneous subarachnoid hemorrhage. Electroencephalogr Clin Neurophysiol 5:41–52, 1953.

83. Walton JN: Subarachnoid Hemorrhage. New York, Churchill Livingstone, 1956.

84. White PT, Bailey AA, Bickford RG: Epileptic disorders in the aged. Neurology 3:674–678, 1953.

85. Winn HR, Richardson AE, O'Brien W, et al: The long term prognosis in untreated cerebral aneurysms: II. Late morbidity and mortality. Ann Neurol 4:418–426, 1978.

86. Yeh HS, Kashiwagi S, Tew JM, et al: Surgical management of epilepsy associated with cerebral arteriovenous malformations. J Neurosurg 72:216–223, 1990.

87. Yeh S, Privitera M: Secondary epileptogenesis in humans with cerebral arteriovenous malformations. Epilepsia 30:683, 1989.

ROBERT W. TEASELL, MD, FRCPC
MARC McRAE, MSc
HILLEL M. FINESTONE, MD, FRCPC

ASPIRATION AND PNEUMONIA FOLLOWING STROKE

From the Department of Physical
    Medicine and Rehabilitation
University of Western Ontario
London, Ontario
Canada

Reprint requests to:
Robert W. Teasell, MD
Department of Physical Medicine
    and Rehabilitation
London Health Sciences Center
339 Windermere Road
London, Ontario N6A 5A5
Canada

Aspiration following stroke has long been regarded as a common source of morbidity with pneumonia, death, and sepsis. Silver et al. and Bounds et al. reported pneumonia to be the second highest cause of death in the initial phase following a stroke.[5,43] Detection of silent and audible aspiration and subsequent adaptive management strategies are regarded as important in the prevention of pneumonia.[23,24,32,47,48,50] This has led to an increasing emphasis on the management of dysphagia and aspiration following stroke.

DYSPHAGIA FOLLOWING STROKE

Incidence of Dysphagia

Dysphagia can be defined simply as "difficulty with swallowing" and is not synonymous with aspiration. Several studies have examined the incidence of dysphagia in acute stroke patients. Gordon et al. studied swallowing in 91 consecutive stroke patients of whom 82 (90%) were studied within 4 days of stroke onset.[16] Dysphagia was defined as an inability to drink 50 ml of water or choking more than once while attempting to drink 50 ml of water on two occasions; 41 patients (45%) with an acute stroke experienced dysphagia based on these criteria, and 37 of 86 (43%) who had a cerebral hemispheric stroke similarly suffered from dysphagia. Similarly, Barer studied swallowing in 357 single cerebral hemispheric stroke patients within 48 hours of symptom onset and found that 105 (29%) had difficulty swallowing a mouthful of water.[4]

Smithard et al. prospectively studied swallowing in 149 consecutive stroke patients.[44] Swallowing status could not be determined in the 28 patients who had a significantly reduced level of consciousness during the first week. In the remaining 121 patients, a standardized bedside swallow assessment was conducted by a physician within 3 days of the stroke. Sixty of the 121 patients (50%) were felt to have an unsafe swallow due to dysphagia.[44] Based on these and other reports, dysphagia following stroke is recognized as quite common, particularly in the acute phase following a stroke.

Pathophysiology of Dysphagia

Dysphagia following stroke is generally a consequence of a delay in the pharyngeal phase of swallowing. Pharyngeal stasis is seen in the valleculae or pyriform sinuses and may be related to pharyngeal paresis, delayed pharyngeal movement of the food bolus, or unilateral pharyngeal paralysis.[7] Dysphagia occurs not only following brain stem and bilateral hemispheric strokes but has also been shown to occur following unilateral hemispheric lesions.[4,7,16,34,40,50] In the case of unilateral hemispheric lesions, there is increasing evidence that swallowing difficulties may be more significant clinically in right versus left hemispheric strokes.[8,40] Dysphagia may become problematic in terms of its potential effect on nutrition, which may in turn affect the rehabilitation potential or length of stay.[15] However, the greatest concern regarding dysphagia clinically is the potential risk of aspiration and pneumonia, and it is this fear that drives clinical management.

ASPIRATION FOLLOWING STROKE

Aspiration is defined as entry of material into the airway below the level of the true vocal cords. Many stroke patients with dysphagia do not aspirate, and the terms are not synonymous. The diagnosis of aspiration should be suspected when the stroke patient has a subjective complaint of trouble with swallowing, an abnormal chest radiograph, congested voice quality, or a delay in voluntary initiation of the swallow reflex and coughing during or after swallowing.[24] Diagnosis is initially established through a clinical assessment that involves an oral motor assessment followed by the introduction of one or several teaspoons of water. If stroke patients are then able to handle this minimal amount of fluid, a small cup of water is carefully introduced.[44] All stroke patients are potential aspirators, but certain identifiable risk factors exist that greatly increase the likelihood of aspiration (Table 1).

TABLE 1.   Risk Factors for Aspiration Poststroke

Brain stem stroke
Difficulty swallowing oral secretions
Coughing/throat-clearing or wet, gurgly voice quality after swallowing water
Choking more than once while drinking 50 ml of water
Weak voice and cough
Wet-hoarse voice quality
Recurrent lower respiratory infections
Low-grade fever or leukocytosis
Auscultatory evidence of lower-lobe congestion
Immunocompromised state

TABLE 2.   Radiologic Evaluation during Videofluoroscopic Modified Barium Swallow

1. Oral Phase

Lips:	Closure
Tongue:	Anterior and posterior motion with consonants; motion and coordination during transport, and manipulation of bolus
Soft palate:	Evaluation and retraction with consonants
Jaw:	Motion
Oral:	Pocketing

2. Pharyngeal Phase

Swallow:	Delay, absence
Peristalsis:	Residue in valleculae, pyriform sinuses, nasopharyngeal regurgitation

3. Laryngeal Function

Elevation of larynx
Penetration into laryngeal vestibule
Aspiration

Cough:	Presence, delay, effectiveness

Vocal cord function

4. Postexamination Chest X-Ray

Chronic changes
Presence of barium in valleculae, pyriform sinuses, tracheobroncheal tree, lungs

Adapted from Bach DB, Pouget S, Belle K, et al: An integrated team approach to the management of patients with oropharyngeal dysphagia. J Allied Health 18:459–468, 1989.

Videofluoroscopic Modified Barium Swallow Studies in Aspiration

Where aspiration is suspected the videofluoroscopic modified barium swallow (VMBS) study is now considered the gold standard in confirming the diagnosis.[45] As awareness regarding aspiration has increased, so has the frequency with which VMBS studies have been performed. A VMBS study examines the oral and pharyngeal phases of swallowing. The patient must have sufficient cognitive and physical skills to undergo testing.[3] The subject is placed in the sitting position in a chair designed to simulate the typical mealtime posture.[3] Radiopaque materials of various consistencies are tried; barium-impregnated thin and thick liquids, pudding, bread, and cookies are routinely used.[3] Various aspects of oral, laryngeal, and pharyngeal involvement are noted during the radiographic examination (Table 2). The VMBS study is then followed by a chest radiograph to document whether any barium was aspirated into the tracheobronchial tree.

Based on anecdotal experience, patients who aspirate more than 10% of the test bolus or who have severe oral or pharyngeal motility problems on VMBS studies are considered at high risk of pneumonia.[32,35] However, it can be difficult to assess whether 10% or more of the test bolus has been aspirated. Nevertheless, the degree of aspiration seen on VMBS is a critical determinant of patient management (Fig. 1). Whether a patient develops pneumonia after aspiration is to some extent dependent on other factors, such as the immune state or general health of the stroke patient.

The VMBS study not only establishes the presence and extent of aspiration but may also establish the mechanism of the swallowing disorder. Aspiration most often results from a functional disturbance in the pharyngeal phase of swallowing related to reduced laryngeal closure or pharyngeal paresis. A VMBS study is recommended in cases in which the patient is experiencing obvious problems maintaining adequate hydration or nutrition, where concern is expressed regarding frequent choking while eating, or in the case of recurrent respiratory infections. Factors such as cognition, a new stroke, depression, an immunocompromised state, and underlying lung disease also must be considered. Definitive criteria for when one should perform a VMBS

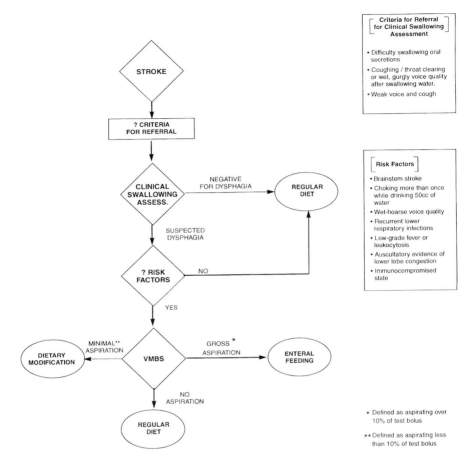

FIGURE 1.   An algorithm for swallowing management of stroke patients shortly after onset. Patients demonstrating potential swallow problems should be referred for a clinical swallowing assessment. Where dysphagia is still suspected and one or more risk factors are present, a videofluoroscopic modified barium swallow study is warranted. Where minimal aspiration is demonstrated consideration should be given toward dietary modification. Where gross aspiration is present, enteral feeding is generally necessary.

study in stroke patients has yet to be determined in a systematic and scientific manner. When the VMBS study is positive for aspiration and there are continuing concerns about aspiration, another VMBS study is generally ordered 1–3 months following the initial VMBS study.

Incidence of Aspiration in Patients Referred for VMBS

Aspiration following stroke was initially studied primarily in select populations of high risk or in dysphagic patients referred for VMBS studies. Veis and Logemann studied 38 consecutive stroke patients with dysphagia or concerns about aspiration who were referred for a VMBS examination within 4 months of stroke onset.[50] Twelve of the 38 patients (32%) aspirated. Horner et al. reported on 47 stroke patients referred for videofluoroscopic swallow examination.[24] The patients were tested an average of 2.9 months poststroke (1–24 months), and 33 of the 47 were evaluated within the first month of their stroke; 24 of the 47 patients (51.1%) aspirated. These initial studies used preselected patients—high-risk cases referred for VMBS assessment—and cannot be considered indicative of the general stroke population. Nevertheless, such studies raised concerns that aspiration was a significant concern in stroke patients many months after stroke onset.

Prospective Studies of Aspiration Poststroke

To better appreciate the clinical significance of aspiration, two prospective studies have been performed on stroke patients. Aspiration occurred in a significant number—albeit smaller than previously thought—of stroke patients shortly following stroke onset. The first study, by Smithard et al., included 121 stroke patients. Videofluoroscopy was performed in 95 patients (77.7%) within a median of 2 days.[44] Twenty of the 95 (21%) aspirated. Interestingly, the same study reported that videofluoroscopy offered no advantage over bedside assessment in determining who would develop a chest infection. The authors noted that because the number of patients was small and because certain patients were not included in the study, "a real effect on outcome may have been missed."

The natural history of aspiration following stroke was also prospectively studied by Kidd et al., who looked at 60 consecutive patients admitted to a teaching hospital with an acute stroke (55 hemispheric and 5 brain stem).[28] Videofluoroscopy identified aspiration in 25 patients (42%) within 72 hours of stroke onset. After 3 months, 14 of the 60 initial subjects had died and 4 were unavailable for follow-up. Videofluoroscopy was not repeated in four patients in whom the initial test had shown no abnormality. The remaining 38 subjects underwent a second videofluoroscopy at 3 months; 16 had aspirated on the initial assessment and 22 had not. Of the 38 subjects, only three (8%) were still aspirating 3 months after stroke onset.[28]

Silent Aspiration

The importance of identifying aspirators, particularly with VMBS studies, was given greater impetus with the reporting that a substantial number of aspirators could not be identified clinically—the so-called silent aspirators. Silent aspiration is defined as "penetration of food below the level of the true vocal cords, without cough or any outward sign of difficulty."[30] Detailed clinical swallowing assessments were shown to underdiagnose or miss these cases of aspiration.[23,24,45] In particular, the presence or absence of a gag reflex failed to distinguish aspirating from nonaspirating stroke patients.[23,24,45] Silent aspirators were considered to be at special risk of developing complications because of the difficulty in identifying them using the clinical assessment alone. Silent aspirators were to be suspected in stroke patients with recurrent lower respiratory infections, chronic congestion, low-grade fever, or leukocytosis.[12]

Silent aspirators accounted for a substantial number of poststroke aspirators when the results of simultaneous clinical assessment and VMBS studies were compared. Kidd et al. found that five of 60 (8%) consecutively admitted acute stroke patients who underwent videofluoroscopy within 72 hours of their strokes were silent aspirators with no outward signs of dysphagia.[28] Logemann reported that even the most experienced clinicians failed to identify about 40% of aspirating patients during a bedside examination.[32]

In the most influential study with regard to silent aspiration, Splaingard and Hutchins studied 107 patients, most of whom had suffered strokes, were admitted to a rehabilitation center, and subsequently were referred for swallowing evaluation.[45] Each patient underwent a careful clinical bedside assessment including a standardized diagnostic feeding routine. Aspiration was suspected if, during the feeding assessment, the clinician noted signs of respiratory distress, choking, coughing, food-tinged secretions in patients with tracheostomies, or a wet-hoarse vocal quality. Patients were then studied within 72 hours of clinical examination by VMBS studies performed by individuals blinded to the results of the clinical assessment. Of the total patient population, 43 (40%) aspirated at least one consistency of food during VMBS studies. Bedside evaluation identified only 18 (42%) of the 43 patients who aspirated on VMBS studies. Of the 25 patients who aspirated on VMBS studies but who were not reported to be aspirators on bedside clinical assessment, 21 (or 20% of the entire sample) did not cough or change clinically at the time aspiration was noted during VMBS studies and were felt to be silent aspirators.[45]

PNEUMONIA AND ASPIRATION

Pneumonia is a consequence of aspiration poststroke, and its prevention has been the primary rationale for diagnosis and management of aspiration.[6,19,22,27] Mortality following a stroke as a consequence of pneumonia (presumably due to aspiration) has been reported as high as 3% within the first 3 months and 6% within the first year.[19,28] Aspiration pneumonia has therefore been regarded as important because it reportedly contributes significantly to morbidity and mortality.[2,16,19,27,32,43,50]

Aspiration alone is not sufficient to cause pneumonia; aspiration of small amounts of saliva occurs during sleep in almost half of normal subjects.[13,26] Pneumonia is most likely to occur when the lung's natural defenses are overwhelmed by excessive or toxic (i.e., gastric contents) aspirate, leading to a localized infection or a chemical pneumonitis. Some of the factors associated with an increased risk of aspiration pneumonia, other than direct dysphagia-related factors due to stroke (see Table 1), include reduced levels of consciousness, a tracheostomy, gastric reflux or emesis, nasogastric tubes (due to mechanical interference with the cardiac sphincter), and a compromised immune system.[13]

Defining Aspiration Pneumonia

Clinical criteria for aspiration pneumonia across studies has proven to be variable.[45] Johnson et al. defined pneumonia as radiographic evidence of segmental consolidation of infiltrates or recorded respiratory difficulty with segmental moist rales on chest auscultation plus two of the following supporting signs or symptoms: temperature elevation above 100°F, white blood cell count greater than 10,000, or evidence of hypoxia.[27] DePaso used similar criteria.[10] Teasell et al. also used similar criteria with a diagnosis of pneumonia based on radiologic evidence of consolidation/infiltration and at least one other feature of either granulocytosis, increased temperature (above 38°C), or shortness of breath.[47] In contrast, Kidd et al. used the concept of a lower respiratory tract infection, which they defined as "the production of sputum in conjunction with the development of crackles on auscultation, with or without the presence of fever or leucocytosis."[28] Smithard et al. defined "chest infection" as the presence of two or more of the following: tachypnea (> 22/min), tachycardia, inspiratory crackles, bronchial breathing, and use of antibiotics.[44] Odderson et al. did not define their criteria for aspiration pneumonia.[38] Obviously, the criteria used for defining pneumonia will influence its incidence, and much of the variability among studies can be accounted for by differences in the inclusion criteria for a diagnosis of pneumonia.

Relationship between Pneumonia and Dysphagia/Aspiration

A relationship between pneumonia and dysphagia/aspiration has been reasonably well established despite variability among studies. Gordon et al. found that seven of 41 (17%) patients with dysphagia developed clinical and chest radiographic evidence of a chest infection within 1 week.[16] In contrast, Horner et al. reported no cases of aspiration pneumonia among 47 stroke patients.[24] Smithard et al. reported that patients with dysphagia on bedside assessment had a higher risk of chest infection (33% vs. 16%; p < .05) and poor nutritional state (p < .001).[44] The criteria for chest infection in this study was very liberal. Johnson et al. reported on a study of 60 stroke patients referred for videofluoroscopic evaluation of poststroke dysphagia drawn from a total population of 304 consecutive patients with acute stroke admitted to hospital.[27] The development of pneumonia correlated well with slower pharyngeal transit time but, surprisingly, not with aspiration as demonstrated on VMBS.[27]

Holas et al. found that aspiration on VMBS studies put stroke patients at much higher risk of developing pneumonia.[22] The risk was 8.36 times greater for those who aspirated 10% or more of barium-impregnated test materials compared with those who aspirated less than 10% or who did not aspirate. The risk was 6.95 times greater for aspirators compared to nonaspirators. Similarly, Schmidt et al. found the odds ratio for developing pneumonia to be 7.6 times greater for those who aspirated during VMBS studies.[42]

In a review of 441 consecutive stroke patients admitted to a rehabilitation unit, Teasell et al. found that only 12 of 441 patients (2.7%) developed pneumonia while hospitalized.[47] The incidence of pneumonia among proven aspirators (on VMBS) was 11.9% but only 0.6% among presumed nonaspirators. Aspirators appeared to have a 20-fold increased risk of developing pneumonia compared to presumed nonaspirators. Brain stem stroke patients were at significantly higher risk of pneumonia.[47]

In their prospective study of 60 acute stroke patients, Kidd et al. reported that 19 (32%) developed a lower respiratory tract infection within the first 14 days.[28] The relatively high incidence of lower respiratory tract infection compared to other studies may have been related to a lower threshold in terms of what constitutes a respiratory infection complication. Of 19 lower respiratory tract infections, 17 (89%) occurred in aspirating patients. Lower respiratory tract infection was significantly more common in aspirating patients (68%) than nonaspirators (6%) (p < 0.0001). The presence of dysphagia, abnormal pharyngeal sensation, and stroke severity were associated with the development of a respiratory infection, but age, sex, or the side of the stroke were not.[28]

Table 3 summarizes factors likely to be associated with aspiration pneumonia. The combination of aspiration seen following stroke, the concern regarding silent aspiration, and the association between aspiration and pneumonia has increasingly led to attempts to diagnose and manage aspiration poststroke.

TABLE 3.   Factors More Likely to be Associated with Aspiration
Pneumonia Following Stroke

Brain stem stroke
Aspiration on VMBS (risk greater if patient aspirates more than 10% of barium-laced test material)
Slower pharyngeal transit time on VMBS
Immunocompromised state or chronic lung disease

VMBS = Videofluoroscopic modified barium swallow

MANAGEMENT OF ASPIRATION POSTSTROKE

The goal of management of the aspirating stroke patient is to prevent pneumonia while ensuring that the patient is receiving adequate hydration and nutrition. Malnutrition may have a significant impact on stroke rehabilitation outcome[14,15] (see chapter entitled "Outcome Predictors and the Effectiveness of Stroke Rehabilitation") but is not the subject of this review.

VMBS Studies and Management Guidelines

The VMBS study is still considered the gold standard in diagnosing aspiration. Patients who aspirate less than 10% of the test bolus on VMBS studies or who have difficulty with high volumes of thin liquids are considered at mild to moderate risk of aspiration, i.e., trace aspirators.[32] In these cases, oral feedings are regarded as appropriate. Before deciding on the appropriateness and type of oral feedings, other factors must be considered such as the patient's respiratory status, the effectiveness of airway clearance, and the type and amount of aspirate.[3] Aspirating more than 10% of the test bolus is generally considered an indication for nonoral (i.e., nasogastric, gastrostomy, jejunostomy tube) feedings; however, the actual risks with oral feedings for this group of patients have not been established.

Dietary Modifications

Although there is some evidence that dietary modifications may affect the incidence of aspiration pneumonia,[17] the effect of the mode of feeding on the rate of respiratory infection has not been definitely established. Dysphagia diets are often determined by the results of the VMBS study. Bach et al. have noted that these diets have three purposes: (1) to decrease the risk of aspiration, (2) to provide adequate nutrients and fluids, and (3) to provide a progressive approach to feeding based on improvement or deterioration of swallowing function.[3] Special diets are based on four distinct consistencies: thick fluids, pureed, minced, and soft chopped. A dysphagia soft diet excludes all hard, small, and stringy food particles.[3] There are three consistencies of meat in the soft diet: soft chopped, minced, and ground. A pureed diet has the consistency of pudding and is generally easier to swallow than a more regular diet.[50] A diet of thick fluids can eliminate all thin liquids. Alternatives to thin liquids such as jelled water or liquids may be required.

The most common dietary modification is avoidance or careful regulation of thin liquids, because they are the most poorly manipulated in transit through the oropharynx and they represent the food consistency most likely to be aspirated. Severely dysphagic patients are often started on no oral feeds and gradually progressed to a pureed diet followed by a soft chopped diet with thick fluids. Patients are eventually allowed thin liquids as it is determined that they can swallow them without aspirating. No randomized controlled studies have demonstrated whether these modified diets influence outcome, but a large multicenter trial has been initiated.[9]

Progressive Management

Over time, particularly in the earlier stages following a stroke, changes to the diet can be made as the patient's dysphagia improves and risk of aspiration lessens. Progression can be determined on clinical swallowing assessment unless the patient is a silent aspirator, detectable only on VMBS study, in which case the clinical examination must be considered unreliable. A repeat VMBS study may be needed to guide management. Special techniques, such as compensatory head and neck postures,[32] double swallowing, or coughing after swallowing[24] may be employed. Many stroke patients, especially those with right hemispheric lesions, are impulsive and

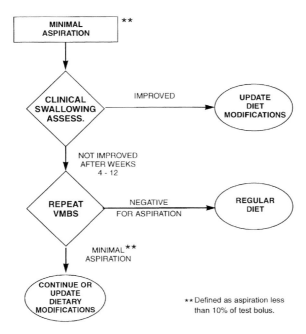

FIGURE 2. An algorithm for continuing management of minimal aspirators poststroke. Regular clinical swallowing assessments would allow the monitoring of swallowing status with regular updating of dietary modification based on clinical status. If there is no improvement after 1–3 months, the videofluoroscopic modified barium swallow study can be repeated.

may attempt to eat and swallow too quickly. Therefore, close supervision with frequent cuing may be necessary.[35] Figures 2 and 3 show progressive management of trace and gross aspirators on VMBS studies.

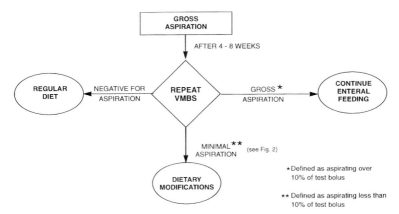

FIGURE 3. For gross aspirators on the initial videofluoroscopic modified barium swallow (VMBS) study, the risk of pneumonia is highest. Therefore, nonenteral feeds should be continued until the VMBS study can be repeated in 4–8 weeks or until the patient clinically demonstrates substantial improvement.

Studies of Efficacy of Dysphagia Therapy

In the only randomized controlled trial looking at the effectiveness of dysphagia therapy, DePippo et al. divided 115 patients into three graded levels of dysphagia therapy.[11] Patients in the first group received a single formal dysphagia treatment session, and family members helped them select the appropriate diet and use compensatory swallowing techniques. For the second group, the therapist prescribed the diet and then reevaluated it every other week. In the final group, the therapist prescribed the diet and saw the patient daily to reinforce recommended compensatory swallowing techniques. Outcome measures of pneumonia, dehydration, calorie-nitrogen deficits, recurrent upper airway obstruction, and death were reviewed until discharge and 1 year poststroke. There was no statistically significant difference between the three groups. The authors concluded that limited patient and family instruction regarding the use of dietary modification and compensatory swallowing techniques was as effective as daily therapist monitoring of dysphagia.[11] Patients were admitted to the study about $4\frac{1}{2}$ weeks poststroke and were in rehabilitation only 2 weeks, which limits the conclusions one can draw from the study.

Odderson et al. looked at the effect of introducing a swallowing management protocol as part of an overall introduction of clinical pathway guidelines for the management of stroke patients.[38] A total of 48 of 124 (39%) acute nonhemorrhagic stroke patients admitted to an urban community hospital failed an initial swallow screen and required intervention. Of these, 19% required gastrostomy tube placement. No patients developed aspiration pneumonia that year, but 6.7% had developed it 2 years previously. However, the authors never defined aspiration pneumonia, and the study was neither randomized nor blinded. Although the control group (those treated a year before the introduction of clinical pathways) were not actually defined, the stroke types were assumed to be similar. The authors concluded that early swallow screening and dysphagia management in patients with acute stroke reduced the risk of aspiration pneumonia and was cost-effective based on increased lengths of stay as a consequence of the pneumonia.[38]

Nonoral Feedings

Nonoral or tube feeding in neurogenic aspiration has become a well-established rehabilitation practice. However, Kidd et al. have noted that the most appropriate time to begin enteral feeds has not been determined.[28] Nasogastric tube feedings have been shown to be less effective and have more side effects than gastrostomy feedings,[25,39] and they are often poorly tolerated. Norton et al. studied 30 stroke survivors, 16 of whom were randomized into a gastrostomy feeds group and 14 into a nasogastric feeds group.[37] The gastrostomy feeds group did better in terms of ability to receive and maintain prescribed feeds, maintain nutrition, earlier discharge from hospital, and mortality. Evidence suggests that use of enteral feedings in a primarily nonstroke population may not actually reduce the incidence of aspiration.[33]

Wanklyn et al. reviewed the records of 37 patients with cerebral infarcts who required a percutaneous gastrostomy.[51] The percutaneous G-tube (PG) was inserted a median of 26 days after stroke onset (range 12–131 days). Patients had a mean age of 74. Assessment was carried out a mean of 12 months poststroke. Complications occurred in 11 cases (30%): five patients developed chest infections (less than 1 week after PG), three developed local infection, two patients experienced inadvertent removal, and one had a perforation. Three patients (8%) died from complications of the PG during the first 5 days after PG insertion; one of the three had suffered perforation with peritonitis and two had developed chest infections.

However, at the time of assessment, 31 patients had died and six were still alive. The median survival from the time of PG was 53 days; only 12 patients survived more than a year. Despite this poor survival, the authors still recommended PG to ensure adequate nutrition. In this study it appeared that only the sickest patients received PG tubes and that the high complication rate may not have been due entirely to the PG tube.

Gastric Versus Jejunal Tube Feedings

Controversy also exists as to whether gastric or jejunal tube feedings are best.[23] However, with jejunal tube feedings there appears to be less risk of aspiration from regurgitation of gastric feeds. Gastric tube feeding is considered an acceptable alternative for recurrent aspiration,[21,31,46] but others consider aspiration to be a contraindication to gastric tube feeding and an indication for jejunal tube feeding.[1,20] Jejunal tube feedings are theoretically safer in high-risk patients, because the pyloric sphincter provides an added defense against reflux of tube feeds.[18,36] Turner has gone so far as to state that gastrostomy is generally reserved for patients with intact swallow reflexes (low risk of aspiration), whereas jejunostomy would be recommended for individuals who lack these swallow reflexes (high risk of aspiration).[49] Bolusing of tube feeds and generally feeding in a more physiologic manner has been reported as an advantage of gastric tube feeding over jejunal tube feeding.[41] At present the issue of gastrostomy versus jejunostomy tubes remains unresolved. With the more recent percutaneous gastrojejunal tube placement techniques, complications of placement appear to be minimized.

FUTURE ISSUES

The issue of aspiration poststroke has received much attention over the past decade. It has been established that aspiration is quite common poststroke. Pneumonia is much less common but occurs significantly more often among diagnosed aspirators. What has not been established is whether diagnostic testing such as VMBS or aggressive management of aspiration makes a difference in the development of complications, especially pneumonia. Among high-risk patients such as those with brain stem strokes, it is likely that the use of VMBS in patients suspected of aspirating clinically will prove to be useful in directing management to prevent future complications. With unilateral hemispheric stroke patients, VMBS is less likely to be useful in diagnosing aspiration leading to pneumonia because of the lesser frequency of both severe aspiration and pneumonia in hemispheric patients. There is some evidence that right hemispheric stroke patients may be at increased risk of complications, but the risk is not as great as in brain stem strokes.[8,47]

A prospective randomized controlled study examining the effect of various management strategies in preventing pneumonia in high-risk individuals or patients suspected of aspirating would be difficult to perform because of concerns regarding the ethics of the control group. Increasing questions about the efficacy of current management strategies should lead to fewer ethical misgivings regarding nontreatment of controls. The cost-effectiveness of various interventions has been discussed but has not been adequately determined in appropriate clinical trials.

CONCLUSION

Aspiration is an important complication in stroke patients. Although VMBS can accurately delineate the presence of aspiration leading to alteration of feedings through dietary modification or tube feedings, there are concerns that it may lack utility in effectively determining who will develop pneumonia. Its role in the management of stroke patients has not been fully defined. Targeting specific high-risk patients who have suspected dysphagia on clinical assessment (see Fig. 1) would seem to be most appropriate. Management of dysphagia and aspiration involves dietary modifications, special compensatory techniques, and nonoral tube feeds. Although these measures have not been demonstrated definitively to prevent complications, they intuitively make sense. Where necessary, gastrojejunal tube feeding is relatively safe and effective as a means of bypassing dysfunctional swallowing mechanics following stroke.

REFERENCES

1. Alzate GD, Coons H, Elliott J, Cary PH: Percutaneous gastrostomy for jejunal feeding: A new technique. AJR 147:822–825, 1986.
2. Arms R, Dines D, Tinstman T: Aspiration pneumonia. Chest 65:136–139, 1974.
3. Bach DB, Pouget S, Belle K, et al: An integrated team approach to the management of patients with oropharyngeal dysphagia. J Allied Health 18:459–468, 1989.
4. Barer DH: The natural history and functional consequences of dysphagia after hemispheric stroke. J Neurol Neurosurg Psychiatry 52:236–241, 1989.
5. Bounds JV, Wiebers DO, Whisnant JP, Okazaki H: Mechanism and timing of deaths from cerebral infarctions. Stroke 12:474–477, 1981.
6. Brown M, Glassenberg M: Mortality factors in patients with acute stroke. JAMA 224:1493–1495, 1973.
7. Chen MYM, Ott DJ, Peele VN, Gelfand DW: Oropharynx in patients with cerebrovascular disease: Evaluation with videofluoroscopy. Radiology 176:641–643, 1990.
8. Daniels SK, Foundas AL, Iglesia GC, Sullivan MA: Lesion site in unilateral stroke patients with dysphagia. J Stroke Cerebrovasc Dis 6:30–34, 1996.
9. Dennis M: The FOOD (Feed or Ordinary Diet) Trial. Presented at the 1997 North American Stroke Meeting, Montreal, Quebec, October 18, 1997.
10. DePaso W: Aspiration pneumonia. Clin Chest Med 12:269–284, 1991.
11. DePippo KL, Holas MA, Reding MJ, et al: Dysphagia therapy following stroke: A controlled trial. Neurology 44:1655–1660, 1994.
12. Elliott J: Swallowing disorders in the elderly: A guide to diagnosis and treatment. Geriatrics 43:95, 1988.
13. Finegold SM: Aspiration pneumonia. Rev Infect Dis 13(suppl 9):S737–742, 1991.
14. Finestone HM, Greene-Finestone LS, Wilson ES, Teasell RW: Malnutrition in stroke patients on the rehabilitation service at follow-up: Prevalence and predictors. Arch Phys Med Rehabil 76:310–316, 1995.
15. Finestone HM, Greene-Finestone LS, Wilson ES, Teasell RW: Prolonged length of stay and reduced functional improvement rate in malnourished stroke rehabilitation patients. Arch Phys Med Rehabil 77:340–345, 1996.
16. Gordon C, Hewer RL, Wade DT: Dysphagia in acute stroke. BMJ 295:411–414, 1987.
17. Groher ME: Bolus management and aspiration pneumonia in patients with pseudobulbar dysphagia. Dysphagia 1:215–216, 1987.
18. Gustke RF, Varma RR, Soergel KH: Gastric reflux during profusion of the proximal small bowel. Gastroenterology 59:890–895, 1970.
19. Hanning C, Wuttge-Hanning A, Hormann M, Hermann I: A cinematographic study of the pathologic mechanism of aspiration pneumonia. Fortschr Rontgenstr 159:260–267, 1989.
20. Hinsdale JC, Lipkowitz GS, Pollock TW, et al: Prolonged enteral nutrition in malnourished patients with nonelemental feeding: Reappraisal of surgical technique, safety and costs. Am J Surg 149:334–338, 1985.
21. Hogan RB, DeMarco DC, Hamilton JK, et al: Percutaneous endoscopic gastrostomy—to push or pull: A prospective randomized trial. Gastrointest Endosc 32:253–258, 1986.
22. Holas MA, DePippo KL, Reding MJ: Aspiration and relative risk of medical complications following stroke. Arch Neurol 51:1051–1053, 1994.
23. Horner J, Massey EW: Silent aspiration following stroke. Neurology 38:317–319, 1988.
24. Horner J, Massey EW, Riski JE, et al: Aspiration following stroke: Clinical correlates and outcome. Neurology 38:1359–1362, 1988.
25. Hull MA, Rawlings J, Murray FE, et al: Audit of outcome of long-enteral nutrition by percutaneous endoscopic gastrostomy. Lancet 341:869–872, 1993.

26. Huxley EJ, Viroslav J, Gray WR, Pierce AK: Pharyngeal aspiration in normal adults and patients with depressed consciousness. Am J Med 64:564–568, 1978.
27. Johnson ER, McKenzie SW, Sievers A: Aspiration pneumonia in stroke. Arch Phys Med Rehabil 74:973–976, 1993.
28. Kidd D, Lawson J, Nesbitt R, MacMahon J: The natural history and clinical consequences of aspiration in acute stroke. Q J Med 88:409–413, 1995.
29. Lazarus BA, Murphy JB, Culpepper L: Aspiration associated with long-term gastric versus jejunal feeding: Critical analysis of literature. Arch Phys Med Rehabil 71:46–53, 1990.
30. Linden P, Siebens AA: Dysphagia: Predicting laryngeal penetration. Arch Phys Med Rehabil 64:281–284, 1983.
31. Llaneza PP, Melendez AM, Roberts R, Dunn GD: Percutaneous endoscopic gastrectomy: Clinical experience and follow-up. South Med J 81:321–324, 1986.
32. Logemann JA: Evaluation and Treatment of Swallowing Disorders. San Diego, College-Hill Press, 1983.
33. Logen R, Weinryb J: Aspiration pneumonia in nursing home patients fed via gastrostomy tubes. Am J Gastroenterol 84:1509–1512, 1989.
34. Meadows J: Dysphagia in unilateral cerebral lesions. J Neurol Neurosurg Psychiatry 36:853–860, 1973.
35. Milazzo LS, Bouchard J, Lund DA: The swallowing process: Effects of aging and stroke. Phys Med Rehabil State Art Rev 3:489–499, 1989.
36. Muller-Lisaner SA, Fimmel CJ, Will N, et al: Effect of gastric and transpyloric tubes on gastric emptying and duodenogastric reflux. Gastroenterology 83:1276–1279, 1982.
37. Norton B, Horner-Ward M, Donnelly MT, et al: A randomized prospective comparison of percutaneous endoscopic gastrostomy and nasogastric tube feeding after acute dysphagic stroke. BMJ 312:13–16, 1996.
38. Odderson IR, Keaton JC, McKenna BS: Swallow management in patients on an acute stroke pathway: Quality is cost effective. Arch Phys Med Rehabil 76:1130–1133, 1995.
39. Park RHR, Allison MC, Lang J, et al: Randomized comparison of percutaneous endoscopic gastrostomy and nasogastric tube feeding in patients with persisting neurological dysphagia. BMJ 304:1406–1409, 1992.
40. Robbins J, Levine RL, Maser A, et al: Swallowing after unilateral stroke of the cerebral hemisphere. Arch Phys Med Rehabil 74:1295–1300, 1993.
41. Rombeau JL, Jacobs DO: Nasogastric tube feeding. In Rombeau JL, Caldwell MD (eds): Clinical Nutrition. Vol 1. Philadelphia, WB Saunders, 1984, pp 261–274.
42. Schmidt J, Holas M, Halvorson K, Reding M: Videofluoroscopic evidence of aspiration predict pneumonia and death but not dehydration following stroke. Dysphagia 9:7–11, 1994.
43. Silver F, Norris J, Lewis A, Hachinski V: Early mortality following stroke: A retrospective review. Stroke 15:492–496, 1984.
44. Smithard DG, O'Neill PA, Park C, et al: Complications and outcome after acute stroke. Does dysphagia matter? Stroke 27:1200–1204, 1996.
45. Splaingard ML, Hutchins B, Sulton LD, Chaudhuri G: Aspiration in rehabilitation patients: Videofluoroscopy vs bedside clinical assessment. Arch Phys Med Rehabil 69:637–640, 1988.
46. Stern JS: Comparison of percutaneous endoscopic gastrostomy with surgical gastrostomy at a community hospital. Am J Gastroenterol 81:1171–1173, 1986.
47. Teasell RW, Marchuk Y, McRae M, Finestone HM: Pneumonia associated with aspiration following stroke. Arch Phys Med Rehabil 77:707–709, 1996.
48. Tobin MJ: Aspiration pneumonia. In Dantzker DR (ed): Cardiopulmonary Critical Care. New York, Grune & Stratton, 1986.
49. Turner WW Jr: Nutritional considerations in the patient with disabling brain disease. Neurosurgery 16:707–713, 1985.
50. Veis S, Logemann J: Swallowing disorders in persons with cerebrovascular accidents. Arch Phys Med Rehabil 66:373–374, 1985.
51. Wanklyn P, Cox N, Belfield P: Outcome in patients who require a gastrectomy after stroke. Age Ageing 24:510–514, 1995.

HILLEL M. FINESTONE, MD, FRCPC
LINDA S. GREENE-FINESTONE, MSc, RD

NUTRITION AND DIET POSTSTROKE

From the Department of Physical
  Medicine and Rehabilitation
University of Western Ontario
London, Ontario
Canada

Reprint requests to:
Hillel M. Finestone, MD, FRCPC
Department of Physical Medicine
  and Rehabilitation
London Health Sciences Center
University Campus
339 Windermere Road
London, Ontario N6A 5A5
Canada

Nutritional and dietary issues play fundamental roles in the rehabilitation of patients who have sustained a stroke. The study of poststroke nutrition is relatively new. The past decade has brought to light new information regarding the high prevalence of the undernourished state in stroke patients and its association with adverse outcomes. Stroke patients are nutritionally vulnerable because they have a large number of neurologic deficits that can contribute to decreased dietary intake and, eventually, malnutrition. This chapter addresses nutritional assessment and also focuses on specific nutritional and dietary concerns of stroke patients and strategies for treatment.

FACTORS CONTRIBUTING TO EATING DIFFICULTIES AND NUTRITIONAL IMPAIRMENT

Dysphagia is common after acute stroke, with incidences ranging from 25–45%.[22,23] Dysphagia also has been observed in 47% of stroke patients on a rehabilitation service 2–3 weeks poststroke.[17] This prevalence declined to 17% by the patients' follow-up examination 2–4 months later.[17] In a study of 43 patients admitted to hospital with a primary diagnosis of dysphagia resulting from neurologic dysfunction, 80% exhibited dysphagia-induced starvation as evidenced by a significant rate of weight loss and markedly abnormal anthropometric examinations. More than 70% exhibited visceral protein depletion. In these patients, untreated dysphagia resulted in the development of malnutrition.[35]

Other neurologic deficits that may adversely affect the stroke patient's ability to self-feed include upper extremity paralysis or paresis, apraxia, agnosia, right and left disorientation, depression, and visual neglect or denial of the paralyzed extremity.[11] Stroke patients sometimes exhibit eating-related behavior problems such as attention-concentration deficit, eating too fast or too slowly, or forgetting to swallow. Strategies for coping with the mental and physical changes affecting food intake, as well as nutritional status, are discussed in the section on treatment.

METABOLIC CONSEQUENCES OF STROKE

In the acute metabolic response to injury, initially there is a decline in energy (caloric) expenditure and increased activity of the sympathetic nervous system, including elevated cortisol output. A hypermetabolic phase follows in which energy expenditure and nitrogen excretion are increased. To meet the demands for tissue fuel and liver synthesis of acute phase proteins, there is an increase in mobilization of amino acids from muscle and free fatty acids from adipose tissue. This hypercatabolism results in net losses from the protein and fat compartments of the body. Some of this loss is obligatory during the stress response. If nutritional requirements can be estimated and provided, protein synthesis will increase. If not, fat and protein will continue to be mobilized to meet exaggerated energy expenditure, and malnutrition may result.[36]

The issue of whether there is an acute phase response to stroke has received some attention, in patients with cerebral infarcts, during the past decade. Davalos et al. reported that levels of 24-hour free urinary cortisol were higher in patients classified as malnourished than in nonmalnourished (p = 0.025).[14] Nonmalnourished and malnourished levels, respectively, were approximately two or three times normal values on admission and decreased to 1 to 1.5 times normal at day 7 (p < 0.001). Irrespective of nutritional status classification, the acute stroke patients experienced a rise and fall in cortisol levels that was consistent with the stress response.

After excluding patients with evidence of infection, Beamer et al. found higher levels of interleukin-6 (IL-6), a regulator of the acute phase response, and interleukin-1 receptor antagonist (IL-1RA), an anti-inflammatory mediator in the acute phase, in patients with acute stroke compared to healthy, community-living controls (p < 0.001).[9] Both IL-6 and IL-1RA were significantly correlated with the C-reactive protein, an acute phase protein, suggesting that there is an acute phase response to brain infarction.

If a hypermetabolic state occurs following some types of stroke, amounts of nutrients required for the maintenance of health would greatly increase. Currently, little data are available on energy and nitrogen output following stroke. In a subset of the Davalos study, lower resting energy expenditure (REE) on day 1 was reported in malnourished patients. These patients also had significantly higher urinary cortisol levels. Reduced REE and elevated cortisol output are characteristic of the initial phase of the stress response.[14] There is some evidence of increased protein catabolism following acute stroke. Mountokalakis and Dellos reported that nitrogen loss, expressed as urea-creatinine ratio, in stroke patients doubled between 4 and 10 days after stroke onset (p < 0.001) before returning to levels similar to the initial levels.[30] Further research is needed in this area.

NUTRITIONAL ASSESSMENT OF THE STROKE PATIENT

Nutritional assessment is used to evaluate nutritional status and establish baseline information, including the identification of nutrient imbalances, excesses, deficiencies, and forms of malnutrition (undernutrition) or overnutrition (obesity). The goal of the assessment is to help the patient attain or maintain a sufficient level of energy and nutrients (normal nutrition status) to reduce the risk of adverse outcomes associated with poor nutrition and promote an optimal level of health.

The development of malnutrition is a process. In the first stage, dietary insufficiency of nutrients progresses from decreased levels in tissue and body fluids to a reduced functional level in tissues and diminished activity in nutrient-dependent enzymes. The latter stages include functional change, clinical symptoms, and signs.

The nutritional assessment may take different forms, ranging from brief screening tools to comprehensive evaluation. Anthropometric and biochemical measurements as well as physical examination and medical and dietary histories are useful in assessing nutritional status. Although dietary intakes can sometimes appear to be adequate on assessment, certain drugs, disease states, or dietary components can affect ingestion, absorption, transportation, utilization, or excretion of nutrients.[21]

The International Classification of Diseases, or ICD-10, classifies malnutrition according to type and degree (E40–E46).[38] Body weight, a primary measure, can be expressed as weight change and weight relative to the number of standard deviations below the mean value of a reference population. Normative measures for Canada and the United States are available.[18,20,29]

Table 1 provides an overview of the common indices used in nutritional assessment as well as indicator levels found in mild, moderate, and severe depletion. Tests are most effectively used in combination or serially. Comprehensive descriptions of parameters of the nutritional assessment are available.[21,26]

Prevalence of Malnutrition in the Stroke Patient

In a study of the nutritional status of acute stroke patients in Sweden, Axelson et al. determined that 16% and 22% of patients were malnourished on hospital admission and discharge, respectively.[7] Male gender, presence of infection, treatment with cardiovascular drugs, and advanced age significantly predicted undernutrition on discharge (median hospital stay 16.5 days, range 12–42 days). Of patients with severe stroke and hospital stays longer than 3 weeks, 56.3% were malnourished.[6] Poor nutritional status was defined as at least two of six nutrition-sensitive parameters below defined lower reference limits.

Protein-energy malnutrition, defined as an abnormal finding in one of three nutrition-sensitive parameters, was observed in 16.3% of 104 patients following acute stroke.[14] This increased to 26.4% by day 7 in the surviving patients and 35% by day 14 in those remaining hospitalized. Notably, triceps skinfold measurements, an estimator of the fat compartment, fell significantly between admission and day 7 ($p = 0.002$). Admission characteristics such as the presence of malnutrition, swallowing difficulties, greater neurologic deficit (Canadian Stroke Scale ≤ 5) (all $p < 0.001$), and higher free urinary cortisol ($p = 0.043$) were associated with the presence of malnutrition 1 week poststroke.

In the above studies, malnutrition was evident in 16% of patients on admission following acute stroke. Therefore, it should be recognized that some stroke patients who are entering the stroke recovery process are already undernourished. New cases of malnutrition also develop, particularly among patients with more severe strokes.[6,7]

An early study of malnutrition in 15 stroke patients on a rehabilitation service found that 3 patients were obese and 9 patients (60%) had significant malnutrition in the form of kwashiorkor (protein malnutrition) or marasmus (protein-calorie malnutrition).[32]

TABLE 1. Selected Indices of Malnutrition in Adults[3,26,33]

Compartment	Indices	Depletion Mild	Depletion Moderate	Depletion Severe	Indications	Practical Limitations
Fat and Protein	% desirable body weight (acutal weight/desirable weight) × 100	80 < 90	70 < 80	≤ 69	Appropriate parameter for healthy populations; Metropolitan Life Insurance Tables (MLIT)—based on disease-free insured population; weight associated with lowest mortality rate	Frame size must be estimated using elbow breadth or wrist circumference/weight ratio; MLIT findings not representative of entire age 25–59 population; elderly not included
	Percentile desirable body weight	10 < 25	5 < 10	< 5	National Health Examination Survey (NHANES I, II) standards presented as percentiles according to age and frame size; identifies risk of depletion and obesity	NHANES I, II—weight not associated with longevity, morbidity or mortality; Loss of body parts must be considered
	% usual body weight (actual weight/usual weight) × 100	85–90	75 < 85	≤ 74	More useful with ill populations in assessing weight change; Will not overlook depletion in the obese	May rely on patient memory
	% weight loss per 1 month / 3 months / 6 months $\dfrac{(usual - actual\ weight)}{usual\ weight} \times 100$	5.0 / 7.5 / 10.0	5.0 / 7.5 / 10.0	> 5.0 / > 7.5 / > 10.0	Severity and significance of weight loss are assessed	Allowances must be made for amputations; Lack of specificity regarding body compartments
Visceral Protein Stores	Serum albumin (gm/L)	28 < 35	21 < 28	< 21	Levels correlate with degree of malnutrition, morbidity and mortality; Inexpensive prognostic indicator; Half-life of about 20 days; therefore useful for long-term monitoring	Relatively large body pool; Hypoalbuminemia not specific to visceral protein depletion; other causes: liver disease, infection, nephrotic syndrome, postoperative states, metabolic stress, fluid imbalances, zinc deficiency, malabsorptive states

Table continues on next page

TABLE 1. Selected Indices of Malnutrition in Adults (Cont.)

Compartment	Indices	Depletion Mild	Depletion Moderate	Depletion Severe	Indications	Practical Limitations
Visceral Protein Stores (cont.)	Serum transferrin (TF) (mg/dl)	150 < 200	100 < 150	< 100	Shorter half-life, 8–10 days; therefore more sensitive to acute changes than albumin. May be calculated from total iron binding capacity (TIBC) e.g., grant equation: $TF = 0.87\ TIBC(mg/dl) + 10$	Other causes of low TF levels: chronic infection, acute metabolic stress, uremia, nephrotic syndrome, increased iron stores, liver disease, overhydration, iron overload, vitamin A deficiency
	Thyroxine-binding prealbumin (TBPA) (mg/dl)	10 < 15	5 < 10	< 5	Sensitive indicator, especially in acute stages of protein energy malnutrition. Useful for measuring short-term changes. Half-life = 2–3 days	Other causes of low TBPA levels: acute metabolic stress, postsurgery, altered nitrogen and energy balance, liver disease, infection, dialysis, inflammation. Limited use in renal failure
	Retinol-binding protein (gm/L)	< 0.3	< 0.3	< 0.3	Reflects acute changes in protein malnutrition. Half-life about 12 hours	Other causes of low levels: vitamin A or zinc deficiency, acute metabolic stress, postsurgery, liver disease, cystic fibrosis, hyperthyroidism
Subcutaneous Fat Stores	Triceps, biceps, subscapular and suprailiac skinfold measurements				Standards and percentile tables should be demographically similar to population surveyed	Requires trained personnel, standardized techniques, and proper calipers to minimize errors
	% of standard = (actual measurement/standard) × 100	> 90	60–90	< 60	Serial measurements can document depletion and repletion	Accuracy is affected by age and muscularity of subject
	Percentile	5–15	5–15	< 5	More beneficial with large populations than with individual hospital patients	Reliability is improved with testing multiple sites because fat distribution is not uniform

Table continues on next page

TABLE 1. Selected Indices of Malnutrition in Adults (Cont.)

Compartment	Indices	Depletion Mild	Depletion Moderate	Depletion Severe	Indications	Practical Limitations
Somatic Protein Stores	Midarm muscle circumference (MAMC) MAMC (cm) = midarm circumference (cm) – [3.14 × triceps skinfold (cm)]				Standards and percentile tables should be demographically similar to population surveyed. Serial measurements allow subject to serve as own standard. More beneficial with large populations than with individual hospital patients	Muscle mass evaluation at a single site may not be indicative of total muscle mass. Measurement error present. In presence of protein-energy malnutrition, values may be within normal limits
	% of standard = (actual measurement/standard) × 100	>90	60–90	<60		
	Percentile	5–15	5–15	<5		
	Creatinine-height index (CHI) % CHI = 100 × actual 24-hour creatinine excretion/expected 24-hour creatinine excretion	80 < 90	60 < 80	<60	Indicator of lean body mass because urinary creatinine excretion is proportionate to muscle mass and released at a constant rate in those with normal renal function	Accurate 24-hour urine collection required. Daily variations and ingestion of meat may influence results. May not be accurate in the elderly because creatinine excretion declines with age. Standards based on medium body frame. Steroids, tobramycin sulphate, Mandol may decrease results
Immuno-competence	Total lymphocyte count (mm³) = % lymphocytes × white blood cells/100	1500 <1800	900 <1500	<900	Screening parameter in noncritical patients. Correlated with albumin in predicting morbidity and mortality postoperatively	Levels increase with infection, leukemia, tissue necrosis. Levels decrease with cancer, metabolic stress, steroid therapy postsurgery, radiotherapy, chemotherapeutic agents, immunosuppressive medications, and other drugs

From Finestone HM, Greene-Finestone LS: Nutrition and diet in neurologic rehabilitation. In Lazar RB (ed): Principles of Neurologic Rehabilitation. New York, McGraw-Hill, 1998, pp 401–431.

TABLE 2. Prevalence and Degree of Malnutrition in Stroke Patients on the Rehabilitation Service

Nutritional Status	Rehabilitation Admission % (n = 49)	Rehabilitation— 1 Month % (n = 32)	Rehabilitation— 2 Months % (n = 9)	2–4 Months of Follow-up % (n = 42)
Malnourished—total	49 (24)	34 (11)	22 (1)	19 (8)
Mild	14 (7)	13 (4)	22 (1)	5 (2)
Moderate	19 (9)	13 (4)	0 (0)	10 (4)
Severe	16 (8)	9 (3)	0 (0)	5 (2)

From Finestone HM, Greene-Finestone LS, Wilson ES, Teasell RW: Malnutrition in stroke patients on the rehabilitation service and at follow-up: Prevalence and predictors. Arch Phys Med Rehabil 75:310–316, 1995; with permission.

Malnutrition was present in 49% of stroke patients admitted to a rehabilitation service 2–3 weeks poststroke in a longitudinal study of 49 stroke patients by Finestone et al.[17] Malnutrition was determined using a combination of anthropometric and biochemical parameters and was assessed 1 and 2 months later in those remaining on the rehabilitation unit and at 2–4 month follow-up in 42 of the patients. For the diagnosis of malnutrition, at least two nutrition-sensitive parameters were required to be below the normal range. Overall, malnutrition declined in prevalence and severity among the remaining patients over time (Table 2). However, some adequately nourished patients became malnourished or severity of malnutrition increased in some of the already malnourished patients.

In this study, significant predictors of malnutrition on admission to the rehabilitation service included the use of tube feeding on the acute service and a history of prior stroke and diabetes mellitus. Tube feedings were effective in reversing malnutrition. On entry to the rehabilitation service, those who were malnourished were more likely to require tube feedings. All malnourished inpatients and home tube-fed outpatients who received tube feedings for at least 1 month attained adequate nutritional status.[17]

The development of malnutrition is a concern in stroke patients. Estimates of the prevalence of undernutrition on a rehabilitation service range from 49–60%.[17,32] The former prevalence (49%) was observed even when patients were on a rehabilitation service of a tertiary care hospital where radiologic swallowing studies, a swallowing team, dietitians, and enteral feedings were readily available.

Functional Outcomes Related to Nutritional Status

Undernutrition is predictive of poorer functional status outcome and reduced functional improvement rate in acute stroke patients and those undergoing rehabilitation. Using the Modified Barthel Index (MBI) to evaluate functional status, Aptaker et al. determined that serum albumin, a nutrition-sensitive, but not specific, marker, was positively associated with higher functional mobility and degree of improvement, decreased complication rate, and higher self-care scores.[4]

Finestone et al. studied the relationship between MBI scores and malnutrition on a rehabilitation service.[16] Malnourished patients consistently demonstrated lower MBI scores than adequately nourished patients at all intervals at which they were evaluated: admission, 1 month, 2 months, and 2–4 months of follow-up. Stroke patients who were malnourished on admission to rehabilitation were significantly more likely to have lower MBI scores 1 month later. It was remarkable that all patients who scored in the dependent range at 1 month had been malnourished on admission for rehabilitation. Length of stay varied with nutritional status. The mean

TABLE 3.   Baseline Daily Fluid Requirements in Adults and Pediatric Patients

Patient Group	Fluid Requirements
Children (< 16 years)	
0.5–3 kg	120 ml/kg
3–10 kg	100 ml/kg
10–20 kg	1,000 ml plus 50 ml/kg each kg over 10 kg
> 20 kg	1,500 ml plus 20 ml/kg each kg over 20 kg
Adults	
Young active (16–30 years)	40 ml/kg
Average adult (25–55 years)	35 ml/kg
Older patients (56–65 years)	30 ml/kg
Elderly (> 65 years)	25 ml/kg

From Blackburn GL, Bell SJ, Mullen JL (eds): Nutritional Medicine, Case Management Approach. Philadelphia, WB Saunders, 1989; with permission.

length of stay was 48.3 days for malnourished stroke rehabilitation patients and 34.1 days for the adequately nourished group (p = 0.006). This contributed to the significantly reduced functional improvement rate (MBI score improvement by discharge/length of stay) of the malnourished group when the patients with initial scores in the dependent range were compared.

Increased dietary intake has been associated with functional outcome gains. In a case series report, Allison et al. described dysphagic stroke patients with recurrent aspiration pneumonia and/or nasogastric tube dislodgement and, consequently, poor dietary intake.[2] Their response to rehabilitation was poor 4–6 months after stroke.[2] When nutritional intake increased after the introduction of gastrostomy feedings, improvements in weight and serum albumin into the normal range and improved response to physiotherapy were noted.

Davalos et al. studied malnutrition following acute stroke and its association with poor clinical outcome, as defined as death or Barthel Index (BI) ≤ 50, at 1 month poststroke.[14] Malnutrition at day 7 more commonly (41%) preceded poor outcome at 1 month than in those with good outcome (14%) (BI > 50, p = 0.003). Complications such as urinary or respiratory tract infections (50% vs. 24%, p = 0.017) and bedsores (17% vs. 4%, not significant) were more common in the malnourished than adequately nourished patients.

Fluid Requirements

The risk of dehydration in stroke patients is often underappreciated. This is particularly true of dysphagic patients receiving all nutrition by mouth, because liquids are often a difficult texture for dysphagic patients to control. Even when fluids are thickened to ease control, patients may be unable to maintain adequate hydration. Alternate methods, such as intravenous administration, may be required.

Table 3 presents general guidelines for the determination of fluid requirements. Fluid requirements should also take into account the effects of age, disease, and medical treatment. Fluid requirements are increased above normal as a consequence of fever, diarrhea, vomiting, excessive sweating, fistula drainage, and during the administration of hyperosmolar formulas.[24]

NUTRITIONAL AND DIETARY CONCERNS

Nutritional Treatment: Step by Step

The following steps outline the nutritional management of stroke patients.[15]

1. Monitor nutritional status by routine ongoing nutritional screenings and/or comprehensive assessments.

2. Provide adequate nutrition to prevent the development of malnutrition or to improve poor nutritional status. Little is known of the metabolic demands and subsequent nutritional needs of patients with stroke. The clinical dietitian should consider food consistency, medical status, age, activity level, food preferences, and ethnic background when planning the diet. A clinical dietitian or dietary technician should perform periodic calculations of energy and protein intake (calorie counts) in patients suspected of eating poorly. A high-energy, high-protein diet would be recommended for patients who are malnourished or at risk of becoming malnourished.

3. In those suspected of dysphagia, a swallowing assessment should be performed by a speech-language pathologist (SLP) who can recommend modifications

TABLE 4. Interventions for Secondary Medical Complications Affecting Food Intake in Patients with Stroke[4,11,27]

Medical Condition	Intervention
Upper extremity hemiparesis or paralysis	Teach patient to use unaffected hand, even if paralyzed one has been dominant
	Consult occupational therapist, use assistive devices to assist in eating skills when appropriate
	Provide opportunities for feeding rehabilitation for as long as progress is noted
	Encourage self-feeding; provide finger foods
	Prevent fatigue
	Maintain human dignity
Disorientation Altered level of consciousness	Give clear, repeated, slow-paced instructions and demonstrations
	Encourage participation of family
	Review medications (antipsychotic and sedative anticholinergic can impair mental status)
	Be nonjudgmental or changes in personality
Altered emotional behavior: depression, irascibility, lability, indifference	Reassure with word or touch
	Medications such as antidepressants and methylphenidate have the side effect of appetite suppression
	Oral supplements may be helpful
	Tube feeds may be helpful in those who refuse to eat
	Lability may not reflect actual emotion
Dysphagia	Dysphagia evaluation, consult speech-language pathologist, clinical dietitian
	Implement dysphagia diet and/or tube feeding
Apraxia	Break down tasks into a familiar set of small steps
	Monitor quantity eaten
	Continually encourage eating
Visuospatial perceptual deficits	Give directions and discussions on unaffected side
	Depending on level of cognition, present food within visual field or train patient to rotate tray to bring attention to the previously "hidden food" and purposefully look to side of "blind spot"
	Remediation and computer-controlled audiovisual-based rehabilitation programs can be useful for improving feeding skills
Denture ill-fit due to facial paralysis or gum shrinkage during denture removal	Dental consultation
	New set of dentures if necessary
	In meantime, liquid nutritional formula and/or soft, pureed diet
Obesity	Reduced-energy diet because excess weight can interfere with mobility and long-term outcome
Decubitus ulcers	Adequate energy and protein

to food and fluid consistencies. A modified barium swallow may be recommended if there are serious aspiration concerns. Regular communication with team members regarding the patient's dietary treatment is essential to the progress and upgrading of the dysphagia diet (see below).

4. Observe patients for signs of dehydration, and monitor fluid balance regularly. This is particularly important for dysphagic patients on exclusively oral diets and those enterally fed using hyperosmolar formulas.

5. If the patient is unable to consume food orally, or is unable to consume sufficient quantities, or the risk of aspiration is high, enteral nutrition should be provided until the swallowing and gag reflexes return and oral intake is adequate. During the transition from enteral to oral intake, both types of feedings may be provided, with the enteral portion gradually decreasing as the oral portion is increased. The adequacy of the oral intake should be verified by calorie counts.

6. Medical complications related to stroke often affect dietary intake. Table 4 describes approaches for coping with secondary problems such as visuospatial perceptual deficits, upper extremity paralysis or paresis, and apraxia.

7. Cognitive changes may produce altered eating behaviors such as attention-concentration deficit/forgetting to eat, combativeness/throwing food, eating too fast or too slowly, forgetting to swallow, or chewing constantly/overchewing food. Table 5 suggests practical strategies for dealing with these situations.

8. When hospital discharge is planned, the type of feeding and quantity of diet should be discussed with the patient and caregivers.

Nutritional Strategies

The diet strategies for patients poststroke fall into five categories: the high-energy, high-protein diet; energy-reduced diet; high-fiber diet; dysphagia diets; and enteral diets.

TABLE 5.   Practical Interventions for Eating-related Problems in Individuals with Stroke

Behavior Problem	Interventions
Attention-concentration deficit/forgets to eat	Remind patient to eat and drink; discuss available foods. Verbally direct client through each step of the eating process. Place utensils in hand.
Eats to fast	Seat with role-models. Set utensils down between bites. Offer food items separately. Offer foods that take time to chew. Use smaller utensil/cup.
Eats too slowly	Monitor eating pace; provide verbal cues: "chew," "take another bite." Serve first to allow ample meal time. Use insulated dishes to maintain proper temperatures. Alter texture if patient has difficulty chewing.
Forgets to swallow	Tell patient to swallow. Observe or feel for swallow before offering next mouthful. Stroke upward on patient's larynx. Check for remaining food at end of meal.
Chews constantly/over-chews food	Tell patient to stop chewing after each bite. Serve soft foods to reduce need to chew. Offer small bites. Carefully remove food from mouth if patient is unable to swallow it.
Will not wake up or get up to eat	Ask why. Discuss time preference for meals; arrange more appropriate nap time. Evaluate medication for possible cause. Evaluate nutritional adequacy of total daily food intake. Have client wash face, clean teeth. Develop a contract identifying patient's mealtime preferences and facility's responsibility.
Refuses to eat	Try placing a small amount of food on lower lip.

Adapted from Consultant Dietitians in Health Care Facilities: Dining Skills: Practical Skills for the Caregivers of Eating-Disabled Older Adults. Chicago, American Dietetic Association, 1994.

The High-Energy, High-Protein Diet

A high-energy, high-protein diet is appropriate for stroke patients demonstrating excessive weight loss, inadequate weight gain, malnutrition, or concurrent skeletal fractures. The rationale behind this diet is that the augmented protein intake supplies the amino acids required for the building, maintenance, and repair of body tissue. Supplemental energy is required to spare the protein from being used as a source of energy. The energy level should be appropriate to maintain body weight or promote weight gain.[33]

The normal adult protein requirement is 0.8 gm/kg of body weight per day.[37] For patients requiring protein repletion, intakes in the range of 1.5–2.0 gm/kg/day are recommended in the absence of renal or hepatic insufficiency.[3] To allow for the proper utilization of protein, the diets should contain 66 kJ (150 kcal) of nonprotein energy for every gram of available nitrogen (or 6.25 gm protein). Nutritional supplements (commercial beverages or puddings) or frequent meals and snacks can be used to augment dietary intake. Food intake should be monitored and nutritional status assessed regularly.

The Reduced-Energy Diet

Following stroke, patients' mobility and, consequently, their energy requirements are frequently reduced. If energy intake exceeds output, weight gain and obesity may occur. This can adversely affect functions such as transfers and ambulation and place extra stress on caregivers. If excess weight is interfering with rehabilitation, weight reduction is advised. A clinical dietitian can recommend a reduced-energy diet that contains age-appropriate levels of nutrients and behavior modification recommendations. Physical activity should be increased when possible, and consideration should be given to whether increased appetite is a side effect of the patient's medications.

The High-Fiber Diet

Constipation, a frequent sequela of stroke, is often related to inadequate hydration or poor intake of dietary fiber. The patient's hydration should be assessed. A daily fluid intake of 1,200–2,000 ml should be encouraged provided there is no medical reason for fluid restriction.[13] Most dysphagia diets and diets based on enteral formulas without added fiber are low in fiber. When commercial fiber supplements such as Metamucil are used, additional fluids are recommended. Dietary sources of insoluble fiber are particularly effective in increasing fecal bulk,[39] and the clinical dietitian can advise on sources of dietary fiber to be increased. Participation in exercise, attention to the urge to defecate, and the establishment of a routine toileting schedule should be encouraged. Whether constipation is a side effect of medications such as antidepressant or narcotic preparations should be evaluated.[13]

Dysphagia Diets

Prescription and Implementation. Based on the results of the bedside assessment and/or the videofluoroscopic examination (modified barium swallow), in which a variety of food and liquid consistencies are used, the physician and SLP make diet recommendations. The clinical dietitian assesses the patient's nutritional status, determines the energy and protein requirements, and helps the patient adapt to the prescribed diet modifications. Together with the SLP, the patient's progress is followed to allow a smooth progression to the highest diet level possible, all the while achieving or maintaining adequate nutritional status.[34] The nursing staff may

TABLE 6. Dietary Considerations for Dysphagia in Patients with Neurologic Disorders

Condition	Dietary Consideration	Rationale
Slow/weak/uncoordinated pharyngeal peristalsis	Include highly seasoned, flavorful, aromatic foods; add sugar, spices	Maximize stimulus for swallow
	Serve food at either very warm or very cold temperatures	Maximize stimulus for swallow
	Include highly textured foods such as diced cooked vegetables, finely chopped raw vegetables in gelatin base, diced canned fruit	Maximize stimulus for swallow
	Maintain semisolid consistencies that form a cohesive bolus	To avoid consistencies that will tend to fall apart in the pharynx
	Avoid sticky or bulky foods	To reduce risk of airway obstruction
	Be cautious with thin liquids (water, juices, milk); iced tart juices or crushed popsicles—banana and vanilla melt slowest (flavor and temperature may stimulate reflex)	They are difficult to control, unpredictable, and may spill into pharynx prior to swallow reflex
	Medium- or spoon-thick liquids may be substituted	
	Thicken thin liquids with nonfat dry milk powder, fruit flakes, or commercial thickeners	
	Small frequent meals	Minimize fatigue; optimize food temperature and total nutrient intake
Weakened or poor oral-muscular control	Maintain semisolid consistencies that form a cohesive bolus	Requires less oral manipulation; purees are difficult to control
	Avoid slippery, sticky foods	
	Avoid thin liquids (see above description of thin liquids and recommendation)	See above rationale
	Small frequent meals	Minimize fatigue; optimize total nutrient intake
Reduced oral sensation	Position food in most sensitive area	Maximize sensation possible
	Do not mix textures (e.g., vegetable soup)	Maximize sensation possible
	Use colder temperatures	Maximize sensation possible
	Use highly seasoned, flavorful foods	Maximize sensation possible
Crycopharyngeal dysfunction	Maintain liquid/pureed diet if no other contraindications present	Liquids and purees will pass into the esophagus more easily
Decreased laryngeal elevation	Limit diet to medium- and spoon-thick liquids, soft solids	Thin liquids easily penetrate larynx
	Avoid sticky or bulky foods or food that will fall apart	Reduce risk of airway obstruction
Decreased vocal cord closure	Avoid thin liquids	Easy, quick laryngeal penetration
	Avoid foods that will fall apart	Reduce risk of small pieces entering larynx after the swallow

Adapted from American Dietetic Association: Handbook of Clinical Dietetics. 2nd ed. New Haven, CT, Yale University Press, 1992.

assist or supervise patients during mealtimes, which can be done in a common dining room to enhance the social atmosphere and allow for regular monitoring of the patient's progress. The occupational therapist (OT) can perform a mealtime evaluation to screen for feeding difficulties. The OT can provide adaptive equipment to

TABLE 7. Examples of Foods and Fluid Consistencies

Consistency	Food Examples
Semisolids that form a cohesive bolus	Hot cereals; quiches; egg; tuna or meat salad; ground meats with gravy; moist, soft meat or fish loaf; soft cheeses; aspic; canned fruit; custard; pudding; finger gelatin; whipped gelatin; cheesecake with sauce
Spoon-thick liquids	Frozen products,* gelatin desserts, pudding, yogurt, pureed fruit
Medium-thick liquids	Blenderized or cream soups, eggnog, nectar, milk shakes or malts, high-protein or high-calorie commercial supplemental formulas
Thin liquids	Water, broth, milk, chocolate milk, coffee, tea, hot chocolate, fruit juices, soda, alcoholic beverages, standard commercial supplemental formulas, vegetable juice
Foods that fall apart	Plain ground meats, dry crumbly breads, crackers, plain rice, thin hot cereals, cooked peas or corn, plain chopped raw vegetables and fruits, thin pureed foods such as applesauce
Sticky or bulky foods	Peanut butter, fresh white bread, plain mashed potatoes, bran cereals, refried beans, raw vegetables and fruits, bananas, chunks of plain meats

* Frozen products such as frozen juices, popsicles, ice chips, ice cream, and sherbet would be restricted if they are allowed to melt to thin liquid in the mouth, thereby becoming a hazard to swallowing.
From American Dietetic Association: Handbook of Clinical Dietetics. 2nd ed. New Haven, CT, Yale University Press, 1992; with permission.

assist with mechanical aspects of feeding. Along with the OT, the physical therapist can help determine any requirements for external support during feeding or the modified barium swallow.[8,15]

The Dysphagia Diet. Patients with stroke commonly exhibit conditions that necessitate dietary modifications (Table 6).

Characteristics of the dysphagia diet include texture modification of food and fluids. Foods may be chopped, minced, or pureed, and fluids may be thickened. Examples of food and fluid consistencies are found in Table 7, and an example of a multistage dysphagia diet is shown in Table 8. Solid foods are assigned to one of five groups, which progress from the easiest to the most difficult foods to swallow.[34]

The dysphagia diet must meet the patient's individual needs depending on degree and site of the oropharyngeal impairment and the patient's own tolerance and preference. The dysphagia diet is nutritionally adequate so long as the patient consumes normal quantities of food at each meal. If oral intake is limited, the dysphagia diet should be complemented by high-energy, high-protein foods. If oral intake remains insufficient, the use of tube feedings should be considered. Vitamin, mineral, and commercial supplements may be offered orally or by tube feeding. Patients may begin the diet at any stage and progress by more than one category at a time according to swallowing ability and tolerance.[34] Regular reassessments are essential in order to upgrade the oral diet as necessary. The diet should have as many normal characteristics as possible, both for psychological reasons[31] and to enhance palatability. Dysphagia diets tend to be low in fiber, making constipation a concern. Fiber supplementation may be necessary.

Liquids are grouped separately into thin, medium-thick, and spoon-thick categories (see Table 7) because patients' ability to swallow them is independent of their ability to swallow solids. For some patients, thin fluids pass through the swallowing tract too quickly to be detected. Thicker fluids can be sensed more readily, but they can accumulate in the back of the pharynx and spill into the trachea. Thin liquids may be thickened with starch, skim milk powder, pureed fruit, infant cereals,

TABLE 8.   Main Features of Solid Food Dysphagia Diet

Five categories that progress in swallowing difficulty from easiest to most difficult:

Stage 1. All pureed foods, smooth hot cereals, strained soups thickened to pureed consistency, creamed cottage cheese, smooth yogurt, and puddings

Stage 2. All foods in previous stage plus soft moist whole foods such as pancakes; finely chopped tender meats, fish, and eggs bound with thick dressing; soft cheeses (e.g., American); noodles and pasta; tender cooked leafy greens; sliced ripe banana; soft breads; soft moist cakes

Stage 3. All foods in previous stages plus eggs any style, tender ground meats bound with thick sauce, soft fish, whole soft vegetables, drained canned fruits

Stage 4. All foods in previous stages plus foods with solids and liquids together (e.g., vegetable soup), all whole foods except hard and particulate foods such as dry breads, tough meat, corn, rice, apples

Stage 5. Regular diet

From Pardoe EM: Development of a multistage diet for dysphagia. J Am Diet Assoc 93:568–571, 1993; with permission.

or commercial thickening agents. Thickened fluids are often suitable for patients unable to tolerate any normal liquids. The fluids must maintain the consistency of a puree until swallowed.[34] General guidelines for the dysphagia diet are found in Table 9.

The adequacy of hydration should be verified by monitoring fluid balance and serum electrolyte levels (see Table 3). If fluid intake is insufficient despite the use of thickened fluids, hydration may need to be supplemented, such as with nasogastric tubes, gastrostomy tubes, or intravenous routes.[15]

ENTERAL NUTRITION

Tube feeding is a method of nutritional support for patients with a functional gastrointestinal (GI) tract. Symptoms such as gastric or intestinal obstruction, paralytic ileus, intractable vomiting, or severe diarrhea preclude its use.

The type of tube feeding and the route of access are dictated by the medical condition and the length of time that the tube feeding is expected to be used. Figure 1, which provides an algorithm for determining the optimal type of feeding, takes

TABLE 9.   Dysphagia Diet: General Guidelines for the Patient

1. Follow American or Canadian Dietetic Association Guidelines for food selection.

2. Eat small, frequent meals instead of three large meals to improve meal tolerance.

3. Follow each meal with oral cleaning to prevent mouth sores and to avoid swallowing any remaining unchewed food.

4. Determine, with the therapist, the best head and/or body posture for swallowing.

5. Sit upright during food ingestions and do not lie down for at least 15–30 minutes afterward; avoid large snacks 1–2 hours before sleep.

6. Place food in middle of mouth or on the unaffected side, if applicable.

7. Concentrate and chew food slowly; ingest foods in small mouthfuls (one half to one teaspoon).

8. Avoid washing food down with liquids.

9. Use liquid thickeners if thin fluids are to be avoided; the dietitian can advise on this.

10. Check the form of medication being used (e.g., liquid, crushed, or whole pills) to ensure that it complies with the swallowing regimen.

Adapted from Ontario Dietetic Association–Ontario Hospital Association Nutrition Care Manual. Don Mills, Ontario, Ontario Hospital Association, 1989.

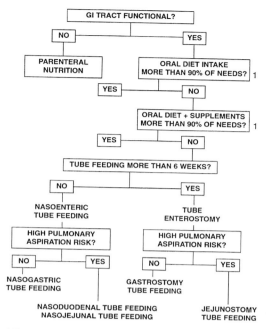

FIGURE 1. Determining the optimal feeding mode. From Hopkins B: Assessment of nutritional status. In Gottschlich MM, Matarese LE, Shronts EP (eds): Nutrition Support Dietetics—Core Curriculum. 2nd ed. Silver Springs, MD, American Society for Parenteral and Enteral Nutrition, 1993, pp 15–65; with permission.

into account clinical factors such as adequacy of oral intake, anticipated duration of enteral support, and risk of aspiration. The VMBS is often used initially to determine whether safe oral feeding is feasible[1] (see chapter entitled "Aspiration and Pneumonia following Stroke").

Classification of Enteral Diets. Tube feedings vary in energy density, osmolarity, lactose content, molecular form of substrate, and cost. A clinical dietitian should be consulted on the optimal formulation to meet the patient's nutritional needs.

Enteral diets can be complete or supplementary. If taken in adequate quantities, complete formulations provide the nutrient and energy requirements for most individuals. Enteral feeding may be categorized as follows.

1. **Polymeric diets** represent the most common category of enteral formula used in neurologically impaired patients. These formulas are appropriate for patients with a functional GI tract. They typically contain intact protein, polyunsaturated fatty acids with or without medium-chain triglycerides, glucose oligosaccharides, or starch. They are complete provided that sufficient volume is administered. Subcategories of the polymeric group include standard, high-nitrogen, fiber-supplemented, concentrated, milk-based, and commercial or homemade blenderized formulas.

Some institutions and individuals blenderize regular food, such as meat, fruits, vegetables, cereal, and oil. Their preparation is labor-intensive and poses a high risk of contamination. Nutrient composition is variable. Blenderized feedings may or may not contain lactose. They supply trace elements and natural sources of fiber.

However, because of their high-viscosity, blenderized feedings require large-bore feeding tubes. Commercially blenderized feeds are bacteriologically safe and provide consistent nutritional composition. They are generally more expensive than other polymeric feeds.

Many polymeric tube feeds are palatable for oral use as well. They may be flavored, unflavored, or bland. Because their viscosity is low, small-bore feeding tubes may be used. They are sterile prior to opening and, once open, are bacteriologically safe provided that protocols for handling are followed. Osmolality varies from isosmolar (300 mOsm/kg water) to high-level osmolar (about 700 mOsm/kg water) in some of the concentrated formulas and milk-based formulas. The energy content of tube feedings is generally 1 kcal, or 4.2 kJ per ml. Concentrated formulas, supplying up to 2.0 kcal, or 8.4 kJ/ml, are indicated in patients with fluid restrictions or limited formula tolerance. Fiber is generally lacking in the standardized feeds, but variations with added fiber are available to promote normal bowel function. High-fiber formulas are useful for long-term feedings. High-nitrogen polymeric formulas are indicated in the presence of malnutrition, a catabolic state, or in those with or at risk of pressure sores.

2. **Partially hydrolysed (or elemental) formulas** contain protein in amino acid or peptide form, carbohydrate as glucose oligosaccharides, and fat as long- or medium-chain fatty acids. This type of feeding is indicated in situations of gut malfunction, including malabsorption, short bowel syndromes, chronic pancreatitis, or bile salt deficiency.[3,33] Examples include Vital HN by Ross, and Vivonex TEN by Sandoz.

3. **Modular, or combined modular, protein, carbohydrate or fat products** can be used to enhance an existing formula, or they can be combined to produce a complete formula for those with specialized nutrient, fluid, or electrolyte needs.[6] Malnourished patients or those in a catabolic state may benefit by the addition of a protein supplement. Examples include Promod by Ross and Casec by Mead Johnson.

4. **Specialized formulas** are available for patients with impaired renal function, compromised pulmonary function, diabetes, and those in critical care.[15]

Routes of Access. Feeding routes may be classified into nasoenteric and enterostomy types. Nasoenteric feeding includes the following routes: nasogastric (tube from nose to stomach), nasoduodenal (tube from nose through pylorus and into duodenum), and nasojejunal (tube from nose through pylorus and into jejunum, usually placed radioscopically).[3] Nasogastric feedings are generally safe, particularly when there is no evidence of reflux or aspiration. Enterostomies can be inserted surgically or percutaneously, often by gastrostomy and jejunostomy. A gastrostomy involves tube placement in the stomach; tube sizes, pliability, and techniques vary. Jejunostomy involves the creation of a jejunal stoma that can be intermittently catheterized via needle catheter placement or direct tube placement. In percutaneous endoscopic gastrostomy or jejunostomy, the feeding tube is percutaneously inserted under endoscopic guidance into the stomach or jejunum. The tube is secured by rubber "bumpers" or an inflated balloon catheter. It is often performed with local anesthesia by a gastroenterologist. If the patient exhibits altered level of consciousness or dysfunction of cranial nerves IX, X, and XII, feedings should be delivered distal to the pylorus.[27] Percutaneous gastrojejunostomy, a procedure favored in the authors' institution, involves the percutaneous insertion of a guidewire and subsequent feeding catheter into the jejunum via the stomach. This is performed by a radiologist, and only local anesthetic is required.[15]

TABLE 10. Possible Adverse Reactions to Tube Feeding

Problem	Possible Causes	Management Strategy
Mechanical complications		
Tube displacement	Coughing, vomiting	Replace tube and confirm placement
	Dislodgement by patient	Replace tube; restrain patient, if necessary, consider alternative feeding route
Tube obstruction or clogging	Inadequate taping of tube	Position tube properly and tape correctly
	Improperly crushed medication	Use liquid medications when possible
	Medications mixed with incompatible formulas	Follow drug nutrient interaction guidelines and flush tube before and after addition of medication
	Formula residue adhering to tube; failure to irrigate properly	Flush tube with 20–50 ml water before starting and after stopping feeding; flush tube at least every 4 hours during continuous infusion*
Gastric retention, aspiration pneumonia	Delayed gastric emptying	Reposition tube into small intestine
	Patient lying flat during infusion	Elevate head of bed to 30° or more during and for 2 hours after infusion
Nasopharyngeal irritation; mucosal erosion; otitis media	Displaced feeding tube	Monitor and confirm tube placement before feeding
	Large-bore vinyl or rubber feeding tubes for prolonged periods	Consider use of soft, small-bore feeding tubes or feeding by tube enterostomy
	Improper positioning or placement	Position tube properly and tape correctly; choose tube of correct size for patient
	Decreased salivary secretions due to lack of chewing; mouth breathing	Keep mouth and lips moist. Allow chewing of sugarless gum, gargling, or sucking on anesthetic lozenges if appropriate
Skin irritation, excoriation and infection at ostomy site**	Leakage of gastric or intestinal secretions from stoma site; site is portal of entry for bacteria	Use appropriate enterostomal therapy. Ensure ostomy catheter anchored via retention device to avoid dislodgement. Treat infection with local and systemic antibiotics—a tube change may also be required
Gastrointestinal complications		
Nausea and vomiting; cramping; distension	Improper location of tube	Periodically confirm tube position
	Rapid increase in rate, volume, or concentration	Return to slower rate and advance by smaller increments. Advance only when tolerated at current rate
	High osmolality	Dilute to isotonic strength if gastric residuals are consistently high. Increase concentration over several days. Consider change to isotonic formula

Table continued on next page

TABLE 10. Possible Adverse Reactions to Tube Feeding (Cont.)

Problem	Possible Causes	Management Strategy
Gastrointestinal complications (cont.)	Delayed gastric emptying	Check gastric residuals every 4–6 hours on continuous feedings or prior to each bolus.
		Monitor for drugs or disease states that may influence gastric or intestinal motility†
	Lactose intolerance	Change to lactose-free formula
	Cold formula	Warm to room temperature before use
	Obstruction	Stop formula feeding immediately
	Excessive fat in formula	Switch to lower-fat formula; reduce fat in modular feedings
Constipation	Inadequate fiber or fluid intake	Monitor intake and output, add free water if intake is not greater than output by 500–1,000 ml/day; use formula with added fiber
	Medications	Evaluate medication side effects, suggest stool softener or bulk-forming laxative
	Inactivity	Increase patient activity if possible
Diarrhea, defined as passage of more than 200 gm of stool per 24 hours or the passage of liquid stools	Protein-energy malnutrition, decreased oncotic pressure due to serum albumin below 3.0 gm/dl	Use isotonic or elemental formula at slow rate initially. If severe, suggest antidiarrhea therapy or parenteral nutrition
	Infectious origin, microbial contamination of formula	Confirm with stool, blood, or formula culture. Review tube-feeding handling and infection control procedures
	Malabsorption of fat or other nutrients	Evaluate for pancreatic insufficiency, use pancreatic enzyme replacements if indicated. Change to low-fat or elemental formula
	Bolus feeding, dumping syndrome	Change to continuous feeding or decrease bolus volume and increase frequency of feeding
	Hyperosmolar formula	Reduce rate and increase gradually, dilute formula or change to isotonic product
	Medication	Consider antidiarrheal agents such as Kaopectate, paregoric, or Lomotil. Change to fiber-containing formula
Metabolic complications		
Hyperosmolar dehydration	Administration of hypertonic formula with inadequate water	Initiate hypertonic feedings at reduced rates, dilute or consider use of isotonic formula

Table continued on next page

TABLE 10. Possible Adverse Reactions to Tube Feeding (Cont.)

Problem	Possible Causes	Management Strategy
Metabolic complications (cont.)		
Fluid overload or overhydration	Refeeding of patients with protein-energy malnutrition, common in patients with cardiac, renal or hepatic disease Prolonged use of over dilute formula	Restrict fluids, use concentrated formula Advance formula concentration as tolerated
Hyponatremia	Congestive heart failure, cirrhosis, hypoalbuminemia, edema, ascites Excess gastrointestinal losses	Apply diuretic therapy; restrict fluids. Use concentrated formula Monitor serum levels and hydration status and replace sodium as needed
Hypernatremia	Dehydration	Assure adequate fluid intake
Hypokalemia	Acidosis, insulin administration, diarrhea, marked malnutrition, diuretic therapy	Monitor electrolytes daily, supplement potassium as needed
Hyperkalemia	Renal insufficiency	Perform frequent biochemical monitoring. Use formula containing low levels of potassium
Other serum electrolyte or mineral abnormalities	Various	Monitor serum levels regularly, making individual adjustments as needed
Essential fatty acid (EFA) deficiency	Formula with low levels of EFA used over prolonged time periods	Provide a minimum of 4% of the caloric intake from EFAs. Add 5 ml safflower oil daily
Glucose tolerance, hyperglycemic hyperosmolar nonketotic coma	Diabetes mellitus or temporary insulin resistance caused by trauma or sepsis	Many need to stop feeding and to rehydrate patient. Monitor blood sugar frequently, making adjustments in insulin dose. Avoid formulas high in simple sugars
Increased respiratory quotient excess CO_2 production, respiratory insufficiency	Overfeeding of calories, especially in the form of carbohydrates	Reduce the respiratory quotient by balancing the calories provided from fat, protein, and carbohydrate. Increase the percentage of calorie provided as fat by using high-fat formula or adding modular fat

* The authors' facility uses a solution of 1 tablet of sodium bicarbonate (300 mg) and 1 pancreolipase capsule mixed with 5–15 ml of water. The solution must be infused via a 5–10-ml syringe to generate adequate pressure.[28]

** From Ideno KT: Enteral nutrition. In Gottschlich MM, Matarese LE, Shronts EP (eds): Nutrition Support Dietetics—Core Curriculum. 2nd ed. Silver Springs, MD, American Society for Parenteral and Enteral Nutrition, 1993, pp 71–103.

† A nuclear medicine gastric emptying study may be helpful.

Adapted from American Dietetic Association: Handbook of Clinical Dietetics. New Haven, CT, Yale University Press, 1992; with permission.

Methods of Enteral Feeding Administration. Continuous drip feedings are delivered by gravity drip or, for better volume accuracy and tolerance, by infusion pump. They are administered at a constant rate, usually over 24 hours. This method reduces the possibility of pulmonary aspiration.

Intermittent infusions are equally divided feedings, infused four to six times throughout the day. They can be given by gravity drip over 30–60 minutes or by infusion pump. Because this type of feeding frees patients from tube feeding equipment between feedings, it is convenient for those undergoing active rehabilitation and those on home tube feeding. It is also used for non–critically ill patients. A cyclic method of intermittent infusion may be used wherein the tube feeding is administered at a high infusion rate over 8–16 hours. This may be helpful in the transition from tube feeding to oral diet, with tube feeding delivered at night and oral diet ingested by day,[27] and it allows for uninterrupted rehabilitation during the day.

Bolus feeding involves the rapid delivery of a feeding into the GI tract by syringe or funnel. It is suited to the rehabilitation patient, those on home tube feeding, and non–critically ill patients. Feeding is usually carried out in less than 15 minutes.

The risk of pulmonary aspiration can be reduced by implementation of a protocol that includes confirming tube placement in the upper duodenum and elevating the patient's head to at least 30° during feeding and for at least 1 hour after feeding.[25] Blue food coloring can be added to feedings (1 ml/500 ml feeding) to detect possible aspiration. Feedings should begin at a slow, continuous rate, and the rate should advance every 8–12 hours until desired volume is achieved. Gastric residuals should be verified every 4 hours; if they measure more than 150 ml, hold feeds for 2 hours. Excessive residue may be a sign of an obstruction or digestive problem. If this continues, reevaluate the feeding regimen. An alternate route may need to be considered. This regimen is rarely required.[15]

Complications of Tube Feeding. Adverse reactions associated with tube feeding are relatively few and can usually be detected and controlled through proper monitoring. Complications associated with tube feeding are usually categorized as mechanical, GI, and metabolic.[10] Mechanical complications include tube blockages and local skin infections at the site of tube insertion. GI complications, such as cramping and diarrhea, are frequent but are easily rectified. Metabolic complications are often related to inadequate monitoring of fluid and electrolyte balance, blood sugars, and renal status. Table 10 describes potential adverse reactions, their causes, and management strategies.[15]

Home Tube Feeding. General considerations include assessing who will administer feedings, compatibility of the tube feeding with the patient's schedule, and type of follow-up.[12] Formula considerations include the adequacy of the formula, tolerance of the feedings, whether it is ready to use or requires preparation, cost, storage space, supplier, method of purchase and delivery, and availability of third-party payment. Equipment considerations include type of pump or gravity drip set, other accessories, whether to rent or lease equipment, expense of equipment, availability of third-party payment, and ease of administration.

Patient instructions should include written guidelines on proper sanitation of feeding and equipment, rate and strength of feedings, time of administration, body position and length of time to remain in position, temperature of feedings, maximum hanging time, maximum time to keep formulas open, amount of fluids to flush between feedings, how to deal with complications, and care of the tube and exit site.

CONCLUSION

Stroke may affect, or be affected by, nutrition and diet. Evidence suggests that about half of all stroke patients are malnourished on admission to the inpatient rehabilitation service. Factors associated with malnutrition include poorer functional outcome and prolonged rehabilitation stay.

A clinical goal of the rehabilitation effort should be to prevent or to identify and treat inadequate nutritional and feeding states. In the future, investigations concerning metabolic demands, stress responses, and specific dietary needs of the stroke patient can influence methods of assessment, nutritional delivery, and therapy. Specific attention to nutritional issues can help patients reach their full rehabilitation potential.

REFERENCES

1. Akpunonu BE, Mutgi AB, Roberts C, et al: Modified barium swallow does not affect how often PEGs are placed after stroke. J Clin Gastroenterol 24:74–78, 1997.
2. Allison MC, Morris AJ, Park RHR, Mills PR: Percutaneous endoscopic gastrostomy tube feeding may improve outcome of late rehabilitation following stroke. J R Soc Med 85:147–149, 1992.
3. American Dietetic Association: Handbook of Clinical Dietetics. 2nd ed. New Haven, CT, Yale University Press, 1992.
4. Aptaker RL, Roth EJ, Reichhardt G, et al: Serum albumin level as a predictor of geriatric stroke rehabilitation outcome. Arch Phys Med Rehabil 75:80–84, 1994.
5. Arego DE, Koch S: Malnutrition in the rehabilitation setting. Nutrition Today July/August:28–32, 1986.
6. Axelsson K, Asplund K, Norberg A, Eriksson S: Eating problems and nutritional status during hospital stay of patients with severe stroke. J Am Diet Assoc 89:1092–1096, 1989.
7. Axelsson K, Asplund K, Norberg A, Alafuzoff I: Nutritional status in patients with acute stroke. Acta Med Scand 224:217–224, 1988.
8. Bach DB, Pouget S, Belle K, et al: An integrated team approach to the management of patients with orolaryngeal dysphagia. J Allied Health 18:459–468, 1989.
9. Beamer NB, Couli BM, Clark WM, et al: Interleukin-6 and interleukin-1 receptor antagonist in acute stroke. Ann Neurol 37:800–804, 1995.
10. Bergstrom LR, Larson DE, Zinsmeister AR, et al: Utilization and outcomes of surgical gastrectomies and jejunostomies in an era of percutaneous endoscopic gastrostomy: A population-based study. Mayo Clin Proc 70:829–836, 1995.
11. Buelow JM, Jamieson D: Potential for altered nutritional status in the stroke patient. Rehabil Nurs 15:260–263, 1990.
12. Chicago Dietetic Association Staff and South Suburban Dietetic Association Staff: Manual of Clinical Dietetics. 3rd ed. Chicago, American Dietetic Association, 1988.
13. Consultant Dietitians in Health Care Facilities/American Dietetic Association: Mental Status, Nutrition Care for Specific Diseases. Practical Interventions for the Caregivers of the Eating-disabled Older Adult. Chicago, American Dietetic Association, 1994.
14. Davalos R, Ricart W, Gonzalez Huix F, et al: Effect of malnutrition after acute stroke on clinical outcome. Stroke 27:1028–1032, 1996.
15. Finestone HM, Greene-Finestone LS: Nutrition and diet in neurologic rehabilitation. In Lazar RB (ed): Principles of Neurologic Rehabilitation. New York, McGraw-Hill, 1998, pp 401–431.
16. Finestone HM, Greene-Finestone LS, Wilson ES, Teasell RW: Prolonged length of stay and reduced functional improvement rate in malnourished stroke rehabilitation patients. Arch Phys Med Rehabil 77:340–345, 1996.
17. Finestone HM, Greene-Finestone LS, Wilson ES, Teasell RW: Malnutrition in stroke patients on the rehabilitation service and at follow-up: Prevalence and predictors. Arch Phys Med Rehabil 76:310–316, 1995.
18. Fitness and Amateur Sport, Canadian Standardized Test of Fitness: Operations Manual. Ottawa, ON, Minister of State, Fitness and Amateur Sport, 1986.
19. Food and Nutrition Board, National Research Council: Recommended Dietary Allowances. 10th ed. Washington, DC, National Academy of Sciences, 1989.
20. Frisancho AR: New standards of weight and body composition by frame size and height for assessment of nutritional status of adults and the elderly. Am J Clin Nutr 40:808–819, 1984.
21. Gibson RS: Principles of Nutritional Assessment. New York, Oxford University Press, 1990.

22. Gordon C, Hewer RL, Wade DT: Dysphagia in acute stroke. BMJ 295:411–414, 1987.

23. Groher ME, Bukatman R: The prevalence of swallowing disorders in two teaching hospitals. Dysphagia 1:3–6, 1986.

24. Health and Welfare Canada Scientific Review Committee: Nutrition Recommendations, The Report of the Scientific Review Committee. Ottawa, ON, Minister of Supply and Services, 1990.

25. Hester DD: Neurologic impairment. In Gottschlich MM, Matarese LE, Shronts EP (eds): Nutrition Support Dietetics—Core Curriculum. 2nd ed. Silver Springs, MD, American Society for Parenteral and Enteral Nutrition, 1993, pp 229–241.

26. Hopkins B: Assessment of nutritional status. In Gottschlich MM, Matarese LE, Shronts EP (eds): Nutrition Support Dietetics—Core Curriculum. 2nd ed. Silver Springs, MD, American Society for Parenteral and Enteral Nutrition, 1993, pp 15–65.

27. Ideno KT: Enteral nutrition. In Gottschlich MM, Matarese LE, Shronts EP (eds): Nutrition Support Dietetics—Core Curriculum. 2nd ed. Silver Springs, MD, American Society for Parenteral and Enteral Nutrition, 1993, pp 71–103.

28. Marcaud SP, Stegall KS: Unclogging feeding tubes with pancreatic enzyme. J Parenter Enter Nutr 14:198–200, 1990.

29. Metropolitan Life Insurance Ideal Weights for Height, 1983. 1979 Build Study, Society of Actuaries and Association of Life Insurance Medical Directors of America. Philadelphia, Recording and Statistical Corporation, 1980.

30. Mountokalakis T, Dellos C: Protein catabolism following stroke [letter]. Arch Intern Med 144:2285, 1984.

31. Nelson RA, Millikan CH, Stollar C, Stone DB: Nutrition and the stroke patient. Dialog Nutr 3(4):1–6, 1979.

32. Newmark SR, Sublett D, Block J, Geller R: Nutritional assessment in a rehabilitation unit. Arch Phys Med Rehabil 62:279–282, 1981.

33. Ontario Dietetic Association and Ontario Hospital Association: Nutrition Care Manual. Don Mills, Ontario, Ontario Hospital Association, 1989.

34. Pardoe EM: Development of a multistage diet for dysphagia. J Am Diet Assoc 93:568–571, 1993.

35. Sitzmann JV: Nutritional support of the dysphagic patient: Methods, risks and complications of therapy. J Parenter Enter Nutr 14:60–63, 1990.

36. Stahl WM: Acute phase protein response to tissue injury. Crit Care Med 15:545–550, 1987.

37. World Health Organization: Energy and Protein Requirements. Report of a Joint FAO/WHO/UNV Expert Consultation. Geneva, WHO, 1985, technical report series 724.

38. WHO Collaborating Centers for Classification of Diseases: ICD-10, International Statistical Classification of Diseases and Health-related Problems. 10th rev. Vol 1. Geneva, World Health Organization, 1992.

39. Wrick KL, Robertson JB, Van Soest PJ, et al: The influence of dietary fiber source on human intestinal transit and stool output. J Nutr 113:1464–1479, 1983.

MICHAEL JOHN BORRIE, MBCHB, FRCPC

URINARY INCONTINENCE AFTER STROKE

From the Division of Geriatric
    Medicine
Department of Medicine
University of Western Ontario
    and
Continence Clinic and Continence
    Outreach Program
Parkwood Hospital
London, Ontario
Canada

Reprint requests to:
Michael John Borrie, MBChB,
    FRCPC
Division of Geriatric Medicine
Parkwood Hospital
801 Commissioners Road East
London, Ontario N6C 5J1
Canada

Urinary incontinence following stroke is common and compounds the physical and psychological insult of the neurologic deficit. It has a negative impact on morale and self-esteem. When incontinence persists, it compromises rehabilitation, influences discharge location, and places undue stress on caregivers at home.[26,33] Remaining or becoming dry is an important positive predictor of discharge within 6 months after stroke.[6] Incontinence following stroke receives varying attention[8,36,58] or may be ignored.[11]

EPIDEMIOLOGY

Following stroke, 44–60% of stroke victims have urinary incontinence.[13,17,50] Of these, 17–22% will have premorbid urinary incontinence.[8,13] At 6 months, 14–19% have persisting urinary incontinence.[5,50] A multivariate analysis including 935 acute stroke patients showed that the significant risk factors for urinary incontinence after stroke include age, severity of stroke, diabetes, and comorbidity of other disabling diseases.[50] It is important to recognize that incontinence from any cause including stroke may be resolved, improved, or better managed in almost all cases. One should never assume that the incontinence is entirely a consequence of the stroke. A clear understanding of the etiology and a thorough assessment of incontinence is critical to successful management.

NORMAL BLADDER AND URETHRA

Normal bladder and urethral function is dependent on neurologic, urologic, psychologic, and mobility factors. A detailed discussion of the neurologic reflexes and pathways is beyond the scope of this chapter and is well reviewed elsewhere.[4,10,15,52] In brief, bladder (detrusor) and urethral functions are coordinated for storage and emptying of urine. The sympathetic nervous system promotes storage of urine by relaxing the detrusor smooth muscle to accommodate urine in the bladder. The sphincter closure pressure is sustained by stimulation of sympathetic alpha-adrenergic receptors located at the internal sphincter. During bladder emptying, sympathetic closure of the internal urethral sphincter is inhibited, and parasympathetic acetylcholine-mediated detrusor contraction occurs. The pelvic floor, including the external urethral sphincter and external anal sphincter, has somatic innervation via the pudendal nerve and is under voluntary control. The sacral reflex arc promoting emptying is facilitated by the pontine micturition center. Input to the pontine micturition center occurs from the spinal cord, cerebellum, basal ganglia, and central cortex. The pontine micturition center is consciously inhibited at a cerebral cortical level from the superiomedial portion of the frontal lobe.[4,15,51] This cortical inhibition of micturition is a learned behavior, usually acquired at a young age, and allows an individual to postpone micturition until the appropriate moment. There are pathways to and from the pontine micturition center from the thalamic nuclei in the basal ganglia. In animals, sensory input occurs from the pelvic floor muscles via the spinal cerebellar tracts. The cerebellum has an inhibitory role on bladder filling and facilitates voiding but has no effect on the striated sphincter.[51]

ETIOLOGY

Detrusor Function

Cortical or basal ganglia lesions, particularly from stroke, generally cause an unstable detrusor.[13,21,28,31] In the immediate poststroke period, acute urinary retention may occur. "Cerebral shock" has been postulated as a neurophysiologic explanation.[15,35] Burney and colleagues studied patients within 72 hours of an acute stroke.[21] They correlated computed tomography (CT) and magnetic resonance imaging (MRI) findings with urodynamic testing, which included simultaneous needle electrode electromyogram (EMG). Forty-seven percent had urinary retention. Of those with areflexia, 81% had hemorrhagic infarcts. The majority of those with frontoparietal and internal capsular lesions had detrusor instability.

Unstable detrusor contractions, confirmed at cystometry, occur with little warning, giving symptoms of urinary urgency and urge incontinence. The bladder volume at which unstable bladder contractions occur can be quite variable. It is usually lower than the volume at which a person would normally have a strong sensation to void. In addition to bladder volume, stimuli such as movement, standing, or anxiety can provoke unstable bladder contractions. The term for the unstable bladder due to a neurologic lesion is *detrusor hyperreflexia*.[1,7] Whether or not a person develops detrusor hyperreflexia following a stroke depends on the site, size, and number of lesions and the time elapsed since the stroke; detrusor hyperreflexia is not an invariable consequence of a stroke.[13,28,31,44,46,56,62]

Theoretically, brain stem strokes below the pons, which are uncommon, could cause a loss of synchronization of the detrusor contraction and relaxation of the external urethral sphincter. This so-called detrusor external urethral dyssynergia is well recognized in individuals with spinal cord injuries. A case series of 53 consecutive inpatients admitted to a rehabilitation unit following brainstem stroke reported on the urodynamic studies that were performed on 9 of the 16 patients who had urinary incontinence. Seven of the 9 had acontractile bladders.[24] There was no mention of EMG studies to determine if detrusor urethral dyssynergia was present. True detrusor urethral dyssynergia in general is absent in the majority of poststroke patients.[31,49]

Urologic, Gynecologic, and Other Factors

Urologic conditions such as urethral strictures in men or women may cause incomplete bladder emptying. These conditions may predate the stroke or occur secondary to an indwelling catheter used during the management of the acute stroke. Benign or malignant prostatic obstruction in older men can predate the stroke and may contribute to urinary retention. Immobility or fecal impaction may precipitate urinary retention in the acute phase following a stroke. Pelvic floor weakness in women may predate the stroke and will be an additional etiologic factor to consider when assessing their incontinence.

In a study of 423 patients, Ween et al. found that those patients with small-vessel strokes had a lower frequency of urinary incontinence compared with patients with more extensive large-vessel stroke or hemorrhages. Urinary incontinence after stroke was closely associated with bowel incontinence, dysphagia, and overall functional level. This suggests that urinary incontinence results from multifocal impairments related to the severity of deficit rather than to the damage to specific cortical mechanisms alone. These findings were consistent with those reported earlier by Wade and Hewer.[61]

Bird and colleagues found that elderly patients with stroke were no more likely to be incontinent than age-matched patients with hip fracture. They deduced that the central nervous system was not causal to the development of urinary incontinence.[9]

Poststroke incontinence will invariably occur during periods of reduced consciousness. Aphasia contributes to incontinence because of the person's inability to convey awareness of bladder fullness and the need to void. Physical restraints for "protection" from poststroke delirium compromises continence by reducing independence for toileting, particularly if the person is aware of his or her need to void. Poststroke depression and amotivation are very real phenomena. Incontinence may contribute to the person's depressed affect or may be a consequence of the feeling of hopelessness. Indwelling urethral catheters are often inserted within the first 24 hours poststroke to monitor the fluid output and to manage incontinence while regular transferring to a commode or bedpan is unrealistic. Urinary retention with overflow urinary incontinence may occur if the catheter is removed before the person is ready functionally or psychologically for a toileting program. Incomplete bladder emptying, defined as postvoid residual (PVR) urine greater than 100 ml, has been demonstrated in 29% of patients admitted to hospital with acute stroke.[9] The mean PVR was 370 ml with a range of 125–750 ml. Reversible factors contributing to pre-stroke incontinence can improve or be eliminated in the acute hospital setting. These include poorly controlled diabetes with osmotic diuresis, alcohol-induced antidiuretic hormone inhibition, or the weak diuretic effect of caffeine excess.

INCONTINENCE ASSESSMENT

Corroborated History

The history of the incontinence and related urinary symptoms is the key part of the assessment that is often overlooked.[27] Corroboration by a relative will determine if factors predating the stroke are important. The history of present symptoms from patient or primary nurse history should categorize the incontinence into the following types: urge, stress, incomplete emptying, mixed stress/urge, functional, and iatrogenic. Prestroke urinary urgency and urge incontinence in men or women may reflect a previous stroke or other neurologic lesion with subsequent detrusor hyperreflexia. The same symptoms could also suggest idiopathic detrusor instability in an older individual or, alternatively, sensory urgency with a stable detrusor. In women, loss of urine with stress maneuvers, such as coughing, laughing, sneezing, walking, jumping, usually without urgency predating the stroke suggests genuine stress incontinence due to internal sphincter incompetence. In men, these symptoms are rare unless they have had prostatic surgery with internal sphincter damage. In women or men, prestroke symptoms of hesitancy, reduced stream, straining, or postmicturition dribbling suggest possible outlet obstruction due to urethral stricture or prostatic obstruction in men.

Nurse or patient observations of frequent, often small voids or loss of urine when moving in the bed could indicate urinary retention. The fact that a person is voiding some urine does not rule out urinary retention. Urinary retention with a history of indwelling catheter poststroke may raise the possibility of a catheter-induced urethral stricture.

In previously continent patients, who now have no warning of urinary loss while awake or asleep, poststroke detrusor hyperreflexia is the likely cause. The symptom of urge incontinence poststroke is an accurate predictor of detrusor hyperreflexia.[42]

Examination

The neurologic signs of the stroke will be evident. Ability to transfer on and off a bedpan with assistance every 2 hours is a critical level of mobility. It is one indication of when an indwelling catheter should be removed. Assessment of affect and the patient's expectations for recovery of motor function and continence is important. Poststroke depression causing amotivation may not be evident until some weeks or months after the stroke. This is well reviewed by Koenig and others.[41] Antidepressant drugs can affect bladder and urethral function and can be used for added advantage when treating depression if the patient is also incontinent.

The Mini-Mental State Examination (MMSE) is commonly used to assess memory and cognitive function.[30] The interpretation of the score on the MMSE is limited in patients with aphasia because it is a very verbal test. Physical findings of urogenital prolapse in women may be relevant if prestroke stress incontinence was present and will influence the final choice of treatment. Perianal sensation is usually intact unless there is a history of long-standing diabetes with sacral neuropathy. If sensation is absent, impaired sacral parasympathetic innervation of the detrusor muscle may cause incomplete bladder emptying due to a poorly contractile or noncontractile detrusor (diabetic cystopathy). Rectal examination will rule out fecal impaction and prostatic enlargement.

Bladder Residual Urine

A true PVR urine test is critical to determine if bladder emptying is complete. The patient must void under optimal circumstances in a private location and in an appropriate position. Although in-out catheterization is the gold standard for determining the PVR urine, portable bladder ultrasound is practical, noninvasive, and cost effective.[22] A sterile culture result from the catheter specimen would rule out urinary tract infection. Two consecutive residual urines of greater than 150 ml suggest a significant degree of incomplete bladder emptying, and physical outlet obstruction should be ruled out by urology assessment with cystoscopy. There is no consensus as to what residual urine volume is definitely abnormal.[34] Most would

TABLE 1. Types of Incontinence (Based on History, Examination, and Postvoid Residual Urine)[8]

History	Findings (May Be Present)	Residual	Pathophysiology (Confirmed by Urodynamics)
Urgency	Signs consistent with specific neurologic disease	Low	Detrusor instability
Stress	Demonstrated during stress	Low	(Genuine) stress incontinence
Overflow/incomplete emptying	Palpable bladder Enlarged prostate Urethral stricture Reduced anal sphincter tone Reduced sacral sensation	High	Outlet obstruction and/or poorly contractile detrusor
Mixed	Variable	Variable	Mixed
Functional	Impaired mobility Impaired mental state Environmental factors	Low	Functional
Iatrogenic	Drugs Restraints	Variable	Iatrogenic (depending on medication)

regard greater than 150 ml abnormal, but it depends to some degree on the volume of urine voided before catheterization.

The core evaluation findings from the history, physical examination, and PVR urine test (Table 1) will establish a working diagnosis for subsequent management. A trial of intervention is appropriate without further detailed investigations in those patients with uncomplicated findings and with low residual urine. This approach is consistent with the recently updated clinical practice guidelines for the management of urinary incontinence.[27]

MANAGEMENT

The assessment and management to this point can be accomplished by trained nurses or physicians who are aware of the need for a thorough assessment of incontinence. A team approach is an effective and rewarding way to deal with incontinence.[58] Philosophically, an approach that emphasizes behavioral interventions that are reversible and without side effects, as a first step, is in the patient's best interests. Drug therapy is reversible but often has side effects, and surgical intervention is irreversible.[12,27] If the patient's goal is realistic for regaining continence, it should be communicated and understood by family, nurses, and physicians so that there is a common purpose toward a successful outcome. Differing expectations will undermine the team effort. There is no evidence from patients and caregivers that incontinence often is not well managed.[33]

Fluid Intake

The total measurable fluid intake should be approximately 1500–1800 ml per 24 hours. Food contains fluid, and the total fluid intake will be higher. There is a common misconception by patients, nurses, and physicians, that the patient should drink 6–8 glasses (1500–2000 ml) of water in addition to everything else they drink. The justification for this is a need to "flush the kidneys," reducing the likelihood of the urinary infection. Some medications such as sulpha-containing antibiotics do require a higher fluid intake to prevent renal sulpha crystal deposition. Usually these medications are time-limited. Patients who receive intravenous fluids or who are on a feeding tube because of dysphagia may have fluid loads greater than 2 L per 24 hours. These volumes will compromise successful bladder management. For those who are able to transfer with assistance, an indwelling periurethral catheter is a reasonable measure until the fluid intake can be reduced to a reasonable level and the ability to transfer has improved. This strategy may preserve morale rather than overwhelm the patient with too broad a rehabilitation focus. The alternative to periurethral or suprapubic catheterization is intermittent catheterization. For men who have an unstable bladder and no urinary retention, an external condom catheter will at least keep them dry until a toileting program can be initiated.

Bladder Charts

Once a patient can transfer without assistance and is catheter-free, and urinary infection is ruled out, a baseline bladder chart should be initiated. A bladder chart should record incontinent (wet) events, voiding frequency, fluid intake, and, if possible, voided urinary volumes for 72 hours.[27] Three days of complete information by the primary bedside nurse, patient, or caregiver at home is of more value than many incomplete days. Compliance with subsequent recording requests is more likely to occur. From the baseline bladder chart, mean wet events and voids per 24 hours can be established for later comparison to determine improvement. The particular pattern of incontinence such as night- or daytime incontinence may be evident.

Approaches to Voiding

Scheduled voiding follows a set schedule of voiding every 2–4 hrs, regardless of sensation of bladder fullness. Such a program needs reinforcement. Normally, people are conditioned to void when their bladder is full, i.e., when they "need to go." Following a stroke the cortical awareness of bladder fullness is often reduced. Nurses will ask patients every 2 hours, "do you need to void?" Patients may indicate "no" because they have no sense of bladder fullness or urgency. Initiation of toileting in response to urgency may not allow sufficient time to void successfully. This is particularly true if poststroke mobility is limited. At the first awareness of urgency, the detrusor muscle is often already contracting. In a nonrandomized, small sample study of 19 poststroke patients treated with scheduled voiding versus drug treatment, 6 of the 13 patients on scheduled voiding were continent on discharge compared with 1 of 6 on drug treatment.[31]

Voiding preventively before the bladder volume reaches the threshold at which an unstable contraction occurs promotes continence. *Habit training* is toileting scheduled to match the patient's voiding habits. This is surprisingly difficult for patients to follow consistently. It is also a challenge for nursing schedules, as demonstrated in one controlled study in nursing home residents.[25] Repeat bladder charts will guide habit training with more frequent voids at times of consistent wet events. *Bladder training*, on the other hand, allows for lengthening the voiding interval as the patient becomes consistently dry.[19] For cognitively impaired patients, "prompted," regular voiding every 2 hours is necessary with more direct cuing such as "now is the time to go to the toilet," with the appropriate level of supervision or physical assistance provided. This technique has been evaluated in nursing home residents.[57]

A retrospective study examined characteristics of 75 patients with poststroke urinary incontinence in a bladder management program.[54] Those who did not achieve continence had difficulty with orientation to time, memory, and problem solving.[54]

Pelvic Floor Exercises

Pelvic floor exercises attributed to Kegel are useful, not only for stress incontinence for which they were originally intended, but also to suppress urgency.[40,55]

Successful implementation depends on the patient's compliance. Teaching how to identify and contract the pelvic floor muscles takes time.[18,29] Asking patients to contract the anal sphincter as though they were trying to prevent the passage of gas or a bowel movement is one technique. Secondly, stopping or slowing the stream of urine by contracting the external urethral sphincter, which is part of the pelvic floor muscles, may be successful. Some patients are not able to successfully slow the stream of urine, let alone stop it. Sometimes patients misunderstand the instructions and try to stop the urine stream every time they void. This is counterproductive, because it may promote incomplete bladder emptying. A third technique for women to identify the pelvic floor muscles is for them to insert a finger into the vagina and feel the circumvaginal muscle contraction during voluntary pelvic floor contractions.

Initially, pelvic floor contractions can be sustained up to 5 seconds. Pelvic floor relaxation after contraction, for a count of 3 seconds, is equally as important. Sets of 5 contractions, five times per day, is a reasonable starting point. A goal of 100 contractions per day (10 sets of 10 exercises) is not always obtainable. It is not clear what is the optimal number of contractions per day. Incorporating pelvic floor exercises after voiding as part of their toileting routine is a strategy that helps patients to remember to do the exercises.

Urge Suppression

Cognitively intact patients who can do effective pelvic floor contractions can use them to suppress a sense of urgency. A series of rapid pelvic floor contractions can be effective to suppress the "urgency wave" of the reflex bladder contraction.[18] Sitting down and resisting the temptation to rush to the toilet in response to the urgency is important because the sudden movement may reinforce the reflex bladder contraction. Once the sensation of urgency has temporarily subsided, toileting can occur and is more likely to be successful without urge incontinence. Pelvic floor exercises for patients with poststroke urinary incontinence have not been rigorously evaluated.

Biofeedback

In subjects with persisting incontinence who have not responded to the above conservative measures, biofeedback offers a further effective but time intensive intervention. Audio and visual biofeedback have been used effectively for a number of years for urinary incontinence.[19,20,47] Patients have to be cognitively intact to retain learning between training sessions and to keep accurate records.

Middaugh reported on 4 patients with poststroke incontinence of 8 months' to 10 years' duration.[47] Visual biofeedback was used during sequential filling of the bladder by a catheter with 20-ml increments of sterile water. The subjects were aware of bladder sensations and monitored the visual display of bladder pressure. With a pressure rise indicating detrusor contraction, they contracted their external anal sphincter and urinary sphincter (pelvic floor contraction) and observed the effect of reflex inhibition of the detrusor contraction. At the same time, they were relaxed and avoided general musculoskeletal tensing or breath holding. During biofeedback sessions, all of the subjects demonstrated unstable detrusor contractions at low bladder filling volumes. They also had impaired bladder sensation of fullness with little time between the first sensation of urgency and detrusor contraction. In addition, they had poor urge control, being unable to stop the stream of urine. A particularly interesting observation in 1 patient was that increased spasticity caused by standing resulted in an uninhibited detrusor contraction at a volume of 300 ml.

When the patient was lying relaxed, uninhibited contractions were not evident up to 600 ml. This observation confirmed that spasticity contributes to detrusor instability. The 4 subjects regained continence after biofeedback sessions every 2–4 weeks over a 3-month period, and they remained continent at 12 months.

Biofeedback did not alter the physiologic parameters of the bladder, such as first sensation of fullness, or maximal cystometric bladder capacity. Biofeedback did heighten the awareness of bladder sensation and helped identify early bladder sensations as a cue to void. It also facilitated use of external sphincter contractions to inhibit voiding reflexes.

Urinary Retention

Urinary retention with overflow incontinence may occur following a stroke, usually in the acute phase.[9] Immobility, fecal impaction, anticholinergic action of medications, and outlet obstruction may all contribute. These can be addressed through the combined team rehabilitation efforts by improving mobility, an appropriate bowel routine, reviewing medications, and ruling out bladder outlet obstruction. Teaching the Credé maneuver combined with pelvic floor relaxation may improve bladder emptying for persisting incontinence due to urinary retention.

Intermittent catheterization, by the patient, a relative, or a health professional, can be taught using a sterile technique in a hospital or, alternatively, using a clean (nonsterile) routine for the home environment. Excellent videocassette-recorded teaching aids are available for instruction of patients or caregivers.[37] The frequency of catheterization should be monitored and adjusted. The voided volume and residual for a total bladder volume of 500 ml should not be exceeded. The frequency of catheterization can be reduced as the residual urine decreases. A portable ultrasound bladder scanner has been evaluated on a stroke rehabilitation unit.[22] Monitoring of the PVRs reduced the need for intermittent catheterization. The correlation of ultrasound measurements with actual catheterized volumes was highly significant (r = 0.983). The implementation of a bladder ultrasound program in a rehabilitation facility is quite feasible.[43]

Stress Incontinence

Prestroke stress incontinence due to sphincter incompetence may be worsened by stroke. Kegel pelvic floor exercises, as described earlier, are the first-line approach. Strengthening the pelvic floor and external urethral sphincter function by conscientious repeated sets of pelvic floor exercises each day often resolves or reduces stress incontinence. If resolution using pelvic floor exercises and the above conservative measures is unsuccessful, further investigation is warranted. This could include combined videofluoroscopy and urodynamic studies and consultation with a urogynecologist or urologist to determine if a vaginal pessary, periurethral collagen, or surgery is appropriate.[23]

Cystometry

Incontinence that persists despite improved mobility and a trial of behavioral interventions requires further investigation. Cystometry using periurethral pressure transducers measures the intravesical pressure as the bladder is filled with carbon dioxide or water. The rate of filling with water may be slow, medium, or rapid, i.e., 10 ml, 50 ml, or more than 100 ml per minute, respectively.[1] Dual channel water cystometry with simultaneous bladder and rectal transducer pressure recordings during filling allows subtraction of intra-abdominal pressure. This yields true intravesical pressure in response to bladder filling and allows detection of lower amplitude, unstable bladder contractions. The detrusor response during cystometry in normal healthy individuals is well described.[3] Water cystometry has the added advantage of demonstrating water leakage during filling caused by sphincter incompetence in the absence of detrusor contractions; this can confirm the diagnosis of genuine stress incontinence. As filling progresses, detrusor instability may also be detected, confirming combined detrusor instability and genuine stress incontinence. The traditional International Continence Society definition of *detrusor instability* is a contraction of greater than 15 cm of water, although it is recognized that unstable detrusor contractions may generate lower pressures.[1] Cystometry using ice water as a provocative test in poststroke patients found that 62.5% had a positive test.[38]

The volume at which an unstable detrusor contraction occurs will reflect the severity of the detrusor instability. The magnitude of the detrusor pressure rise measured in centimeters of water clarifies contractility of the detrusor muscle. Sensory urgency with a stable detrusor can be confirmed. The first sensation of fullness and urgency is reported by the patient. However, filling proceeds to maximal cystometric bladder capacity (often 500 ml) without detrusor contraction despite provocative maneuvers such as standing or coughing. Confirmation of sensory urgency supports continued behavioral interventions rather than adding medications, particularly in the elderly.

A combined cystometrogram and EMG (skin or needle electrode) can provide additional information about the external urethral sphincter. This investigation could be helpful in a patient in whom detrusor–external urethral sphincter dyssynergia is suspected. Burney et al. caution that pseudodyssynergia (voluntary contraction of the external sphincter) during involuntary detrusor contraction can occur during the urodynamic study.[21] The person performing the urodynamic study should report to the interpreter any observations of the patient's responses during the study.

Pharmacologic Therapy

PRESCRIBING PRINCIPLES

In most instances, drugs should be considered as an adjunct therapy implemented only after an adequate trial of behavioral interventions. Before commencing medications, bladder charts will establish a new baseline of incontinent events or voiding frequency reflecting the effect of behavioral interventions. This new reference point determines if further improvement occurs in response to the addition of medication. Stating the expected outcomes from medication aids in future decisions about increasing, decreasing, or stopping medications. The main drawback of drugs is their side effect profile, which is often underestimated particularly in the elderly. Following stroke, the potential for adverse medication effects is increased, particularly in those who are on multiple medications or who have cognitive impairment. The potential for side effects is a strong justification for cystometric confirmation of detrusor hyperreflexia before commencing medication. The common medications used for poststroke detrusor hyperreflexia have varying degrees of anticholinergic action and include flavoxate, oxybutynin, propantheline, and imipramine. Tolterodine is a new anticholinergic agent.[2]

There is no advantage to beginning with the maximum dose, regardless of age. Because of likely side effects, the patient may lose confidence that medication will help. For outpatients, a gradual titration can occur over 4–6 weeks. The goal is to arrive at the lowest dose with the optimal effect and fewest side effects. Once an optimal drug effect occurs, there is no need to continue increasing the dose. Likewise, if an increased dose results in intolerable side effects, the drug should be reduced to the level at which the desired action occurred without intolerable side effect. If at that point the desired effect is not present, the medication should be stopped. In inpatients with close monitoring, titration can occur more quickly. After 6 months at an optimal dose, step-wise reduction is worth trying. Continued recovery from the stroke and continued reinforcement of behavioral intervention may negate any benefit from the drug. If symptoms of detrusor hyperreflexia reappear at a lower dose, the indication for continuing the drug is confirmed. The anticholinergic effect, when optimal, decreases detrusor contractility and symptoms of urgency and frequency of voiding, and allows greater postponement of voiding. Common side effects include excessive dry mouth, confusion, postural hypotension, urinary retention, constipation, blurred vision, and nausea. Patients may also note a reduction in the strength of the urinary stream. For the medication to be effective, it is preferable that patients have some awareness of bladder sensations. For the cognitively impaired, the potential for increased confusion from the central anticholinergic action of medications far outweighs any perceived beneficial effect on incontinence, and anticholinergic medications are not recommended. There are a few double-blind trials of the use of anticholinergic drugs for detrusor instability due to various disorders but none in patients who exclusively have detrusor hyperreflexia following stroke.[53]

Drug Doses and Choices

Flavoxate, which has a direct smooth muscle relaxing action and little anticholinergic effect, may be worth trying first because of the lower potential for anticholinergic side effects. It can be started with 200 mg daily and increased by 200 mg per day each week to 200 mg four times a day at week 4. A higher maximum dose of 400 mg three times a day has been shown to be well tolerated.[48] Propantheline, a quaternary ammonium compound, has variable absorption among individuals. Propantheline is said not to cross the blood-brain barrier, and this is a theoretical advantage in those who have potential for confusion. Propantheline is significantly cheaper than oxybutynin or flavoxate. Propantheline can be titrated from 7.5 mg twice daily up to 30 mg three times a day as a maximum over 6 weeks using 15-mg increments each week. Oxybutynin can be titrated by 2.5 mg (half a tablet) each week, up to a maximum of 5 mg three times a day by week 6. Tolterodine is a new anticholinergic agent. It is said to have less influence on the salivary gland function and is, therefore, less likely to cause a dry mouth. Titration can begin using 1-mg tablets and increased up to 2 mg twice a day.

Imipramine is a more complex drug with anticholinergic alpha-agonist and antidepressant properties. Given this profile, imipramine might theoretically be useful for persisting poststroke incontinence in a patient with detrusor hyperreflexia, depression, and some genuine stress incontinence. It should be avoided in male patients with incipient urinary retention due to prostatic obstruction. Imipramine can be titrated over 6 weeks beginning at 10 mg per day and increasing by 10 mg per day each week up to 20 mg three times a day. Poststroke depression has been treated successfully with nortriptyline, although delirium did occur in some subjects.[45] If symptomatic detrusor hyperreflexia is present as well, amitriptyline may have an additional advantage because it has a strong anticholinergic effect compared with nortriptyline. Titration of amitriptyline by 10 mg per week would be a reasonable frequency of increase in the young and every other week up to a maximum dose of 70 mg in the elderly. Amitriptyline should be avoided if there is any cognitive impairment.

For patients with poorly contractile detrusor due to partial bladder denervation and atonic decompensated bladders, bethanechol may improve detrusor contractility. Most experience is anecdotal, and the effectiveness of bethanechol is controversial.[59] Bethanechol, 10 mg three times a day and increasing by 10 mg three times a day each week up to 50 mg three times a day maximum, would be a reasonable trial. This would usually be used as an adjunct to intermittent catheterization. Failure of the residual urine to decrease, excessive sweating, asthmatic attacks, congestive heart failure, and abdominal cramps are all reasons to discontinue bethanechol.

Containment

Resolution of incontinence will not be a realistic goal for every poststroke patient. Impaired mobility, cognitive impairment, unawareness of bladder sensation, and severe detrusor instability are likely the most important factors contributing to persistent incontinence. Many aids to voiding are available and include a variety of male and female urinals, slipper pans, commodes, and adaptions to the toilet itself, such as raised toilet seats and bars. The range of personal incontinence products for containment is extensive. Pads range in size, absorbency, construction, cost, and availability and are disposable or reusable. Pads that contain small volumes of urine are more commonly disposable, but small reusable pads are increasingly becoming available, usually at medical supply stores. Larger reusable bed pads or diapers for daytime or nighttime incontinent episodes are available in reusable or disposable formats. Some reusable bed sheets with very high absorbency draw urine away from the skin and allow undisturbed sleep. Reusable products are more environmentally friendly despite laundering and are more cost effective over the long-term. Some waste management companies are offering hospitals contracts to recycle disposable diapers and pads. The cost effectiveness of these approaches has not been prospectively evaluated. Cost of incontinence within the community and institutions can be substantial, and maintaining mobility is potentially one way to reduce costs.[14]

Catheters

When transfers are difficult, male external condom catheters for day, night, or 24-hour use are worth trying depending on the patient's preference and whether he will leave the external catheter attached. Skin care must be meticulous for this to be successful. Female external catheters are being developed. Long-term indwelling catheters are only indicated with significant persisting retention where attempts for resolution of incontinence have failed and intermittent catheterization is impractical. The patient or caregiver needs to be involved in the decision and to be aware of the risks. Risks include chronic urinary bacteriuria, bladder spasms, leakage around the catheter, and bladder stones or catheter balloon calcification. Catheter care protocol should be followed with regular changes.[16] Latex catheters are cheaper, but if allergy to latex rubber is a problem, the more expensive inert silicon should be used.

OUTCOMES

In a 12-month follow-up study of 235 first-time stroke patients younger than 75 years of age and previous disability, urinary incontinence within 24 hours was the best single predictor of persisting disability.[60] It had a sensitivity of 60% and a specificity of 78%.[60] Five multivariate models designed to predict the outcome of stroke have been evaluated prospectively. They showed no advantage over state of urinary continence in predicting good or poor outcomes.[32] Incontinence as a predictor following stroke has been associated with a poor outcome.[39,61,62]

Urinary incontinence is associated with more severe deficits early in the recovery phase. It negatively influences functional improvement and disposition. Urinary incontinence on admission is associated with higher risk of death, poorer Functional Independence Measure (FIM) change score, FIM efficiency, and discharge to nursing home. Persisting urinary incontinence on discharge has been associated with a low admission FIM (< 60), severe hemiparesis, concomitant bowel incontinence, and dysphagia.[62] Age, gender, site of the lesion, and comorbidities were not associated with persisting urinary incontinence. Urinary tract infection was associated with urinary incontinence on admission but had no bearing on recovery of incontinence. Continence, either remaining dry or regaining continence, has been reported as a positive predictor for survival, recovery, and final discharge.[5,62] Barer reported that only 3% of patients who were continent at day 1 died in the first month.[5] Those who regained continence in the first month were most likely to be home within 6 months of the stroke. This relationship between continence and a good outcome was independent of age or gender. Barer suggested that a return of continence preceded other areas of functional improvement, and that it may be linked to other prognostic factors such as motivation and self-respect.

This raises the possibility that a more rapid return of continence may facilitate return of other functions, possibly through improved motivation and self-esteem. Strategies to help patients with poststroke cognitive impairment achieve continence warrants further evaluation.[54] These could be compared with a standard bladder management program with end-points relating to continence, function, motivation, self-esteem, quality of life, and impact of incontinence.[33,63]

CONCLUSION

Urinary incontinence following stroke is common and is a predictor of poor functional recovery. It is not a necessary consequence of stroke. In virtually all patients, incontinence can be resolved, improved, or better contained. An accurate history, physical examination, and residual urine will determine the prestroke and poststroke factors contributing to incontinence. Detrusor instability is the most common bladder abnormality after a stroke.

Once mobility is not a limiting factor, management of persisting incontinence should focus first on reversible behavioral interventions that do not have side effects. This includes fluid management, bladder charts, scheduled toileting, habit training, prompted voiding, pelvic floor exercises, urge suppression, and biofeedback. Anticholinergic medications for detrusor instability can be used as an adjunct to behavioral interventions. Titration of medication doses will determine the lowest possible dose with the maximum effect and fewest side effects. Persisting stress incontinence, not responding to behavioral interventions, can be evaluated further with urodynamic studies to determine if vaginal pessaries, periurethral collagen injections, or surgery is appropriate. Sterile or clean intermittent catheterization is the preferred management of urinary retention. Containment of incontinence can be very effective using an innovative range of incontinence products.

Resolving or improving incontinence will improve morale, facilitate rehabilitation, reduce time to discharge from hospital, and enhance quality of life.

REFERENCES

1. Abrams P, Blaivas JG, Stanton SL, Anderson JT: Standardization of the terminology of the lower urinary tract function. Urodyn 7: 403–427, 1988.
2. Appell RA: Clinical efficacy and safety of tolterodine in the treatment of overactive bladder: A pooled analysis. Urology 50:90–96, 1997.

3. Bagley NA, O'Shaughnessy EJ: Urodynamic evaluation of voluntary detrusor response in healthy subjects. Arch Phys Med Rehabil 66:160–163, 1985.

4. Bhatia NN, Bradley WE: Neuroanatomy and physiology: Innervation of the urinary tract. In Raz S (ed): Female Urology. Philadelphia, WB Saunders, 1983, pp 12–32.

5. Barer DH: Continence after stroke: Useful predictor or goal of therapy? Age Ageing 18:183–191, 1989.

6. Barer DH, Mitchell JRA: Predicting the outcome of acute stroke: Do multivariate models help? Q J Med 70:27–39, 1989.

7. Bates P, Bradley WE, Glen E, et al: The standardization of terminology of lower urinary tract function. J Urol 121:551–554, 1979.

8. Benbow S, Sangster G, Barer D: Incontinence after stroke. Lancet 338:1602–1603, 1991.

9. Bird MR, McCrory PR, Doinnan GA: Urinary incontinence in elderly patients with acute stroke and hip fracture. Med J Aust 167:415, 1997.

10. Blaivas JG: The neurophysiology of micturition: A clinical study of 550 patients. J Urol 127:958–963, 1982.

11. Bliss MR, McLaren E, Exton-Smith AN: Mattresses for preventing pressure sores in geriatric patients. Med Bull Min Health 25:238–268, 1966.

12. Borrie MJ, Bawden ME, Kartha AS, Kerr PS: A nurse/physician continence clinic triage approach for urinary incontinence: A 25-week randomized trial. Neurourol Urodyn 11:364–365, 1992.

13. Borrie MJ, Campbell AJ, Caradoc-Davies TH, Spears GFS: Urinary incontinence after stroke: A prospective study. Age Ageing 15:177–181, 1986.

14. Borrie MJ, Davidson HA: Incontinence in institutions: Costs and contributing factors. Can Med Assoc J 147:322–328, 1992.

15. Bradley WE, Rockswold GL, Timm GW, Scott FB: Neurology of micturition. J Urol 115:481–486, 1976.

16. Brechtelsbauer DA: Care with an indwelling urinary catheter. Postgrad Med 92:127–132, 1992.

17. Brocklehurst JC, Andrews K, Richards B, Laycock PJ: Incidence and correlates of incontinence in stroke patients. J Am Geriatr Soc 33:540–542, 1985.

18. Burgio KL, Pearce K, Lulco AJ: Staying Dry: A Practical Guide to Bladder Control. Baltimore, Johns Hopkins University Press, 1989.

19. Burgio KL, Burgio LD: Behavior therapies for urinary incontinence in the elderly. Clin Geriatr Med 2:809–827, 1986.

20. Burgio KL, Whitehead WE, Engel BT: Urinary incontinence in the elderly: Bladder-sphincter biofeedback and toileting skills training. Am Int Med 104:507–515, 1985.

21. Burney TL, Senapati M, Desai S, et al: Effects of cerebrovascular accident on micturition. Urol Clin North Am 23:483–490, 1996.

22. Chan H: Noninvasive bladder volume measurement. Am Assoc Neurol Nursing 25:309–312, 1993.

23. Chancellor MB, Blaivas JG: Diagnostic evaluation of incontinence in patients with neurological disorders. Compr Ther 17:37–43, 1991.

24. Chua K, Kong KH: Functional outcome in brain stem stroke patients after rehabilitation. Arch Phys Med Rehabil 77:194–197, 1996.

25. Colling J, Ouslander J, Hadley BJ, et al: The effects of patterned urge response toileting (PURT) on urinary incontinence among nursing home residents. J Am Geriatr Soc 40:135–141, 1992.

26. Ebrahim S, Nouri F: Caring for stroke patients at home. Int Rehabil Med 8:171–173, 1987.

27. Fantl JA, Newman D, Colling J, et al: Urinary Incontinence in Adults: Acute and Chronic Management Clinical Practice Guideline. Number 2, 1996 Update. Rockville, MD, U.S. Department of Health and Human Services, Public Health Service Agency for Health Care Policy and Research, 1996.

28. Feder M, Heller L, Tadmor R, et al: Urinary continence after stroke: Association with cystometric profile and computerised tomography findings. Eur Neurol 27:101–105, 1987.

29. Ferguson K, McKey PL, Bishop KR, et al: Stress urinary incontinence: Effect of pelvic muscle exercise. Obstet Gynecol 73:671–675, 1990.

30. Folstein MF, Folstein SE, McHugh PR: Mini-mental state: A practical method for grading the cognitive state of patients with the clinician. J Psych Res 12:189–198, 1975.

31. Gelber DA, Good DC, Laven LJ, Verhulst SJ: Causes of urinary incontinence after acute hemispheric stroke. Stroke 24:378–382, 1993.

32. Gladman JRF, Harwood DMJ, Barer DH: Predicting the outcome of acute stroke: Prospective evaluation of five multivariate models and comparison with simple methods. J Neurol Neurosurg Psychiatry 55:347–351, 1992.

33. Greveson G, James O: Improving long-term outcome after stroke—The views of patients and carers. Health Trends 23:161–162, 1991.

34. Grosshans CL, Passadori Y, Peter B: Urinary retention in the elderly: A study of 100 hospitalized patients. J Am Geriatr Soc 41:633–638, 1993.

35. Hald T, Bradley WE: The nervous control of the urinary bladder. In Hald T, Bradley WE (eds): The Urinary Bladder: Neurology and Urodynamics. Baltimore, Williams & Wilkins, 1982, pp 48–57.
36. Henriksen T: Incontinence after stroke. Lancet 338:1335, 1991.
37. Intermittent Catheterization for Men or Women [videocassette]. Santa Barbara, CA, Schorr Communications, 1992. Available at no charge to health care professionals from Mentor Medical Systems Canada, Ltd., 1-800-668-6069.
38. Ishigooka M, Hashimoto T, Hayami S, et al: Ice water test in patients with overactive bladder due to cerebrovascular accidents and bladder outlet obstruction. Urol Int 58:84–87, 1997.
39. Jongbloed L: Prediction of function after stroke: A critical review. Stroke 17:765–776, 1986.
40. Kegel AH: Progressive resistance exercises in the functional restoration of the perineal muscles. Am J Obstet Gynecol 56:238–248, 1948.
41. Koenig JG, Studenski S: Post-stroke depression in the elderly. J Gen Intern Med 3:508–517, 1988.
42. Kong KH, Chan KF, Lim AC, Tan ES: Detrusor hyperreflexia in strokes. Ann Acad Med 23:319–321, 1994.
43. Lewis NA: Implementing a bladder ultrasound program. Rehabil Nursing 20:215–217, 1995.
44. Linsenmeyer TA, Zorowitz RD: Urodynamic findings in patients with urinary incontinence after cerebrovascular accident. Neurol Rehabil 2:23–26, 1992.
45. Lipsey JR, Robinson RG, Pearlson GD, et al: Nortriptyline treatment of post-stroke depression: A double-blind study. Lancet 1:297–300, 1984.
46. Maru A: Cystometry and urethral pressure profilmetry after the cerebral stroke. Jpn J Urol 71:171–183, 1980.
47. Middaugh SJ, Whitehead WE, Burgio KL, Engel BT: Biofeedback in treatment of urinary incontinence in stroke patients. Biofeedback Self-Regul 14:3–19, 1989.
48. Milani R, Scalambrino S, Carrera S, et al: Comparison of flavoxate hydrochloride in daily dosages of 600 versus 1200 mg for the treatment of urgency and urge incontinence. J Int Med Res 16:244–248, 1988.
49. Motola JA, Badlani GH: Cerebrovascular accidents: Urological effects and management. Clin Geriatr Med 6:55–68, 1990.
50. Nakayama H, Jorgensen HS, Pedersen PM, et al: Prevalence and risk factors of incontinence after stroke. The Copenhagen Stroke Study. Stroke 28:58–62, 1997.
51. Nishizawa O, Ebina K, Sugaya K, et al: Effect of cerebellectomy on reflex micturition in the decerebrate dog as determined by urodynamic evaluation. Urol Int 44:152–156, 1989.
52. Opitz JL, Thorsteinsson G, Schutt AH, et al: Neurogenic bladder and bowel. In DeLisa JA (ed): Rehabilitation Medicine Principles and Practice. Philadelphia, JB Lippincott, 1988, p 492.
53. Ouslander JG, Sier HC: Drug therapy for geriatric urinary incontinence. Clin Geriatr Med 2:789–807, 1986.
54. Owen DC, Getz PA, Bulla S: A comparison of characteristics of patients with completed stroke: Those who achieve continence and those who do not. Rehabil Nurs 20:197–203, 1995.
55. Palmer MH: Pelvic muscle rehabilitation: Where do we go from here? J Wound Ostomy Continence Nurs 24:98–105, 1997.
56. Reding MJ, Winter SW, Hochrein SA, et al: Urinary incontinence after unilateral hemispheric stroke: A neurologic-epidemiologic perspective. J Neurol Rehabil 1:25–60, 1987.
57. Schnelle JF, Newman DR, White M, et al: Maintaining continence in nursing home residents through the application of industrial quality control. Gerontol 33:114–121, 1993.
58. Silbert PL, Stewart-Wynne EG: Incontinence after stroke. Lancet 339:1602, 1992.
59. Sondra LP, Gershon C, Diokno AC, Lapides J: Urological neurology and urodynamics: Further observations on the cystometric and uroflowmetric effects of bethanechol chloride on the human bladder. J Urol 122:775–777, 1979.
60. Taub NA, Wolfe CDA, Richardson E, Burney PGJ: Predicting the disability of first-time stroke sufferers at 1 year. 12-month follow-up of a population-based cohort in southeast England. Stroke 25:352–357, 1994.
61. Wade DT, Hewer RL: Functional abilities after stroke: Measurement, natural history and prognosis. J Neurol Neurosurg Psychiatry 50:177–182, 1987.
62. Ween JE, Alexander MP, D'Esposito M, Roberts M: Incontinence after stroke in a rehabilitation setting: Outcome associations and predictive factors. Neurology 47:659–663, 1996.
63. Wyman JF, Harkins SW, Choi SC, et al: Psychosocial impact of urinary incontinence in women. Obstet Gynecol 70:378–381, 1987.

K. J. MILLER, MSc, PT
S. J. GARLAND, PhD, PT
G. F. KOSHLAND, PhD, PT

TECHNIQUES AND EFFICACY OF PHYSIOTHERAPY POSTSTROKE

From the School of Physical
Therapy (KJM, SJG)
and Department of Physiology
(SJG)
University of Western Ontario
London, Ontario
Canada
and
Department of Physiology (GFK)
University of Arizona
Tucson, Arizona

Reprint requests to:
K. J. Miller, MSc
School of Physiotherapy
University of Melbourne
Parkville, Victoria 3052
Australia

Traditionally, rehabilitation following stroke has focused on the symptoms of abnormal synergistic movement and spasticity that typically follow a cerebrovascular accident (CVA). As a result, physiotherapeutic interventions have been based on neurophysiologic principles that relied predominantly on the use of physical interventions to facilitate normal movement patterns and improve function. These approaches, including proprioceptive neuromuscular facilitation,[89a] and approaches proposed by Bobath[6] and by Brunnstrom,[79a] are in widespread use in neurorehabilitation. Studies comparing the effectiveness of the approaches on patients in the subacute phase (2–8 weeks poststroke) or chronic phase (more than 3 months poststroke) have demonstrated that patients improved regardless of the type of intervention.[38] However, the studies were methodologically weak and had small sample sizes and little control for experimenter bias or cointerventions. Although scientific evidence to support a particular neurophysiologic approach as a whole is sparse, this chapter discusses the rationale and efficacy of specific facilitatory techniques.

More recently therapists have acknowledged that while spasticity and synergistic movements are important foci of treatment, they have been overemphasized at the expense of recognizing weakness as a prominent concern in stroke patients.[46,62] Several lines of evidence have prompted renewed interest in strengthening techniques for stroke patients. First, spastic muscles

PHYSICAL MEDICINE AND REHABILITATION: State of the Art Reviews—
Vol. 12, No. 3, October 1998. Philadelphia, Hanley & Belfus, Inc.

473

can be weak, because muscles with hyperactive stretch reflexes demonstrate atrophy.[39] Second, while dorsal rhizotomies performed in neurologically impaired children (cerebral palsy) have reduced spasticity, the children often did not improve functionally because of weakness.[2,22] These observations suggested that simply relieving spasticity would not ensure normal movement. In addition, the muscle force produced by patients could not be correlated with the degree of spasticity.[70,81] Finally, evidence that resistive exercise increased spasticity is lacking, and, in fact, a few studies have demonstrated that strengthening regimens have little detrimental effect.[47] This issue is addressed first in this chapter.

Another recent trend in physical therapy concerns the increased emphasis on motor learning principles. Studies have shown that specific exercises and the environment in which they are performed, combined with how tasks are learned, make a difference to motor performance and functional recovery. Moreover, modern imaging in normal subjects has revealed cortical adaptations following specific exercises or learning of motor tasks.[29,56,91] This has suggested that exercise and learning may be able to encourage and sculpt neural changes for recovery of stroke. With this trend in mind, this chapter discusses the approach of the forced-use paradigm.

STRENGTHENING

Weakness as a Symptom of Stroke

Weakness has been defined as inadequate capacity to generate normal levels of muscle force.[5] Unilateral weakness following stroke has been described extensively.[8,17,19,20,32,63,81] Deficits have ranged from 38–70% in the strength of affected knee, elbow extensor, flexor muscle groups, and in muscles about the shoulder and the trunk compared to the nonparetic side.[8,17,19,63,70,81] In addition, the muscles on the nonparetic, or unaffected, side of the body have been shown to have significantly reduced peak torques compared to those of age-matched healthy subjects.[17,90]

Reductions in muscle force associated with CVAs have been attributed to a variety of modifications and adaptations of the motor system. The immediate weakness and flaccidity may be attributed to a loss of central drive or descending command resulting from a widespread decrease in blood flow and neurotransmitter levels, as well as edema in cortical areas subserving motor function.[75] Although some volitional movement is usually recovered, the residual weakness is attributed to continued diminished central drive and transsynaptic changes of targets of corticospinal neurons.[33,36,80]

Long-term changes, such as disuse atrophy, arise from decreased or absent activation of spinal motoneurons, particularly type II motor units.[23] Investigators have suggested that the type II motor units undergo transsynaptic degeneration or remain functionally inactive as a result of the reduced activation.[33] Some of the remaining type II motor units may transform into hybrid fatiguable units that have slower twitch contraction times.[93] Further, hemiplegic weakness has been associated with reduced firing rates[77,84] and altered recruitment of motor units.[44] Selective atrophy of type II muscle fibers accompanied by a predominance and hypertrophy of type I muscle fibers following CVA is described widely.[33,36,50,80] Thus, hemiplegic weakness has been associated strongly with loss or inactivation of the larger force-generating type II motor units. Correlational evidence suggests that less type II fiber atrophy may be present in individuals who display a high level of functional recovery or are more active following stroke.[50,80] Given that the release of many trophic factors often depends on activity of neurons, these studies indirectly support the premise that eliciting activity immediately after stroke might prevent or diminish motoneuron degeneration and later disuse atrophy.

Assessment of Strength Following Stroke

The assessment of strength in persons with central nervous system lesions is controversial in rehabilitation.[9,10,78] However, reliability is not the contentious element of strength assessment following stroke. High intrarater reliability has been reported when strength of the hemiplegic side has been evaluated using handheld dynamometers; with intraclass correlation coefficients (ICCs) ranging from 0.88–0.99.[8,76] Interrater reliability of handheld dynamometry muscle strength assessments of persons with neurologic impairments have yielded Pearson Product Moment correlations of 0.84–0.94 for six muscle groups.[16,76] Finally, ICCs of 0.94 to 0.99 have been documented with repeated measures of hemiparetic peak knee extension torque using isokinetic dynamometers.[15,20]

While investigators and therapists do not dispute the reliability of strength measurements in patients following CVA, many question the validity and clinical inferences that can be made from these measures. The high reliability of strength measures has been attributed to the limited and stereotypic movements exhibited by patients who have poor recovery of motor control following stroke.[76,78] Bohannon and Smith have described how therapists stabilized patients to try to limit the influence of synergies on required movements for strength assessment.[19] Other studies are restricted to patients with adequate recovery of isolated motor control.[20,21,37] For instance, Gowland et al. do not recommend resisted strengthening exercises for an extremity until it has reached stage 4 of motor recovery on the Chedoke-McMaster Stroke Assessment Impairment Inventory.[49] By stage 4, spasticity would be decreasing and the patient would be capable of selected isolated movements out of synergy.

Probably the most controversial aspect of strengthing is the relationship of strength to spasticity and the much-disputed problem of "subtraction paresis," namely, reduced agonist muscle force output due to opposing force created by spastic antagonist muscles.[59] Some investigators report that subtraction paresis plays a significant role in strength assessment,[6,59] but others say that this phenomena is insignificant, particularly when strength is assessed isometrically.[9,18] Evidence suggests that static strength deficits are significantly correlated with spasticity of the agonist muscle rather than antagonist muscle.[13] Inadequate activation of the agonist muscle rather than increased antagonist activity has been associated with the inability to produce adequate force[32] or to perform movement tasks[48] in the upper extremity.

On further investigation of the influence of spasticity on voluntary movements, investigators found that while strong reflex responses to stretch were observed in the passive arm muscle, there was little difference in the responses to stretch between paretic and nonparetic limbs under active conditions.[53] Furthermore, the influence of "spastic" antagonist muscle activity on torque development was weak, and this finding has been confirmed in ambulant stroke patients.[1] Stretch reflexes of the ankle plantarflexor muscles were evoked either at rest or under conditions that simulated ambulation. Although two thirds of the stroke patients had evidence of elevated resting tonic stretch reflexes, the stretch reflexes elicited in the active condition were not different than in the normal control subjects. The authors concluded that "it seems inappropriate to routinely reduce or inhibit the reflex response to improve functional movement in stroke rehabilitation."[1] Clearly, assessments of muscle tone performed with a passive muscle may be inaccurate indicators of the influence of that muscle tone on movement.

Patients with hemiparesis can still modulate force within their available submaximal range of force production. When isometric forces were graded from 5–40% of maximal voluntary contractions, patients were able to increase electromyographic (EMG) activity in conjunction with increased force.[44,84] In general, a linear relationship between force and EMG was maintained regardless of severity of impairment based on scores from the Fugl-Meyer or Ashworth assessments. Moreover, this linear relationship has been observed in patients tested as early as 1 week following CVA and as late as 23 years after CVA. These findings imply that patients may be able to increase the central drive to the neuromuscular apparatus for submaximal contractions despite an inability to activate maximally the muscles of the paretic limb. Furthermore, patients were able to maintain the linear relationship of EMG-to-force regardless of the level of weakness. The slope of the linear relationship varied between patients, suggesting that the type of strength deficit may differ between categories of stroke patients.

To date, it is evident that measures of strength should not be used in isolation to determine status, change, capacity, or outcome for individuals following stroke. While reliability of strength measures has been well established in patients with stroke, the validity and clinical utility of such measures need further research. The present authors suggest that measuring strength at submaximal levels, as well as at maximal levels used in manual muscle tests, may give insight to differences between patients and their outcomes.

Relationships Between Strength and Functional Activities Following Stroke

Numerous correlational studies have been carried out to describe the interrelationships between strength and the functional capabilities of individuals following stroke (Table 1). Positive, statistically significant correlations between the strength of specific muscle groups and a variety of functional attributes have been reported.[7,11–15,20,21,63,83] Results should be viewed carefully given the uncertainties associated with the validity of strength assessment in these patients. Furthermore, correlation studies do not infer causation. Calculation of the coefficient of determination (r^2) can be useful in revealing what proportion of the variance in functional activities can be accounted for by strength variables.

Efficacy of Strengthening Following Stroke

A few studies have investigated the effectiveness of muscle strengthening interventions in improving the force-generating capabilities of hemiplegic limbs following stroke, and all of them have sought to connect any improvements in strength with enhancement of functional abilities. Strengthening paradigms have incorporated both isokinetic and isotonic protocols. Most of these studies have been nonrandomized and self-controlled.

ISOKINETIC TRAINING REGIMENS

Recent studies have investigated the efficacy of isokinetic lower extremity muscle training programs in improving maximal voluntary strength and functional mobility.[37,81] Subjects had experienced their CVA at least 9 months prior to commencing the strengthening programs. While the extent of motor recovery was not reported per se by Sharp and Brouwer,[81] all subjects were identified as community-dwelling stroke survivors who were able to ambulate independently with (9/15) or without (6/15) the assistance of a gait aid. Motor recovery was examined by Engardt

TABLE 1. Relationships between Muscle Strength and Functional
Activities Following Stroke

Functional Activity	Muscle Strength Measure(s) (Paretic Side)	Correlation/Relationship
Upper Extremity Function		
Measured by the Motricity Index, Frenchay Arm Test, Motor Club Assessment, 9 Hole Pegtest	Hand grip strength	r = 0.79–0.90[83]
Hand to mouth movement, graded on a 3-point ordinal scale	Isometric elbow flexor force*	r_s = 0.85[21]
Sitting Balance		
Rated on a 4-point ordinal scale	Isometric trunk forward flexor* and side flexor* force	r_s = 0.46–0.54 (final)[7]
Chair to Mat Transfer		
Rated on a 3-point ordinal scale	Isometric hip flexor,* extensor* and abductor,* knee flexor and extensor, ankle plantarflexor and dorsiflexor force	r_s = 0.30–0.64 (final)[12]
Static Standing Balance		
Rated on a 4-point ordinal scale	Isometric hip flexor,* extensor* and abductor,* knee flexor* and extensor,* ankle plantarflexor* and dorsiflexor* force	r_s = 0.47–0.84 (final)[11] Bohannon, 1989)
Gait Speed		
Comfortable pace	Isometric hip flexor, extensor* and abductor, knee flexor* and extensor, ankle plantarflexor* and dorsiflexor* force	r = 0.25–0.65[14]
	Peak concentric isokinetic knee extensor torque+	r = 0.21–0.72[15,20,63]
	Peak concentric isokinetic knee flexor torque+	r = 0.43–0.72[63]
Maximal pace	Peak concentric isokinetic knee extensor torque+	r = 0.31–0.76[20,63]
	Peak concentric isokinetic knee flexor torque*	r = 0.55–0.70[63]
Cadence		
Comfortable pace	Isometric hip flexor, extensor* and abductor,* knee flexor* and extensor,* ankle plantarflexor* and dorsiflexor* force	r = 0.25–0.65[14]

r = Pearson Product Moment Correlation Coefficients
r_s = Spearman Rho Correlation Coefficients
+ p ≤ .05 only at 1 isokinetic angular velocity or in 1 gender
* p ≤ 0.05
(final) - correlation between final assessment findings

and colleagues.[37] The subjects were able to ambulate independently with (12/20) or without (8/20) assistive devices, and they scored 3–6/6 on the gait subsection of the Motor Assessment Scale (MAS). Their mean physical performance on the Fugl-Meyer scale was 79.5/100 (range 68–97). Most of the subjects had relatively low tone in the lower extremity tone as rated on the Ashworth scale for evaluation of spasticity.

Both groups of investigators studied concentric regimens.[37,81] Improvements in the peak concentric isokinetic torque of the paretic muscles at each of the training velocities were reported following the two training protocols. Functionally, both studies reported improvements in gait velocity ($p < .05$) and Engardt's group observed a larger swing-to-stance ratio with the paretic leg ($p < 0.05$) during gait.[37] Subjects in Sharp and Brouwer's study reported a 25% ($p < .05$) improvement in their physical abilities immediately following the study, as measured by the Human Activity Profile.[40,81] No statistically significant changes were reported in the Timed Up and Go test or a timed stair climb following strength training.[81] The body weight distribution of the subjects did not change transitions between sitting and standing.[37]

On follow-up 4 weeks following the concentric isokinetic training study, Sharp and Brouwer found that while improved peak muscle torques were still evident in the affected lower extremity, most were no longer statistically significant compared to baseline values.[81] Only quadriceps torque continued to improve following cessation of the strengthening program. Despite the apparent detraining effect on muscle strength, functional measures of gait velocity and overall physical activity continued to improve 4 weeks after the strength training program was completed. No changes were seen in the timed Up and Go test or in stair-climbing ability.

The use of eccentric muscle strengthening protocols with stroke survivors has been studied by only one group of investigators. Engardt and colleagues concurrently studied and compared the efficacy of maximal eccentric and concentric isokinetic knee extension training regimens.[37] They reported significant improvements in the peak eccentric isokinetic torque of paretic knee extensor muscles ($p < 0.01$) at each of the training velocities. In contrast to the group performing concentric training, no improvements were seen in gait velocity or in the swing-to-stance ratio of the paretic limb following 6 weeks of eccentric training. However, a significant improvement in body weight distribution as measured by force platforms was cited during transitions between sitting and standing ($p < 0.05$).

Sharp and Brouwer found no change in lower extremity spasticity following the reciprocal flexion/extension concentric protocol when the paretic lower extremity was evaluated using a pendulum test.[3,81] However, Engardt and colleagues reported that, at concentric isokinetic angular velocities of 120° and 180°/sec, antagonist EMG activity was significantly greater ($p < 0.05$) in the concentrically trained individuals than in those who underwent the eccentric training protocol.[37] No differences were observed between the training groups when isokinetic knee extension movements were tested at various angular velocities. Differences in the reported spasticity between the protocols employed by Sharp and Brouwer and by Engardt et al. may be attributable to the methods of evaluating spasticity and the higher angular velocities used for isokinetic testing by Engardt and colleagues.

ISOTONIC TRAINING REGIMENS

Two studies have investigated the efficacy of isotonic lower extremity training protocols in improvement of maximal voluntary muscle strength and functional capabilities following stroke.[54,73] In contrast to the isokinetic studies, the subjects in these studies were inpatient rehabilitation patients who had strokes less than 3 months prior to entry in the training programs. All of the patients investigated by Nugent et al. were able to stand with or without assistance, and 32 of 44 were able to ambulate unaided.[73] All 77 patients in the study by Inaba and colleagues required assistance to walk.[54]

The training protocol and the evaluation of outcome differed greatly between the two studies. Nugent and colleagues employed a weight-bearing exercise (WBE) in which patients stood with the paretic lower extremity on a wooden block 5–12 cm in height and lifted their nonparetic leg from the floor by actively extending the paretic hip and knee.[73] The study was nonrandomized and self-controlled. The investigators sought to determine if there was a dose-response relationship between the WBE with walking outcome as measured by the MAS. Overall, the number of repetitions of the WBE did correlate with the MAS walking score (r = 0.45, p < 0.01). There was a stronger relationship between the outcome measures for patients with initial MAS scores of 1–3 than for those who were more independent (MAS scores of 4–5).

Inaba and colleagues used an Elgin table to strengthen progressively the same combined hip and knee extension movement of the paretic lower extremity in a supine position using an open kinetic chain approach.[54] The study was a randomized, controlled study in which patients were assigned to one of three treatment groups. The control group received daily functional training and selective stretching, the second group received the same regimen with addition of daily active exercises (reciprocal exercises without resistance), and the third group received daily progressive resisted exercises on the Elgin table in addition to the treatment received by the control group.[34] Investigators compared performance in activities of daily living, using a nonstandardized assessment, and lower extremity extension strength between treatment groups after 1 and 2 months of intervention. Following 1 month of treatment, the progressive strengthening group made significant gains in paretic lower extremity strength (p = 0.02) and activities of daily living (p < 0.05) over the other intervention groups. There were no statistically significant differences between the treatment groups following 2 months of intervention.

Future Directions

In general, the studies suggest that strength in stroke patients can be improved and that strengthening can improve functional independence. However, more research using randomized, controlled designs is needed regarding strengthening for individuals following strokes. To date, most subjects in strengthening studies are in the chronic phase, have had reasonable motor recovery, and have had relatively low levels of spasticity prior to training. Research needs to address the validity of outcome strength measures and which patients might best respond to this form of intervention. Further work on distinguishing differences among patients is needed for (1) correlations of outcome and functional level, (2) relationship of degree of spasticity and strengthening, (3) specific deficits of strength, revealed by EMG-force relationships, (4) determination of the effectiveness of strengthening in acute versus subacute periods following stroke, and (5) establishment of the most effective strengthening protocols.

FACILITATION TECHNIQUES

Diminished or Lack of Volitional Movement as a Symptom of Stroke

Patients are often unable to move their affected side immediately following a stroke, and they often continue to be unable to activate voluntarily certain muscle groups. Although different recovery rates seem to be correlated with the initial degree of impairment,[55] almost all stroke patients have some level of inability to activate muscles volitionally. Therapeutic procedures designed to produce voluntary or reflexive movement would be useful, and techniques that increase the likelihood of recruiting a full range of motor unit types would be appropriate.

Eliciting Volitional Movement

Traditionally, facilitatory approaches progress from segmental reflex levels, to reactions and postural responses, to volitional control and higher activation levels. Any facilitation technique has the challenge that an activation that is elicited through segmental reflexes or resistive procedures must be translated into intentional control. For patients who remain flaccid and unable to activate muscles, available approaches remain focused on the facilitation techniques of quick stretch/tapping, vibration, or brushing. Although these techniques are used infrequently by physiotherapists, presumably because of the popularity of other approaches such as NDT, they may be useful for keeping muscles and motoneurons viable and active. Early activation is better than no activation, given the rapid adaptive changes of neurons and the motor system to injury.

QUICK STRETCH AND TAPPING

Quick stretching of the muscle or tapping the muscle or tendon will evoke monosynaptic reflexes. Many of the traditional neurophysiologic approaches to neurologic rehabilitation have incorporated this phenomenon. Clearly, these reflex activations will be of short duration and must be timed to coincide with a voluntary movement to augment the motor command. Reports that tapping decreases reflex excitability,[4] as determined by H-reflex amplitude, could be contaminated by the fact that the muscle is lengthening during the tapping. Increases in muscle length cause reductions of the amplitude of single motor units as well as H-reflexes.[41,45] Thus, the reduction of amplitude evident during the manual muscle tapping could stem from a peripheral source (orientation of muscle fibers underneath the surface recording electrode) rather than reflex excitability in the spinal cord.

VIBRATION

Vibration is known to evoke strong stimulation of Ia afferents, especially with frequencies about 100 Hz. If vibration is applied during voluntary movement, unloading of the muscle spindles during the movement may decrease the effectiveness of the vibration.[24] Thus, if vibration is applied during an active contraction, unloading of the muscle spindles may be prevented by maintaining the muscle in a steady, lengthened position. The effectiveness of vibration also may be improved by applying the stimulus for a minute or more. The tonic vibration reflex (TVR) that is elicited by prolonged vibration in normal humans results in an increase in muscle tension that develops progressively over 20–60 seconds and lasts 2 seconds after the vibration is stopped; the onset of the TVR is appreciably shorter in spastic hemiparesis.[61] Vibration has been reported to result in powerful muscle contraction in patients exhibiting muscle weakness.[51]

LIGHT TOUCH AND BRUSHING

Light touch, applied by brushing the skin overlying the muscle to be facilitated, has augmented the TVR in normal and hemiparetic subjects.[65,82] Although contrary conclusions were drawn by Mason,[64] the stimulus was applied to such a small area (1 cm²) that it is not surprising that the amount of facilitation was low. Garland and Hayes found that brushing increased ankle dorsiflexion range of motion and tibialis anterior EMG activity in hemiplegic subjects with foot drop, particularly if the muscle was warmed up through a series of practice contractions.[42] The ability of hemiplegic subjects to produce a maximal voluntary contraction was facilitated following cutaneous stimulation.[66] Given that cutaneous stimulation was found to decrease the recruitment threshold of high-threshold motor units,[43] this is a possible mechanism for improving function in hemiparetic patients.

Efficacy of Facilitation Techniques

There is evidence to demonstrate short-term positive responses to facilitation techniques in stroke patients. The main criticism of facilitation techniques is the lack of studies to demonstrate their effectiveness in improving functional clinical outcomes after stroke. For instance, although Garland and Hayes found an improvement in ankle dorsiflexion,[42] it is not known if this improvement in range of motion affected more functional activities, such as ambulation. Similarly, although maximal voluntary force has been found to be augmented by vibration or brushing in weak patients, the long-term improvements of motor control following repeated applications of facilitation techniques remain unknown.

Future Directions

Given the necessity for encouraging early movement because of potential transsynaptic degeneration and motor unit-type transformation, facilitation of muscle activation is critical. The available research is sparse with regard to the carryover of muscle activity that is produced with the assistance of facilitatory reflexes to the volitional activation of muscle. However, if initial flaccidity persists, it may be best to achieve muscle activity via reflex or functional electrical stimulation rather than to leave the patient with paretic limbs whose motoneurons and muscles remain quiescent for extended times.

FORCED USE OF THE AFFECTED UPPER EXTREMITY

Learned Disuse as a Symptom of Stroke

Three studies describe encouraging results with the use of slings or splints to restrain the nonparetic upper extremity of persons who have suffered strokes (Table 2).[74,89,92] Because the nonparetic extremity was restrained, patients were forced to use their paretic upper extremity exclusively. The studies were based on successful use of this behavioral technique with monkeys who underwent deafferentation of a single forelimb.[57,87] As observed in patients after stroke, the animals stopped using the affected limb following the deafferentation procedure. However, if the intact limb was restrained for at least 3 days, the animals persisted in using the deafferented limb functionally following removal of the restraint.[57]

Debate has ensued concerning why forced use of the affected limb might be successful in improving function following stroke. The popular theory of "learned nonuse" proposes that poor use of the affected limb is a learned phenomenon related to the aversive consequences of early attempts to manipulate the paretic limb following stroke.[85,86] Individuals learn that it is simply easier and faster to compensate by using the unaffected limb for most activities. Taub has suggested that restraint of the unaffected limb changes the contingencies for reinforcement; the individual must overcome learned nonuse of the affected limb to perform daily activities.[85,86] He has suggested that the concentrated use of the affected extremity improves the strength and control of the limb. Others have advocated the "unmasking" theory—the strengthening of previously unused or dormant synaptic connections through repetition and practice during restraint.[92]

TABLE 2.   Studies of Forced Use of Affected Upper Extremities Following Stroke

Study Design	Subjects	Restraint Intervention	Control Intervention	Outcome
Single case (A-B-A design)[74]	n = 1 18 mos post-CVA	Unaffected arm restrained in a sling through-out the day for 1 wk. Daily passive range of motion for restrained limb	No control group	18 functional tasks were rated for time and quality (0–5 ordinal scale) Trend for reduction in time to complete 18 tasks with each assessment up to 2 wks following the intervention; time to complete tasks increased slightly 4 wks following intervention but remained well below baseline values. No change in quality of upper limb movements following restraint
Nonrandom-ized self-controlled[92]	n = 25 (16 CVA) ≥ 1 yr post-CVA	Unaffected arm restrained in a sling that enclosed fingers during waking hrs for 2 wks. Sling removed 30 min/day to exercise restrained limb	No control group	21 functional tasks were rated for time or force and quality Improved performance of all tasks during the 2nd wk of forced use; change was significant from baseline in 8/21 tasks (p < .05) Improved performance continued in all 21 tasks; change was significant from baseline in 19/21 tasks (p < 0.05) 1 year following intervention
Randomized controlled trial[89]	Total n = 9 4 restraint group; 5 control group) ≥ 1 yr post-CVA (range 1–18 yrs)	Unaffected arm restrained in a sling and resting hand splint. Received active rehabilitation of affected limb for 7 hrs every weekday	Verbally encouraged to use affected limb Self range of motion exercises 15 min/day. 2 sessions of passive physical therapy (passive ROM, assessment)	4 measures were evaluated: 1. Emory Motor Function Test 2. The Arm Motor Activity Test 3. Passive ROM Mean performance on measures 1 and 2 were significantly faster for the restraint group; performance time decreased 30% for the restraint group and increased 2.2% for the control group following intervention. Quality of movement improved on measures 1 and 2 following restraint (p < 0.003). No significant change in passive ROM following intervention 4. Motor Activity Log Marked improvement on Motor Activity Log in restraint group during intervention, with retention or some continued improvement up to 2 yrs following intervention; only small to moderate improvements observed in the control group following intervention

CVA = cerebrovascular accident
ROM = range of motion

Motor Learning and Cortical Adaptations

Evidence in animals and humans suggests that cortical reorganization occurs following central nervous system lesions[30,71] and that this reorganization may be influenced by postlesion experiences to benefit recovery.[27,30,72] However, Koslowski and Schallert have suggested that if an overuse program is started within the first week after the lesion that the size of the lesion increases, creating further areas of damage and loss of function.[60] To what extent these studies may be generalized to forced use interventions used more than a year after a stroke remains to be investigated.

It appears that although practice and repeated use can promote cortical reorganization, the specific kind of practice, and particularly the kind of learning of a motor skill, can specifically affect cortical reorganization. Motor learning as it applies to individuals with neurologic impairments has received greater attention by physiotherapists, particularly with the advent of the Motor Relearning Program approach to treatment.[26] There is a large body of literature pertaining to the acquisition of motor skills by healthy, young, "normal" subjects. Advanced brain imaging and stimulation techniques have revealed cortical adaptations following motor learning in healthy humans[29,56] and may be useful in documenting functional reorganization of the brain in patients recovering from stroke.[25,28] Nudo et al. demonstrated the benefits of rehabilitation-like exercise in adult squirrel monkeys recovering from an ischemic brain infarct.[72]

Although it is not known whether the motor learning principles (e.g., practice schedule, feedback mode) that were developed using normal subjects can be applied to the treatment of stroke patients, limited evidence does support its use with stroke patients. Hanlon et al. tested patients with chronic hemiparesis resulting from stroke using random or blocked practice schedules.[52] As in normal subjects, the random and blocked practice groups performed equally well during the acquisition phase, but the random practice group had superior retention and transfer of skill. Eckhouse et al. had two groups of chronic stroke patients perform arm-reaching tasks.[35] The task was performed best in the group that received audio and visual feedback of their performance. Another form of feedback commonly used in stroke physiotherapy is EMG biofeedback. Two meta-analyses by Moreland and colleagues concluded that EMG biofeedback was an effective adjunct to stroke physiotherapy in the lower limb but not in the upper limb.[68,69]

Efficacy of Forced-Use Paradigms

Several clinical studies have examined outcomes after implementation of a forced-use protocol.[79] Restrained subjects were encouraged verbally to use their affected limbs during the forced-use phase of two studies,[74,92] while Taub et al. gave subjects active daily intervention to facilitate use of the affected upper extremity.[89] Preliminary results by Taub et al. indicate that restraint in combination with "shaping," in which desired movements of the affected extremity were trained in smaller successive approximations, might be more effective in improving the motor function of paretic limb than forced use alone.[88]

In terms of selecting patients who might benefit from a forced-use paradigm, all subjects in these studies had sufficient volitional control to overcome their flexion synergies to complete functional tasks with their affected upper extremity.[92] Subjects in two of the studies were capable of isolated but impaired movements of their paretic wrists and fingers, and they did not have serious cognitive deficits or excessive spasticity.[74,88] Successful application of a forced-use paradigm appears to be possible despite a lengthy time since stroke.[74,88,92] However, no published literature has indicated the efficacy of this approach earlier in the rehabilitation process.

Future Directions

The limited number of studies of forced-use paradigms suggest that this technique has significant potential. An advantage of the technique is that it may target adaptations at cortical levels of the motor system, where the initial damage occurs.

Disadvantages, however, arise in the difficulty in applying this practice in the modern pressures of medical practice. Forced-use would delay the teaching of compensatory strategies using the nonparetic limbs to gain functional independence. With shorter hospitalizations, treatment may be directed toward progressing patients quickly toward functional improvements. Further work is needed to demonstrate the effectiveness of forced use before it can be supported. This may be achieved by designing treatment approaches that incorporate forced use with other techniques that directly facilitate and strengthen the affected limbs.

CONCLUSION

Recent advances in motor control research are shifting the focus of physiotherapy following stroke. Addressing lack of movement or force production at an early stage of rehabilitation is now of prime concern. This does not mean inappropriate muscle activation due to spasticity is ignored but suggests a more balanced view of movement problems that are the sequelae of stroke. There are indications that early intervention could reduce motoneuron loss and subsequent disuse atrophy in paretic muscles. Physiotherapeutic interventions that facilitate muscle activation, strengthen muscles, and encourage use of paretic limbs via forced-use paradigms are receiving greater attention. These techniques are based on new knowledge from basic sciences and have been shown to demonstrate some effectiveness. Future research must examine the neurophysiologic effects and the efficacy of these treatments during the first days and weeks following cerebrovascular insult. Given the present health care climate, such studies must confirm that early interventions reduce rehabilitation time and improve the functional independence of patients following stroke.

REFERENCES

1. Ada L, Vattanasilp W, O'Dwyer NJ, Crosbie J: Does spasticity contribute to walking dysfunction after stroke? J Neurol Neurosurg Psychiatry 64:628–635, 1998.
2. Adams J, Cahan LD, Perry J, Beeler LM: Foot contact pattern following selective dorsal rhizotomy. Ped Neurosurg 23:76–81, 1995.
3. Badj T, Vodovnik L: Pendulum testing of spasticity. J Biomed Eng 6:9–16, 1984.
4. Belanger AY, Morin S, Pepin P, et al: Manual muscle tapping decreases soleus H-reflex amplitude in control subjects. Physiother Can 41:192–196, 1989.
5. Bennett SE, Karnes JL: Neurological Disabilities: Assessment and Treatment. Philadelphia, Lippincott-Raven, 1998.
6. Bobath B: Adult Hemiplegia: Evaluation and Treatment. 2nd ed. London, Heinemann, 1978.
7. Bohannon RW: Recovery and correlates of trunk muscle strength after stroke. Int J Rehabil Res 18:162–167, 1995.
8. Bohannon RW: Lateral trunk flexion strength: Impairment, measurement, reliability and implications following unilateral brain lesions. Int J Rehabil Res 15:249–251, 1992.
9. Bohannon RW: Is the measurement of muscle strength appropriate in patients with brain lesions? A special communication. Phys Ther 69:225–230, 1989.
10. Bohannon RW: Author's response. Phys Ther 69:235–236, 1989.
11. Bohannon RW: Correlation of lower extremity strengths and other variables with standing performance in stroke patients. Physiother Can 41:198–202, 1989.
12. Bohannon RW: Determinants of transfer capacity in patients with hemiparesis. Physiother Can 40:236–239, 1988.
13. Bohannon RW: Gait performance of hemiparetic stroke patients: Selected variables. Arch Phys Med Rehabil 68:777–781, 1987.
14. Bohannon RW: Strength of lower limb related to gait velocity and cadence in stroke patients. Physiother Can 38:204–206, 1986.
15. Bohannon RW, Andrews AW: Correlation of knee extensor muscle torque and spasticity with gait speed in patients with stroke. Arch Phys Med Rehabil 71:330–333, 1990.
16. Bohannon RW, Andrews AW: Interrater reliability of hand-held dynamometry. Phys Ther 67:931–933, 1987.

17. Bohannon RW, Cassidy D, Walsh S: Trunk muscle strength is impaired multidirectionally after stroke. Clin Rehabil 9:47–51, 1995.

18. Bohannon RW, Larkin PA, Smith MB, Horton MG: Relationship between static muscle strength deficits and spasticity in stroke patients with hemiparesis. Phys Ther 67:1068–1071, 1987.

19. Bohannon RW, Smith MB: Assessment of strength deficits in eight paretic upper extremity muscle groups of stroke patients with hemiplegia. Phys Ther 67:522–525, 1987.

20. Bohannon RW, Walsh S: Nature, reliability, and predictive value of muscle performance measures in patients with hemiparesis following stroke. Arch Phys Med Rehabil 73:721–725, 1992.

21. Bohannon RW, Warren ME, Cogman KA: Motor variables correlated with the hand to mouth maneuver in stroke patients. Arch Phys Med Rehabil 72:682–684, 1991.

22. Buckon CE, Sienko TS, Aiona MD, Piatt JH: Assessment of upper-extremity function in children with spastic diplegia before and after selective dorsal rhizotomy. Dev Med Child Neurol 38:967–975, 1996.

23. Burke RE: On the central nervous system control of fast and slow twitch motor units. In Desmedt JE (ed): New Developments in Electromyography and Clinical Neurophysiology. Vol 3. Basel, Karger, 1973, pp 69–94.

24. Burke D, Hagbarth K-E, Lofstedt L, Wallin BG: The responses of human muscle spindle endings to vibration during isometric contraction. J Physiol (Lond) 261:695–711, 1976.

25. Cao Y, D'Olhaberriague L, Vikingstad EM, et al: Pilot study of functional MRI to assess cerebral activation of motor function after poststroke hemiparesis. Stroke 29:112–122, 1998.

26. Carr JH, Shepherd RB: A Motor Relearning Programme for Stroke. London, Heinemann, 1982.

27. Castro-Almancos MA, Garci-Segura LM, Borrell J: Transfer of function to specific area of the cortex after induced recovery from brain damage. Eur J Neurosci 4:853–863, 1992.

28. Chollet F, DiPiero V, Wise RJ, et al: The functional anatomy of motor recovery after stroke in humans: A study with positron emission tomography. Ann Neurol 29:63–71, 1991.

29. Classen J, Liepert J, Wise SP, et al: Rapid plasticity of human cortical movement representation induced by practice. J Neurophysiol 79:1117–1123, 1998.

30. Cohen LG, Brasil-Neto JP, Pascual-Leone A, Hallett M: Plasticity of cortical motor output organization following deafferentation, cerebral lesions and skill acquisition. In Devinsky O, Beric A, Dogali M (eds): Electrical and Magnetic Stimulation of the Brain. New York, Raven Press, 1993, pp 187–200.

31. Cohen LG, Celnik P, Pascual-Leone A, et al: Functional relevance of cross-modal plasticity in blind humans. Nature 389:180–184, 1997.

32. Colebatch JG, Gandevia SC, Spira PJ: Voluntary muscle strength in hemiparesis: Distribution of weakness at the elbow. J Neurol Neurosurg Psychiatry 49:1019–1024, 1986.

33. Dattola R, Girlanda P, Vita G, et al: Muscle rearrangement in patients with hemiparesis after stroke: An electrophysiological and morphological study. Eur Neurol 33:109–114, 1993.

34. Delorme TL, Watkins AL: Progressive Resistance Exercise. New York, Appleton-Century-Crofts, 1951.

35. Eckhouse RH Jr, Morash RP, Maulucci RA: Sensory feedback and the impaired motor system. J Med Syst 14:93–105, 1990.

36. Edstrom L: Selective changes in the red and white muscle fires in upper motor lesions and parkinsonism. J Neurol Sci 11:537, 1970.

37. Engardt M, Knutsson E, Jonsson M, Sternhag M: Dynamic muscle strength training in stroke patients: Effects on knee extension torque, electromyographic activity and motor function. Arch Phys Med Rehabil 76:419–425, 1995.

38. Ernst E: A review of stroke rehabilitation and physiotherapy. Stroke 21:1081–1085, 1990.

39. Fenichel GM, Daroff RB: Hemiplegic atrophy: Histological and etiological considerations. Neurology 14:883–890, 1964.

40. Fix AJ, Daughton DM: Human Activity Profile. Professional Manual. 3rd ed. Odessa, FL, Psychological Assessment Resources, 1988.

41. Garland SJ, Gerilovsky L, Enoka RM: Association between muscle architecture and quadriceps femoris H-reflex. Muscle Nerve 17:581–592, 1994.

42. Garland SJ, Hayes KC: Effects of brushing of electromyographic activity and ankle dorsiflexion in hemiplegic subjects with foot drop. Physiother Can 39:241–247, 1987.

43. Garnett R, Stephens JA: The reflex responses of single motor units in human first dorsal interosseous muscle following cutaneous afferent stimulation. J Physiol (Lond) 303:351–364, 1980.

44. Gemperline JJ, Allen S, Walk D, Rymer WZ: Characteristics of motor unit discharge in subjects with hemiparesis. Muscle Nerve 18:1101–1114, 1995.

45. Gerilovsky L, Tsvetinov P, Trenkova G: Peripheral effects on the amplitude of monopolar and bipolar H-reflex potentials from the soleus muscle. Exp Brain Res 76:173–181, 1989.

46. Giuliani CA: Strength training for patients with neurological disorders. Neurol Rep 19:29–33, 1995.

47. Giuliani CA, Light KE, Rose DK: Effects of an isokinetic exercise program in gait patterns of patients with hemiparesis. Neurol Rep 4:23–24, 1993.

48. Gowland C, deBruin H, Basmajian JV, et al: Agonist and antagonist activity during voluntary upper-limb movement in patients with stroke. Phys Ther 72:624–633, 1992.

49. Gowland C, VanHullenaar S, Torresin W, et al: Treatment. In Gowland C, VanHullenaar S, Torresin W, et al (eds): Chedoke-McMaster Stroke Assessment: Development, Validation and Administration Manual. Hamilton, ON, Chedoke-McMaster Hospitals and McMaster University, 1995, pp 9.25–9.30.

50. Hachisuka K, Umezu Y, Ogata H: Disuse muscle atrophy of lower limbs in hemiplegic patients. Arch Phys Med Rehabil 78:13–18, 1997.

51. Hagbarth K-E: The effect of muscle vibration in normal man and in patients with motor disorders. In Desmedt JE (ed): New Developments in Electromyography and Clinical Neurophysiology. Vol 3. Karger, Basel, 1973, pp 428–443.

52. Hanlon RE: Motor learning following unilateral stroke. Arch Phys Med Rehabil 77:811–815, 1996.

53. Ibrahim IK, Berger W, Trippel M, Dietz V: Stretch-induced electromyographic activity and torque in spastic elbow muscles. Brain 116:971–989, 1993.

54. Inaba M, Edberg E, Montgomery J, Gillis MK: Effectiveness of functional training, active exercise, and resistive exercise for patients with hemiplegia. Phys Ther 53:28–35, 1973.

55. Jorgensen HS, Nakayama H, Raaschou HO, et al: Outcome and time course of recovery in stroke. Part II: Time course of recovery. The Copenhagen Stroke Study. Arch Phys Med Rehabil 76:406–412, 1995.

56. Karni A, Meyer G, Jezzard P, et al: Functional MRI evidence for adult motor cortex plasticity during motor skill learning. Nature 377:155–158, 1995.

57. Knapp HD, Taub E, Berman AJ: Movements in monkeys with deafferented forelimbs. Exp Neurol 7:305–315, 1963.

58. Knutsson E, Martensson A: Dynamic motor capacity in spastic paresis and its relation to prime mover dysfunction, spastic reflexes and antagonist co-activation. Scand J Rehabil Med 12:93–106, 1980.

59. Knutsson E, Martensson A, Granberg L: The effects of concentric and eccentric training in spastic paresis. Scand J Rehabil Med 24(27 suppl):31–32, 1992.

60. Kozlowski DA, Schallert JT: Use-dependent exaggeration of neuronal injury after unilateral sensori-motor cortical lesions. J Neurosci 16:4776–4786, 1996.

61. Lance JW, Burke D, Andrews CJ: The reflex effects of muscle vibration. In Desmedt JE (ed): New Developments in Electromyography and Clinical Neurophysiology. Vol 3. Karger, Basel, 1973, pp 444–462.

62. Light KE: Clients with spasticity: To strengthen or not to strengthen. Neurol Rep 15:19–20, 1991.

63. Lindmark B, Hamrin E: Relation between gait speed, knee muscle torque and motor scores in post-stroke patients. Scand J Caring Sci 9:195–202, 1995.

64. Mason C: One method for assessing the effectiveness of fast brushing. Phys Ther 65:1197–1202, 1985.

65. Matyas T, Spicer S: Facilitation of TVR by cutaneous stimulation in hemiplegics. Am J Phys Med 59:280–287, 1980.

66. Matyas T, Spicer S: Facilitation of the maximum voluntary contraction in hemiplegia by concomitant cutaneous stimulation. Am J Phys Med 65:125–134, 1986.

67. McComas AJ, Sica REP, Upton ARM, Aguilera N: Functional changes in motoneurons of hemiparetic patients. J Neurol Neurosurg Psychiatry 36:183–193, 1973.

68. Moreland JD, Thomson MA, Fuoco AR: Electromyographic biofeedback to improve lower extremity function after stroke: A meta-analysis. Arch Phys Med Rehabil 79:134–140, 1998.

69. Moreland J, Thomson M: Efficacy of electromyographic biofeedback compared with conventional physical therapy for upper-extremity function in patients following stroke: A research overview and meta-analysis. Phys Ther 74:534–545, 1994.

70. Nadeau S, Gravel D, Arsenault AB, et al: Dynamometric assessment of the plantarflexors in hemiparetic subjects: Relations between muscular, gait and clinical parameters. Scand J Rehabil Med 29:137–146, 1997.

71. Netz J, Lammers T, Homber V: Reorganization of motor output in the non-affected hemisphere after a stroke. Brain 120:1579–1586, 1997.

72. Nudo RJ, Wise BM, SiFuentes F, Milliken GW: Neural substrates for effects of rehabilitative training on motor recovery after ischemic infarct. Science 272:1791–1794, 1996.

73. Nugent JA, Schurr KA, Adams RD: A dose-response relationship between amount of weight-bearing exercise and walking outcome following cerebrovascular accident. Arch Phys Med Rehabil 75:399–402, 1994.

74. Ostendorf CG, Wolf SL: Effect of forced use of the upper extremity of a hemiplegic patient on changes in function. Phys Ther 7:1022–1028, 1981.
75. Paczynski R, Chung YH, Diringer MN: Pathophysiology of ischemic injury. In Fischer M (ed): Stroke Therapy. Boston, Butterworth-Heinemann, 1995, pp 29–55.
76. Riddle DL, Finucane SD, Rothstein JM, Walker ML: Intrasession and intersession reliability of hand-held dynamometer measurements taken on brain-damaged patients. Phys Ther 69:182–194, 1989.
77. Rosenfalck A, Andreassen S: Impaired regulation of force and firing pattern of single motor units in patients with spasticity. J Neurol Neurosurg Psychiatry 43:907–916, 1980.
78. Rothstein JM, Riddle DL, Finucane SD: Invited commentary. Phys Ther 69:230–235, 1989.
79. Russo SG: Hemiplegic upper extremity rehabilitation: A review of the forced-use paradigm. Neurol Rep 19:17–22, 1995.
79a. Sawner K, LaVigne J: Brunnstrom's Movement Therapy in Hemiplegia: A Neurophysiological Approach. 2nd ed. Philadelphia, JB Lippincott, 1992.
80. Scelsi R, Lotta S, Lommi G, et al: Hemiplegic atrophy. Morphological findings in the anterior tibial muscle of patients with cerebral vascular accidents. Acta Neuropathol (Berl) 62:324–331, 1984.
81. Sharp SA, Brouwer BJ: Isokinetic strength training of the hemiparetic knee: Effects on function and spasticity. Arch Phys Med Rehabil 78:1231–1236, 1997.
82. Spicer S, Matyas T: Facilitation of TVR by cutaneous stimulation. Am J Phys Med 59:223–231, 1980.
83. Sunderland A, Tinson D, Bradley L, Langton Hewer R: Arm function after stroke. An evaluation of grip strength as a measure of recovery and a prognostic indicator. J Neurol Neurosurg Psychiatry 52:1267–1272, 1989.
84. Tang A, Rymer WZ: Abnormal force: EMG relations in paretic limbs of hemiparetic human subjects. J Neurol Neurosurg Psychiatry 44:690–698, 1981.
85. Taub E: Somatosensory deafferentation research with monkeys. In Ince L (ed): Behavioral Psychology and Rehabilitation Medicine. Baltimore, Williams & Wilkins, 1980, pp 371–401.
86. Taub E: Movement in nonhuman primates deprived of somatosensory feedback. Exerc Sport Sci Rev 4:335–374, 1977.
87. Taub E, Berman J: Movement and learning in the absence of sensory feedback. In Freedman SJ (ed): The Neuropsychology of Spatially Oriented Behavior. Homewood, IL, Dorsey Press, 1968, pp 173–192.
88. Taub E, Crago JE, Burgio LD, et al: An operant approach to rehabilitation medicine: Overcoming learned nonuse by shaping. J Exp Anal Behav 61:281–293, 1994.
89. Taub E, Miller NE, Novack TA, et al: Technique to improve chronic motor deficit after stroke. Arch Phys Med Rehabil 74:347–354, 1993.
89a. Voss DE: Proprioceptive Neuromuscular Facilitation: Patterns and Techniques. 3rd ed. Philadelphia, Harper & Row, 1985.
90. Watkins MP, Harris AB, Kozlowski BA: Isokinetic testing in patients with hemiparesis: A pilot study. Phys Ther 64:184–189, 1984.
91. Weinstein CJ, Grafton ST, Pohl PS: Motor task difficulty and brain activity: Investigation of goal-directed reciprocal aiming using positron emission tomography. J Neurophysiol 77:1581–1594, 1997.
92. Wolf SL, Lecraw DE, Barton LA, Jann BB: Forced use of hemiplegic upper extremities to reverse the effect of learned nonuse among chronic stroke and head-injured patients. Exp Neurol 104:125–132, 1989.
93. Young JL, Mayer RF: Physiological alterations of motor units in hemiplegia. J Neurol Sci 54:410–412, 1982.

ROBERT W. TEASELL, MD, FRCPC
JOHN D. HEITZNER, MD, FRCPC

THE PAINFUL HEMIPLEGIC SHOULDER

From the Department of Physical
Medicine and Rehabilitation
University of Western Ontario
London, Ontario
Canada

Reprint requests to:
Robert W. Teasell, MD
Department of Physical Medicine
and Rehabilitation
London Health Sciences Center
339 Windermere Road
London, Ontario N6A 5A5
Canada

Hemiplegia is a common clinical consequence of a focal cerebral insult resulting from a vascular lesion (i.e., hemorrhagic or ischemic stroke). Good shoulder function is a prerequisite for successful transfers, maintaining balance, performing activities of daily living, and effective hand function.[40] Shoulder pain has been estimated to occur in up to 84% of hemiplegic stroke patients and can result in significant disability in and of itself.[35,38] Pain can occur as early as 2 weeks poststroke but usually occurs 2–3 months poststroke.[38] Although many etiologies have been proposed for hemiplegic shoulder pain, increasingly it appears to be a consequence of spasticity and the sustained hemiplegic posture.

CAUSES OF HEMIPLEGIC SHOULDER PAIN

Possible sources of hemiplegic shoulder pain are listed in Table 1. Factors most frequently associated with shoulder pain are shoulder (glenohumeral) subluxation,[18,34,41,43] shoulder contractures or restricted shoulder range of motion,[2,6,17–19,40] and spasticity, particularly of the subscapularis and pectoralis muscles.[6,8,33,34] Other suggested causes of shoulder pain include reflex sympathetic dystrophy (RSD),[11,14,37] depression,[41] and injury to the rotator cuff musculotendinous unit.[35,36]

Shoulder Subluxation

PATHOPHYSIOLOGY

Shoulder subluxation is best defined as changes in the mechanical integrity of the glenohumeral joint causing a palpable gap between the

TABLE 1.   Potential Causes of Hemiplegic Shoulder Pain

Anatomic Site	Mechanism

Muscle	Rotator cuff tear
	Muscle imbalance
	    Subscapularis spasticity
	    Pectoralis spasticity

Bone	Humeral fracture
Joint	Glenohumeral subluxation
Bursa	Bursitis
Tendon	Tendinitis
Joint capsule	Frozen or contracted shoulder (adhesive capsulitis)
Other	Shoulder-hand syndrome (reflex sympathetic dystrophy)

acromion and humeral head. The most reliable clinical measurement device of the subacromial space used in clinical research is calipers.[5] The glenohumeral joint is multiaxial and has a range of motion that exceeds that of other joints in the body. To achieve this mobility, the glenohumeral joint must sacrifice stability. Stability is achieved through the rotator cuff, a musculotendinous sleeve that maintains the humeral head in the glenoid fossa, while at the same time allowing shoulder mobility. During the initial period following a stroke, the hemiplegic arm is flaccid or hypotonic. Therefore, the shoulder musculature, in particular the rotator cuff musculotendinous sleeve, cannot perform its function of maintaining the humeral head in the glenoid fossa, and there is a high risk of shoulder subluxation.

Shoulder subluxation is a very common problem in hemiplegic patients. During the initial flaccid stage of hemiplegia, the involved extremity must be adequately supported, or the weight of the arm will result in shoulder subluxation. Improper positioning in bed, lack of support while the patient is in the upright position, and pulling on the hemiplegic arm when transferring the patient all contribute to glenohumeral subluxation. Down and lateral subluxation commonly occurs secondary to prolonged downward pull on the arm against which hypotonic muscles offer little resistance.[10] The resulting mechanical effect is overstretching of the glenohumeral capsule (especially its superior aspect) and flaccid supraspinatus and deltoid muscles (Fig. 1).[1,42]

SCAPULAR ROTATION

Other factors seem to play a role in subluxation of the glenohumeral joint. Basmajian and Bazant[1] proposed that, in the normal state, subluxation of the humeral head was prevented by upward angulation of the glenoid fossa and the upper part of the shoulder capsule, the coracohumeral ligament and supraspinatus muscle. They hypothesized that after a hemiplegic stroke the upward angulation of the scapula would be lost. Cailliet[7] added that, in the flaccid stage, the scapula assumed a depressed and downwardly rotated position as the paretic serratus anterior and the upper part of the trapezius muscles no longer support the scapula. The combination of flaccid supportive musculature (in particular the supraspinatus muscle) and a downwardly rotated scapula was presumed to predispose the head of the humerus to undergo inferior subluxation relative to the glenoid fossa.

Prevost et al., using a three-dimensional x-ray technique, actually studied the movement of the scapula and humerus in 50 stroke patients.[39] They compared the

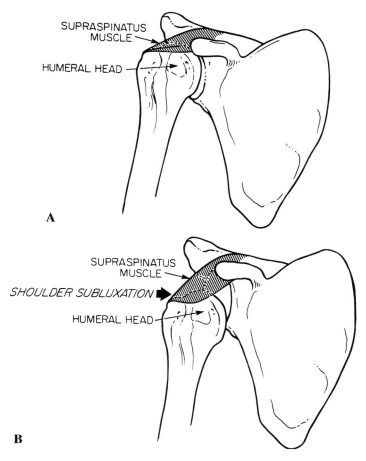

FIGURE 1. *A*, Normal shoulder. The humeral head is maintained in the glenoid fossa by the supraspinatus muscle. *B*, Shoulder subluxation. During the initial phase of hemiplegia, the supraspinatus muscle is flaccid. The weight of the unsupported arm can cause the humeral head to sublux downward out of the glenoid fossa.

affected shoulder to the nonaffected shoulder and were able to demonstrate a difference between the affected and nonaffected shoulders in terms of the vertical position of the humerus (i.e., degree of subluxation) in relation to the scapula. The orientation of the glenoid fossa was also different; however, they found that, with the subluxed shoulder, the glenoid fossa was actually facing less downward. No significant relationship was noted between the orientation of the scapula and the severity of subluxation. They concluded that the scapular position was not an important factor in the occurrence of inferior subluxation in hemiplegia,[39] and this viewpoint now prevails.

PAIN IN SHOULDER SUBLUXATION

Shoulder subluxation may be associated with several conditions including shoulder pain,[18,34,41,43] frozen shoulder, and brachial plexus traction injury[25] although evidence of the latter is lacking.[26] It has long been assumed that, if not corrected, a pattern of traction on the flaccid shoulder will result in pain, decreased range of motion, and contracture. However, not all patients with a subluxed hemiplegic shoulder experience shoulder pain, and it remains controversial as to whether it is a common cause of hemiplegic shoulder pain.[16,34,42] In 1990, Bohannon and Andrews reported shoulder subluxation was not a cause of shoulder pain.[4]

Shoulder subluxation occurs frequently in association with the initially flaccid hemiplegic shoulder. Flaccid supporting shoulder musculature and not scapular rotation appears to account for subluxation occurring. Shoulder subluxation may be a cause of hemiplegic shoulder pain, but this has never been definitely established, with some authors suggesting otherwise. Nevertheless, ensuring that the hemiplegic arm is adequately supported during the initial stage following a stroke may help prevent shoulder subluxation, and this has become an important component of early poststroke care.

Spasticity

Spasticity is defined as a disorder of motor function characterized by a velocity-sensitive increase in resistance to passive stretch of muscles accompanied by hyperactive tendon reflexes and often associated with a clasp-knife phenomenon. Spasticity is one component of the upper motor neuron (UMN) syndrome and is the inevitable accompaniment of hemiplegia and an incomplete motor recovery. Under normal circumstances, a delicate balance exists between facilitating and inhibiting influences on both alpha and gamma motor neurons, which together maintain appropriate control of skeletal muscle length and strength of contraction at the spinal cord level. After a stroke, input from one or more of the supraspinal suppressor areas will decrease or stop entirely. The balance of control over the muscle tips in favor of facilitation, and spasticity results. Spasticity develops only if there is loss of input from both pyramidal and extrapyramidal motor systems. Spasticity presents as increased tone and reflexes on the involved side of the body.

Van Ouwenaller et al. looked at various factors in 219 patients followed for 1 year after a stroke and identified a much higher incidence of shoulder pain in spastic (85%) than in flaccid (18%) hemiplegics.[47] They identified spasticity as "the prime factor and the one most frequently encountered in the genesis of shoulder pain in the hemiplegic patient," but they were unsure of the etiology of the subsequent shoulder pain.[47] In contrast, Bohannon et al. conducted a statistical analysis of 50 consecutive hemiplegic patients (36 with shoulder pain) and asserted that "spasticity . . . was unrelated to shoulder pain."[3] Nevertheless, evidence that spasticity, spastic muscle imbalance in particular, is a cause of hemiplegic shoulder pain is growing.

SPASTIC MUSCLE IMBALANCE

Hemiplegia following stroke is characterized by typical posturing reflecting hypertonic muscle patterns. Flexor tone predominates in the hemiplegic upper extremity and results in scapular retraction and depression as well as internal rotation and adduction of the shoulder. This posture is the consequence of ablation of higher centers and subsequent release of motor groups from pyramidal and extrapyramidal control. In stroke recovery, this "synergy pattern" of muscles is inevitable where recovery is incomplete. One consequence of this is the development of spastic muscle imbalance about the shoulder joint.

Clinically, the internal rotators of the shoulder predominate after a stroke involving that arm, and external rotation is one of the last areas of shoulder function to recover. Hence, during recovery, motor units are not appropriately recruited or turned off; the result is simultaneous cocontraction of agonist and antagonist muscles. A shortened agonist in the synergy pattern becomes stronger, and the constant tension of the agonist can become painful. Stretching of these tightened spastic muscles causes more pain. Shortened muscles inhibit movement, reduce range of motion, and prevent other movements, especially at the shoulder where external rotation of the humerus is necessary for arm abduction greater than 90°. Muscles that contribute to spastic internal rotation or adduction of the shoulder include the subscapularis, pectoralis major, teres major, and latissimus dorsi muscles. However, two muscles in particular have been implicated as most often being spastic and leading to muscle imbalances: the subscapularis and pectoralis major muscles.

Subscapularis Spasticity Disorder. The subscapularis muscle originates on the undersurface of the scapula and inserts on the lesser tuberosity of the humerus as well as on the capsule of the shoulder joint (Fig. 2). It is a major internal rotator of the shoulder.[22] The subscapularis muscle also participates in arm abduction and extension from a flexed position.[13] In normal individuals, nerve impulses to the subscapularis are inhibited during arm abduction; the muscle then relaxes and allows the humerus to externally rotate, thus preventing impingement of the greater tuberosity on the acromion.[12] As part of the typical flexor synergy pattern in spastic hemiplegics, internal rotators, including the subscapularis muscle, are tonically active. This limits shoulder abduction, flexion, and external rotation.

Bohannon et al. found limitation of external rotation of the hemiplegic shoulder was the factor that most correlated with hemiplegic shoulder pain.[3] Hecht specifically linked this problem to the subscapularis muscle when he noted, "The subscapularis muscle is the primary cause of shoulder pain in spastic hemiplegia where external rotation is most limited. Although other muscles may contribute to spasticity, pain, and functional contracture, the subscapularis is the keystone of the abnormal synergy pattern."[21] The subscapularis spasticity disorder is characterized by

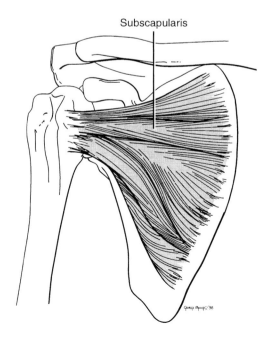

FIGURE 2. The subscapularis muscle. The subscapularis muscle is a major internal rotation of the shoulder. As part of the typical flexor synergy pattern in spastic hemiplegics, the subscapularis is tonically active limiting not only external rotation but also shoulder abduction and flexion.

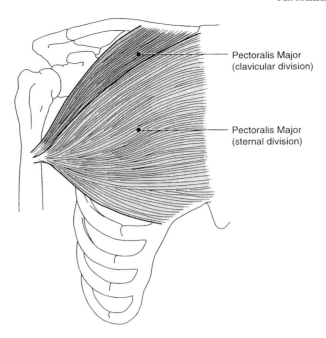

Pectoralis Major
(clavicular division)

Pectoralis Major
(sternal division)

FIGURE 3.   The pectoralis major muscle. The pectoralis major muscle serves to adduct, internally rotate and forward flex the arm at the shoulder.

motion being most limited and pain being reproduced on external rotation. A tight band of spastic muscle is palpated in the posterior axillary fold. In support of this, Inaba et al. reported external rotation was the most painful and limited movement of the hemiplegic shoulder.[23]

Pectoralis Spasticity Disorder.   The pectoralis major muscle serves to forward flex, adduct, and internally rotate the arm (Fig. 3). Hecht has reported on a subset of hemiplegic patients with greater limitations in abduction (and flexion) than on external rotation.[21] In these patients, a spastic pectoralis major muscle appears to be problematic. This disorder is characterized by motion being most limited and pain produced on abduction. A tight band of spastic muscle can be palpated in the anterior axillary fold.[21] It is also noteworthy that the pectoralis major muscle is a synergist of the subscapularis muscle.

FROZEN OR CONTRACTED SHOULDER

A frozen or contracted shoulder is frequently identified as a source of pain in the spastic hemiplegic shoulder.[3,15,17–19,40] Risk et al. performed shoulder arthrography in 30 patients with a painful hemiplegic shoulder.[40] Twenty-three patients demonstrated only capsular constriction typical of a frozen shoulder. The study strongly suggests a frozen or contracted shoulder is, at the very least, associated with hemiplegic shoulder pain. The presence of a frozen or contracted shoulder likely occurs as a consequence of the spastic muscle weakness or imbalance mentioned above, although its presence may be simply an association with no etiologic significance to pain. Alternatively, contracted shoulder muscles may be the final mechanism by which spastic muscle imbalance leads to shoulder pain.

While shoulder subluxation is not always associated with shoulder pain, spasticity generally is. The problem of hemiplegic shoulder pain appears to be due to a combination of spastic muscle imbalance and a frozen contracted shoulder. However, overaggressive stretching of the shoulder through an aggressive stretching program may simply aggravate pain (see Management of the Painful Hemiplegic Shoulder that follows) because it does not address the issue of spastic muscle imbalance.

Rotator Cuff Disorders

Because shoulder pain in a nonstroke population is so often associated with rotator cuff disorder, it should not be surprising that rotator cuff disorders would be seen as a potentially common cause of hemiplegic shoulder pain. However, Risk et al. failed to demonstrate any evidence of rotator cuff tears on arthrography in 30 patients with hemiplegic shoulder pain.[40] A similar study reported a 33% incidence of rotator cuff tears in painful shoulder after strokes.[36] Rotator cuff partial tears are common, and it is always difficult to determine whether they were present premorbidly, even in previously asymptomatic patients. Joynt diagnosed 67 stroke patients as having hemiplegic shoulder pain.[24] Of these patients, 28 received a subacromial injection of 1% lidocaine; approximately 50% obtained moderate or marked relief of pain and improved range of motion. However, this study provides only very indirect evidence implicating rotator cuff disorders as a possible cause of hemiplegic shoulder pain. Generally, hemiplegic shoulder pain is not commonly associated with rotator cuff disorders.

Shoulder-Hand Syndrome

Shoulder-hand syndrome is a form of sympathetically mediated pain involving the hemiplegic upper extremity. Davis et al. reported that 1 out of every 8 stroke victims was diagnosed with this form of upper extremity RSD.[14] Shoulder-hand syndrome is characterized by hand pain and swelling, exquisite tenderness or hyperesthesia, protective immobility, trophic skin changes, and vasomotor instability of the involved upper extremity.

PATHOPHYSIOLOGY

Shoulder-hand syndrome has been associated with lesions of the premotor area of the brain. The etiology of shoulder-hand syndrome is unknown; the sympathetic nervous system has often been implicated, largely because of the associated vasomotor changes. Theoretical peripheral and central etiologies have been proposed. Peripheral etiologic theories suggest trauma to the peripheral nerves. One of these theories postulates ephaptic conduction between efferent sympathetic nerves and afferent somatic nerves with depolarization of the latter being perceived as pain. Numerous central etiologic theories have also been proposed. For example, it has been postulated that there is a disruptive autonomic nervous control from higher central nervous system (CNS) centers, which directly affect the internuncial pool of the spinal cord with decreased inhibition of the sympathetic neurons of the lateral horn. Pain, either from contractures or shoulder subluxation, may stimulate the internuncial pool of the spinal cord resulting in an abnormal sympathetic response.

CLINICAL DIAGNOSIS

Shoulder-hand syndrome generally presents initially with pain in the shoulder followed by a painful, edematous hand and wrist. Frequently, there is decreased range of motion at the shoulder and hand while the elbow joint is spared.[14] Passive

TABLE 2.   Clinical Criteria for Reflex Sympathetic Dystrophy (RSD)

Diagnosis	Criteria
Definite RSD	Pain in an extremity
	Vasomotor instability
	Edematous extremity
	Dystrophic skin changes
Probable RSD	Pain and tenderness in an extremity
	Vasomotor instability
	Extremity swelling
Possible RSD	Vasomotor instability
	Edematous extremity

Adapted from Kozin F, Genant HK, Bekerman C, McCarty DJ: The reflex sympathetic dystrophy syndrome. II. Roentgenographic and scintigraphic evidence of bilaterality and of periarticular accentuation. Am J Med 60:332–338, 1976; Kozin F, Ryan LM, Carrera GF, et al: The reflex sympathetic dystrophy syndrome (RSDS). III. Scintigraphic studies, further evidence for the therapeutic efficacy of systemic corticosteroids, and proposed diagnostic criteria. Am J Med 70:23–30, 1981; and Kozin F: Two unique shoulder disorders: Adhesive capsulitis and reflex sympathetic dystrophy syndrome. Postgrad Med 73:207–216, 1983.

flexion of the wrist, metacarpophalangeal (MCP) joints, and proximal interphalangeal (PIP) joints is painful and limited because of edema over the dorsum of the fingers. As time progresses, the extensor tendons become elevated, and collateral ligaments shorten. If untreated, it is thought that shoulder-hand syndrome will usually eventually progress to a dry, cold, bluish, and atrophied hand. The pain may resolve spontaneously after several weeks.

Kozin proposed clinical criteria to assist in the diagnosis of RSD (Table 2).[30] Other authors insist that only allodynia (pain resulting from nonnoxious stimuli) and hyperalgesia (increased sensitivity to noxious stimuli) need be present to diagnose RSD.[45] Shoulder-hand syndrome usually presents within 3 months and rarely later than 5 months after the patient suffers a stroke.[14] The clinical presentation of RSD remains highly variable.[27–29,44]

DIAGNOSTIC TESTS

Routine radiographs of the involved upper extremity may demonstrate a patchy, periarticular demineralization (Sudeck's atrophy) as early as 3–6 months after the onset of clinical signs. The most sensitive diagnostic test is the technetium diphosphonate bone scan, which demonstrates increased periarticular uptake (mostly at the shoulder and wrist) in the affected upper extremity. Bone scan abnormalities appear earlier than the x-ray changes. Tepperman et al. found 25% of hemiplegic patients demonstrated evidence of RSD in the involved upper extremity although only two thirds went on to develop the clinical syndrome.[46] Temporary resolution of symptoms with sympathetic blockade is considered diagnostic despite potential difficulties with the technique in terms of diagnostic validity. Thermography, in controlled studies, has failed to consistently diagnose RSD and is not considered a valid test.

TREATMENT OF SHOULDER-HAND SYNDROME

Prevention of shoulder problems and aggressive early treatment are recommended to prevent the development of a nonfunctional painful upper extremity. The various treatment options are outlined in Table 3. Therapy consists of vigorous physiotherapy with a focus on range of motion exercises. A 1–2-week course of high-dose corticosteroids or sympathetic blocks either in the form of stellate ganglion

TABLE 3. Treatments for Shoulder-Hand Syndrome

Prevention • Extremely early range of motion exercises • Avoid shoulder subluxation	**Splints** • Resting splint of hand and wrist (controversial)
Exercise • Prevention and treatment of upper extremity contractures • Active exercise if possible • Frequent passive range of motion	**Medication** • Analgesics • Nonsteroidal anti-inflammatory drugs • High-dose oral corticosteroids (10-day course and then taper)
Modalities • Interferential deep heat therapy • Heat/cold modalities especially contrast baths • Hand desensitization program • Transcutaneous electrical nerve stimulation	**Injections** • Stellate ganglion sympathetic block • Guanethidine block **Surgical** • Sympathectomy

blocks or guanethidine local venous blocks may be tried in persistent disabling cases. A surgical sympathectomy may be considered if stellate ganglion sympathetic blocks are consistently effective but symptoms recur. There is no definitive therapeutic intervention for RSD, a point that is reflected by the large number of suggested treatments. Shoulder-hand syndrome that presents longer than 6 months without appropriate treatment has a poor prognosis.[32]

MANAGEMENT OF THE PAINFUL HEMIPLEGIC SHOULDER

Management of the painful hemiplegic shoulder is difficult, and response to treatment is frequently unsatisfactory.[40] Early passive shoulder range of motion is an important prophylactic treatment. Supporting and protecting the involved shoulder in the initial flaccid stage is also regarded as important. Treatment involves analgesics, nonsteroidal anti-inflammatory drugs (NSAIDs), physical modalities (local heat and cold), transcutaneous electrical nerve stimulation, and local steroid injections. Surgical procedures are rarely used.

Positioning

Carr and Kenney did an extensive review on positioning the stroke patient.[9] It is generally agreed that the affected upper extremity should be placed in various positions such as having the shoulder protracted, arm brought forward, spine straight, and fingers extended. Controversy still surrounds the degree of positioning of the arm in the forward position while in the sitting and lying postures. In particular, the numbers and height of the pillows to be used for positioning were not consistent from one study to another.

Slings

Arm slings are often used in the initial stages following a stroke, but they do have some disadvantages. They encourage flexor synergies, inhibit arm swing, contribute to contracture formation, and decrease body image causing the patient to further avoid using that arm. However, a sling remains the best method of supporting the flaccid hemiplegic arm while the patient is standing or transferring.

Zorowitz et al. measured the ability of four ambulatory shoulder supports to correct shoulder subluxation in stroke patients during their acute inpatient rehabilitation.[48] The four supports tested were the single-strap hemi-sling, the Bobath roll, the Rolyan humeral cuff sling, and the Cavalier support. The single-strap hemi-sling significantly eliminated the vertical asymmetry of subluxation. The Rolyan humeral cuff sling significantly reduced total subluxation asymmetry. The authors concluded that, "any of the supports tested, except the Cavalier support, may correct the vertical asymmetry of glenohumeral subluxation but that only the single-strap hemi-sling corrects vertical asymmetry to any significant degree. Lateral displacement of the humeral head does not appear to result from the subluxation itself but may be caused by application of supports such as the Bobath role or Cavalier support. Total asymmetry is significantly reduced only with the use of the Rolyan humeral cuff sling."[48]

As tone returns to the shoulder muscles, the risk of shoulder subluxation decreases and slings can then be withdrawn. Slings tend to accentuate the adduction and internal rotation posture and may contribute to shortening of tonically active muscles. There is as yet no definitive evidence that slings prevent or reduce long-term shoulder subluxation and its potential consequences.

Pulleys and Overaggressive Therapy

Kumar et al. analyzed 28 hemiplegic patients who met study criteria and who were randomly assigned to one of three exercise groups.[31] Pain developed in 8% of patients who underwent range of motion by a therapist, in 12% of the group that used a skateboard, and in 62% of the overhead pulley group (p = 0.014). The three groups did not differ in terms of the side of involvement (p = 0.57), extent of hemiplegia (p = 0.25), or presence of subluxation (p = 0.84). The authors concluded that use of the overhead pulley had the highest risk of developing shoulder pain and should be avoided during rehabilitation of stroke patients.[31]

Injections

As mentioned earlier, Joynt conducted a study of 67 stroke patients diagnosed with hemiplegic shoulder pain.[24] Twenty-eight received a subacromial injection of 1% lidocaine. Of these 28, approximately 50% obtained moderate or marked relief of pain and improved range of motion. However, the study was neither controlled nor blinded.

Motor Blocks and Surgery as Treatment for Muscle Imbalance

Hecht described 13 patients with spastic hemiplegia, limited range of motion, and painful shoulders who had percutaneous phenol nerve blocks applied to the nerves supplying the subscapularis muscle.[20] Patients' ages ranged from 22–76 years (mean 46 years), and the duration of hemiplegia ranged from 2–13 months. Immediate and significant (p < 0.01) improvements in range of motion were observed in abduction (21°), flexion (40°), and external rotation (38°). Relief of pain was also noted with the previously painful movement.[20]

Caldwell et al. eliminated internal rotation and adduction forces by surgically transecting the subscapularis and pectoralis tendons in 13 patients who presented with pain, limited range of motion, and spasticity.[8] Marked increases in range of motion with reductions in pain were reported in 10 patients—with 4 developing active abduction in the postoperative period. No dislocations occurred. A subsequent follow-up study of 50 patients who were similarly treated showed improvement in 88%.[6]

Hecht noted that some patients needed blocks to both the subscapularis and the pectoralis muscles.[21] "Botulinum toxin can be used instead of phenol when the patient cannot tolerate phenol, when sensation is so spared that phenol injection is too painful, when the physician is more comfortable with localizing motor points using that technique, and when a slower onset of shorter duration of action is desired."[21] A prospective review was conducted of 20 patients who either had both a subscapular or a pectoralis major block or had such a good response to the first block that the second block was not felt to be necessary. Eighty-five percent benefited from the subscapularis block, 55% benefited from pectoralis major block, and 45% demonstrated improved active range of motion following the block.[21]

CONCLUSION

Hemiplegia is a common sequela of stroke, and a painful hemiplegic shoulder frequently develops as a consequence. The majority of these problems have their origins in the spasticity and sustained postures that are characteristic of the hemiplegic upper extremity. Shoulder subluxation does not appear to cause pain, but spastic muscle imbalance, particularly sustained internal rotation due to a hyperactive subscapularis muscle, appears to be highly correlated with the development of hemiplegic shoulder pain. The painful hemiplegic shoulder can add significantly to the patient's overall level of disability and may be at least partially avoided with therapeutic intervention. However, once established, this problem can be very difficult to treat.

REFERENCES

1. Basmajian JV, Bazant FJ: Factors preventing downward dislocation of adducted shoulder joint: Electromyographic and morphological study. J Bone Joint Surg 41A:1182–1186, 1959.
2. Bloch R, Bayer N: Prognosis in stroke. Clin Orthop 131:10–14, 1978.
3. Bohannon RW, Larkin PA, Smith MB, Horton MG: Shoulder pain in hemiplegia: Statistical relationship with five variables. Arch Phys Med Rehabil 67:514–516, 1986.
4. Bohannon RW, Andrews AW: Shoulder subluxation and pain in stroke patients. Am J Occup Ther 44:507–509, 1990.
5. Boyd EA: Clinical measures of shoulder subluxation: Their reliability. Can J Public Health 83(suppl 2):524–528, 1992.
6. Braun RM, West F, Mooney V, et al: Surgical treatment of the painful shoulder contracture in the stroke patient. J Bone Joint Surg 53A:1307–1312, 1971.
7. Cailliet R: The Shoulder in Hemiplegia. Philadelphia, FA Davis, 1980.
8. Caldwell CB, Wilson DJ, Brown RM: Evaluation and treatment of the upper extremity in the hemiplegic stroke patient. Clin Orthop 63:69–93, 1969.
9. Carr EK, Kenney FD: Positioning of the stroke patient: A review of the literature. Int J Nurs Stud 29:355–369, 1992.
10. Chaco J, Wolf E: Subluxation of the glenohumeral joint in hemiplegia. Am J Phys Med Rehabil 50:139–143, 1971.
11. Chu DS, Petrillo C, Davis SW, Eichberg R: Shoulder-hand syndrome: Importance of early diagnosis and treatment. J Am Ger Soc 29:58–60, 1981.
12. Codman EA: The Shoulder. Boston, Thomas Todd Co, 1934.
13. Cole TM, Barry DT, Tobis JS: Measurement of musculoskeletal function. In Kottke FJ, Lehmann JF (eds): Krusen's Handbook of Physical Medicine and Rehabilitation. Philadelphia, WB Saunders, 1990, pp 20–71.
14. Davis SW, Pestrillo CR, Eischberg RD, Chu DS: Shoulder-hand syndrome in a hemiplegic population: A 5-year retrospective study. Arch Phys Med Rehabil 58:353–355, 1977.
15. Eto F, Yoshikawa M, Ueda S, Hirai S: Post-hemiplegic shoulder-hand syndrome with special reference to related cerebral localization. J Am Ger Soc 28:13–17, 1980.
16. Fitzgerald-Finch OP, Gibson II: Subluxation of the shoulder in hemiplegia. Age Ageing 4:16–18, 1975.
17. Fugl-Meyer AR, Jaasko L, Leyman I, et al: The post-stroke hemiplegic patient. I. A method for evaluation of physical performance. Scand J Rehabil Med 7:13–31, 1975.
18. Grossens-Sills J, Schenkman M: Analysis of shoulder pain, range of motion, and subluxation in patients with hemiplegia. Phys Ther 65:731, 1985.
19. Hakuno A, Sashika H, Ohkawa T, Itoh R: Arthrographic findings in hemiplegic shoulders. Arch Phys Med Rehabil 65:706–711, 1984.
20. Hecht JS: Subscapular nerve block in the painful hemiplegic shoulder. Arch Phys Med Rehabil 73:1036–1039, 1992.
21. Hecht JS: The role of spasticity in hemiplegic shoulder pain and what to do about it. Presented at the 57th Annual Assembly of the American Academy of Physical Medicine and Rehabilitation, Orlando, FL, November 17, 1995.

22. Hollinshead WH, Jenkins DB: Functional Anatomy of the Limbs and Back. Philadelphia, WB Saunders, 1981.
23. Inaba MK, Piorkowski M: Ultrasound in treatment of painful shoulder in patients with hemiplegia. J Phys Ther 52:737–741, 1972.
24. Joynt RL: The source of shoulder pain in hemiplegia. Arch Phys Med Rehabil 73:409–413, 1992.
25. Kaplan PE, Meredith J, Taft G, Betts HB: Stroke and brachial plexus injury: A difficult problem. Arch Phys Med Rehabil 38:415–418, 1977.
26. Kingery WS, Date ES, Bobobo CR: The absence of brachial plexus injury in stroke. Am J Phys Med Rehabil 72:127–175, 1993.
27. Kozin F, McCarty DJ, Sims J, Genant HK: The reflex sympathetic dystrophy syndrome. I. Clinical and histologic studies: Evidence for bilaterality, response to corticosteroids and articular involvement. Am J Med 60:321–331, 1976.
28. Kozin F, Genant HK, Bekerman C, McCarty DJ: The reflex sympathetic dystrophy syndrome. II. Roentgenographic and scintigraphic evidence of bilaterality and of periarticular accentuation. Am J Med 60:332–338, 1976.
29. Kozin F, Ryan LM, Carrera GF, et al: The reflex sympathetic dystrophy syndrome (RSDS). III. Scintigraphic studies, further evidence for the therapeutic efficacy of systemic corticosteroids, and proposed diagnostic criteria. Am J Med 70:23–30, 1981.
30. Kozin F: Two unique shoulder disorders: Adhesive capsulitis and reflex sympathetic dystrophy syndrome. Postgrad Med 73:207–216, 1983.
31. Kumar R, Metter EJ, Mehta AJ, Chew T: Shoulder pain in hemiplegia. The role of exercise. Am J Phys Med Rehabil 69:205–208, 1990.
32. Lieberman JS: Hemiplegia: Rehabilitation of the upper extremity. In Kaplan PE, Cerullo LJ (eds): Stroke Rehabilitation. Stoneman, MA, Butterworth Publishers, 1986, pp 95–117.
33. Moskowitz E: Complications in the rehabilitation of hemiplegic patients. Med Clin North Am 53:541–559, 1969.
34. Moskowitz E, Goodman CR, Smith E, et al: Hemiplegic shoulder. N Y State J Med 69:548–550, 1969.
35. Najenson T, Yacubovich E, Pikelini S: Rotator cuff injury in hemiplegic patients. Scand J Rehabil Med 3:131–137, 1971.
36. Nepomuceno CS, Miller JM III: Shoulder arthrography in hemiplegic patients. Arch Phys Med Rehabil 55:49–51, 1974.
37. Perrigot M, Bussel B, Pierrot Deseilligny E, Held JP: L'epaule de l'hemiplegique. Ann Med Phys 18:175–187, 1975.
38. Poduri KR: Shoulder pain in stroke patients and its effect on rehabilitation. J Stroke Cerebrovasc Dis 3:261–266, 1993.
39. Prevost R, Arsenault AB, Dutil E, Drouin G: Rotation of the scapular and shoulder subluxation in hemiplegia. Arch Phys Med Rehabil 68:786–790, 1987.
40. Risk TE, Christopher RP, Pinals RS, et al: Arthrographic studies in painful hemiplegic shoulders. Arch Phys Med Rehabil 65:254–255, 1984.
41. Savage R, Robertson L: Relationship between adult hemiplegic shoulder pain and depression. Physiotherapy Can 34:86–90, 1982.
42. Shahani BT, Kelly EB, Glasser S: Hemiplegic shoulder subluxation [abstract]. Arch Phys Med Rehabil 62:519, 1981.
43. Shai G, Ring H, Costeff H, Solzi P: Glenohumeral malalignment in hemiplegic shoulder. Scand J Rehabil Med 16:133–136, 1984.
44. Steinbrocker D: Shoulder-hand syndrome: Present perspective. Arch Phys Med Rehabil 49:388–395, 1968.
45. Tahmoush AJ: Causalgia: Redefinition as a clinical pain syndrome. Pain 10:187–197, 1981.
46. Tepperman PS, Greyson ND, Hilbert L, et al: Reflex sympathetic dystrophy in hemiplegia. Arch Phys Med Rehabil 65:442–447, 1984.
47. Van Ouwenwaller C, Laplace PM, Chantraine A: Painful shoulder in hemiplegia. Arch Phys Med Rehabil 67:23–26, 1986.
48. Zorowitz RD, Idank D, Ikai T, et al: Shoulder subluxation after stroke: A comparison of four supports. Arch Phys Med Rehabil 76:763–771, 1995.

J. B. ORANGE, PhD
ANDREW KERTESZ, MD, FRCPC

EFFICACY OF LANGUAGE THERAPY FOR APHASIA

From the School of Communication
  Sciences and Disorders (JBO)
  and
Department of Clinical Neurological
  Sciences (AK)
University of Western Ontario
London, Ontario
Canada

Reprint requests to:
J. B. Orange, PhD
School of Communication Sciences
  and Disorders
University of Western Ontario
London, Ontario N6G 1H1
Canada

The question of whether language therapy is useful for individuals with aphasia has been debated for several decades. There are long-standing controversies about whether therapy for individuals with aphasia helps the recovery of language beyond levels achieved spontaneously after brain injury. Other questions remain as to which language-based treatments are more effective than others and whether language therapy provided by speech-language pathologists is of greater benefit than therapy provided by trained and untrained volunteers. Despite these controversies and questions, there is a considerable body of literature that addresses the overall utility of language therapy for aphasia. A smaller collection of research explores the differential effects of various types of language-based interventions for individuals with aphasia. This chapter provides an overview of the studies that examine the usefulness of language therapy for aphasia. The discussion first informs readers about different levels of usefulness (i.e., efficacy, effectiveness, efficiency) and then addresses several important methodologic challenges of conducting studies on the efficacy of language therapy for aphasia. A summary of findings from selected studies is presented. Prognostic factors for recovery of language also are presented, which may help clinicians make informed decisions about referrals of individuals with aphasia to speech-language pathologists for language assessment and therapy. The chapter concludes with a discussion of issues for future research on efficacy studies of language therapy for individuals with aphasia.

APHASIA

Definitions of aphasia have evolved over the past 150 years. Early conceptualizations were that aphasia resulted from impairment of localized, discrete, and interconnected neural centers responsible for discrete language functions. Early 20th century perspectives stressed the cognitive underpinnings of the language impairments. More current views focus on cognitive, neurolinguistic, and psycholinguistic modular- and process-oriented disruptions of language. Aphasia is generally described as an impairment of language as a result of focal brain damage to the language dominant cerebral hemisphere.[19] Some researchers believe that language is lost rather than impaired,[9] suggesting that language is best recovered by relearning the rule-based systems of language, including grammar, syntax, phonology, and semantics. Kertesz[38] clinically described aphasia as a ". . . neurologically central disturbance of language characterized by paraphasias, word finding difficulty, and variably impaired comprehension, associated with disturbance of reading and writing, at times with dysarthria, non-verbal constructional, and problem-solving difficulty and impairment of gesture."[38] The following definition of aphasia proposed by McNeil is a comprehensive conceptualization:

> Aphasia is a multimodality physiological inefficiency with, greater than loss of, verbal symbolic manipulations (e.g., association, storage, retrieval, and rule implementation). In isolated form it is caused by focal damage to cortical and/or subcortical structures of the hemisphere(s) dominant for such symbolic manipulations. It is affected by and affects other physiological, information processing, and cognitive processes to the degree that they support, interact with, or are supported by the symbolic deficits.[50]

The language impairment of aphasia is distinct from the language and cognitive-communication problems associated with nonlanguage dominant hemisphere damage,[80] dementia,[54] and traumatic brain injury.[84] Widespread use of the term *aphasia* in its broadest denotation—of language impairments following brain injury—is common among physicians and some health care professions[2,17] but is not always accepted by speech-language pathologists.[8] Determining a suitable definition of aphasia is not a moot academic exercise. Au and colleagues note, "How one defines aphasia determines how it should be studied."[2] The conceptualizations of aphasia have important bearing on the design, methodology, analyses, and interpretations of findings from studies on the usefulness of language therapy for aphasia. A detailed discussion of the relative merits of the different conceptualizations and descriptions of aphasia is beyond the scope of this chapter. Readers should be cognizant, however, of the sometimes disparate views of aphasia and how the different definitions may influence interpretations of findings from studies of the efficacy of language therapy for aphasia in general, or of specific language interventions.

Efficacy, Effectiveness, and Efficiency

Before discussing efficacy studies of language therapy, a clarification of terminology is warranted. The term *efficacy* is often used to describe whether a particular therapeutic intervention works. Efficacy refers to the proven effects of treatment or changes (usually statistically significant) in performance.[11,58] A widely accepted definition of efficacy is, "The extent to which a specific intervention, procedure, regimen or service produces a beneficial result under ideal conditions. Ideally, the determination of efficacy is based on the results of a Randomized Control Trial."[42]

Effectiveness, on the other hand, is "a measure of the extent to which a specific intervention, procedure, regimen or service, when deployed in the field in routine circumstances, does what it is intended to do for a specified population."[42] Measures of treatment effectiveness reflect actual changes in behavior or performance. That is, effectiveness refers to functional, meaningful, and clinically significant changes. Research trials that show treatment effectiveness generally lack the rigorous designs and methodologic criteria of a randomized clinical (control) trial (RCT) but nonetheless often provide evidence that the intervention has a positive influence on a person's performance in daily life. The functional effects would be observable and measurable in terms of the individual's disability (i.e., functional consequence of an impairment) and handicap (i.e., social consequences of an impairment or disability).[93]

The final term, *efficiency*, is defined by Last as "the effects or end results achieved in relation to the effort expended in terms of money, resources, and time. The extent to which the resources used to provide a specific intervention, procedure, regimen or service of known efficacy and effectiveness are minimized. A measure of the economy (or cost in resources) with which a procedure of known efficacy and effectiveness is carried out."[43] Measures of the efficiency of language therapy for aphasia, for example, would show which of two or more therapeutic approaches works best or whether services provided by a speech-language pathologist are more efficient than services provided by family or trained volunteers.

The literature on the usefulness of language therapy for individuals with aphasia is composed primarily of effectiveness and efficiency studies that span the past 35 years, but works appear sporadically from the 1920s to the 1960s.[67] Numerous large, medium, and small group investigations, case studies, and well-controlled single-subject experiments show the positive benefits of language therapy on recovery profiles.[29] Several studies that closely resemble an RCT protocol provide unequivocal evidence for the efficiency of language therapy for different severity levels and types of therapy.[21,48,73,89,90] More recently, investigators have published effectiveness studies showing improvement in everyday communication skills[4] and studies showing the efficiency of different therapy approaches, such as melodic intonation therapy[74] and the usefulness of computers on language recovery.[34] The interest in effectiveness studies has evolved only over the past 15 years due to focused interest in discourse (i.e., two or more connected sentences) and functional communication (i.e., everyday communication such as conversation), and a concomitant development of sophisticated models of discourse processing and functional communication. The number of published efficacy, effectiveness, and efficiency studies, however, is surprisingly low considering the surge in interest in determining the usefulness of language therapy for individuals with aphasia during the late 1970s and throughout the 1980s and the renewed interest in the mid 1990s.

Methodologic Challenges

Conducting efficacy, effectiveness, and efficiency trials is a complex process requiring the simultaneous control of several crucial factors. The low number of studies to date is due largely to design and methodology challenges such as controlling numerous subject variables and spontaneous recovery, defining a control group, specifying the nature of the treatment, and the lack of standardized measures for functional communication.[67]

Numerous criteria must be taken into account when selecting subjects with aphasia for an efficacy study (Table 1). Individuals with aphasia are a heterogeneous group whose language profiles differ based on factors such as cause, time since onset, type, severity level, and size and site of lesion. Kertesz and McCabe, for example, showed that the type of aphasia changes over the course of recovery.[41] Thus,

TABLE 1.   Selection Criteria for Efficacy Studies of Patients with Aphasia

Age (at present and at onset)

Sex

Handedness

Education level (years of formal school and consideration for employment-related experiences)

Socioeconomic status

Premorbid primary language proficiency (and in other spoken and written languages)

Etiology (occlusive versus hemorrhagic stroke, tumor, infection, trauma)

First or previous aphasia-related etiologies

Time postonset

Site(s) and size of lesion

Severity of language impairment

Sensory status (hearing and vision problems)

Associated medical, neurologic, and psychiatric conditions (e.g., diabetes, Parkinson's disease, apraxia, depression)

Adapted from Rosenbek JC, LaPointe LL, Wertz RT: Aphasia: A Clinical Approach. Austin, TX, ProEd, 1989.

it is impossible to hold constant the type of aphasia over the total period of the efficacy study. Conducting an efficacy trial requires that independent variables such as those in Table 1 must be controlled for and matched in a corresponding group to ensure that the measured changes in the dependent variables are due to the therapeutic interventions and not to spurious effects from uncontrolled subject characteristics or changes in aphasia classification.

The time at which language treatment is initiated after onset is an important consideration in determining the efficacy of the intervention. Spontaneous recovery refers to the improvements in language without therapy that may occur up to 6 months or longer following brain injury;[13] most spontaneous recovery is believed to occur within the first 3 months.[41] Using a control group that does not receive language therapy is the most effective way to account for spontaneous recovery but does create ethical objections related to withholding treatment during a critical period. Shewan and Kertesz measured differences in performance in the treatment and control groups (i.e., control subjects self-selected not to receive therapy) during and after most of the spontaneous recovery had occurred; however, their control group was not randomized.[73] Wertz et al. coped with the ethical problems of control groups by studying treated and randomized control patients after the effects of spontaneous recovery are presumed to be over (i.e., 3–6 months following onset),[89] and by deferring treatment.[90]

One of the single most contentious issues in the research on efficacy of language therapy for aphasia is establishing a control group wherein random assignment to treated and untreated groups occurs immediately after onset. The random assignment of subjects to treated and untreated groups is one of the features of an RCT, the gold standard by which scientists measure the efficacy of therapeutic interventions. However, it is considered ethically unacceptable to assign subjects randomly to a no-treatment group when doing so may jeopardize their recovery. The approach adopted by Shewan and Kertesz did not include randomized controls, and Wertz et al. did not study treatment in the early stages of spontaneous recovery.[73,89] One of the studies that used randomized controls after onset has been criticized for mixing etiologies and providing treatment for less than 2 hours per week.[44] At present, only Wertz et al.[90] have successfully resolved the issue of using a randomized control group to the satisfaction of aphasiologists.

Approaches to treating aphasia include language-oriented therapy,[72] melodic intonation therapy,[74] and simulation approaches.[70] Other variations include whether therapy is provided in a group or individual setting, by a speech-language pathologist or a trained volunteer, and how often therapy is provided. Holland and Wertz noted that all language therapies for aphasia are not equal.[32] Many of the efficacy studies on language therapy for aphasia have not controlled the type or degree of treatment very well or clearly defined the nature of treatments, leaving unanswered questions regarding the methodology and the final interpretation of findings.

A more recent methodologic challenge concerning the effectiveness of language therapy and aphasia is the relative dearth of standardized measures of functional communication. None of the current commonly used standardized language batteries, such as the Western Aphasia Battery[39] or the Boston Diagnostic Aphasia Examination,[24] were designed to measure functional communication. Two measures of functional communication standardized for individuals with aphasia include the Communication Activities of Daily Living (CADL)[28] and the recently published American Speech-Language-Hearing Association's Functional Assessment of Communication Skills for Adults,[23] but both have limitations with external validity. CADL is undergoing revision to make it more comprehensive and valid. Several nonstandardized questionnaires and checklists exist that address everyday language and communication performances of individuals with aphasia. Examples include the Functional Communication Profile,[69] the Communicative Effectiveness Index,[45] the Pragmatic Protocol,[63] and the Profile of Communicative Appropriateness.[59] The utility of these measures in efficacy studies is limited by the lack of a standardized protocol of administration and scoring and a lack of psychometric properties. Researchers in language efficacy and aphasia are left with few standardized measures of functional communication other than observational outcomes to document changes in performance.

USEFULNESS OF LANGUAGE THERAPY

Several comprehensive reviews of the efficacy, effectiveness, and efficiency of language therapy for aphasia have appeared in the literature over the past 15 years.[22,29,31,58,65,66,71,87,88] Many of the reviews provide a temporally based summary of studies describing good and bad designs, interpreting positive and negative findings, and critiquing subject selection criteria, outcome measures, and other methodologic issues. Most reviews have been qualitative narrative summaries wherein each of the authors has concluded that therapy is beneficial despite mixed findings from a few studies and no effects from a minority of others. More recently, meta-analyses by Robey[65,66] and, to a lesser extent, the meta-analysis by Whurr, Lorch, and Nye[92] provide empirical evidence of the positive effects of language therapy for individuals with aphasia. Robey, Whurr et al., and other reviewers uncovered hundreds of large, moderate, and small group studies, case studies, and single-subject trials. The meta-analysis selection criteria used by Robey and by Whurr et al. reduced the number of studies they analyzed down to 21,[65] 45,[92] and 55.[66] The following section discusses findings from selected efficacy, effectiveness, and efficiency studies, including an overview of the results from Robey's meta-analyses.

Efficacy Studies

Most efficacy studies on language therapy for aphasia involve group studies in which large groups of subjects (60 or more), moderate sized groups (10–60), or

TABLE 2. Summary of Selected Group Efficacy Studies of Language Therapy and Aphasia

Study	Sample Size	Aphasia Types	Treatment Type	Outcome
Vignolo[83]	68	Several types	Traditional language therapy based on Schuell et al.'s (1964) stimulation approach, minimum of 1 session per week to 20 sessions in 40 days	No significant difference between treated versus untreated groups; group treated earlier (prior to 6 mo postonset) and longer (for more than 6 mo) better performance than group treated later and for shorter periods
Sarno et al.[68]	31	Severe global aphasia	3 nonrandomized groups; programmed therapy group from 3–144 mo (Schuell et al.'s stimulation therapy); nonprogrammed therapy group from 3–72 mo (social interaction); no-treatment group followed 18–72 mo	No significant differences between treated versus untreated groups
Basso et al.[7]	281	239 strokes: 137 acute (< 2 mo postonset); 86 subacute (2–6 mo); 58 chronic (> 6 mo)	162 received traditional stimulation therapy at least 3 times/week for not less than 5 mo; 119 untreated controls (not randomly assigned)	Significantly greater number of treated subjects improved versus untreated; earlier treated group (acute) improved significantly more than chronic treated group; weak inverse relationship between age and improvement
Lincoln et al.[44]	191	Unilateral and bilateral, single and multiple strokes, brain tumors, dementia	Type not reported; random assignment to treated group and untreated controls; treatment twice/week for 24 weeks	No significant differences in improvement between treated and untreated groups
Shewan and Kertesz[71]	100	Occlusive or stable hemorrhagic stroke; global Broca's, Wernicke's, anomic, and conduction; all 2–4 weeks postonset for assessment and < 7 weeks for therapy	Random assignment to treatment groups but self-selected to control group; therapy 3 hr/week until recovered or 12 mo; 1 group received language-oriented therapy; 1 group stimulation-facilitation therapy; 1 group stimulation therapy by nurse; 1 group untreated controls	SLP-treated groups significantly improved compared to controls; nurse-treated group approached significance

Table continued on next page

small groups (< 10) participated.[29] Several of the group studies include control subjects based on true random assignment to treated and untreated groups, control subjects on waiting lists, or control subjects who are unavailable for treatment (i.e., self-selected no treatment. Table 2 summarizes representative findings from frequently cited group efficacy studies. These studies illustrate the range of designs,

TABLE 2 (Cont).   Summary of Selected Group Efficacy Studies of Language Therapy
and Aphasia

Study	Sample Size	Aphasia Types	Treatment Type	Outcome
Wertz et al.[90]	121	Several types; well-controlled selection criteria with single occlusive infarct	Subjects randomly assigned; 1 group received stimulation and stimulus-response therapy by SLPs for 8–10 hr/week for 12 weeks followed by 12 weeks no therapy; 1 group received home treatment by trained volunteer 8–10/week for 12 weeks followed by 12 weeks no treatment; 1 group deferred therapy for 12 weeks followed by 12 weeks stimulation and stimulus-response therapy by SLPs	Therapy–no therapy group significantly better at 12 weeks than deferred therapy group after 12 weeks of no therapy but no significant difference at 24 weeks; deferred therapy group improved following 12 weeks of therapy; no significant differences between SLP and volunteer therapy groups at 12 weeks
Poeck et al.[62]	68	All vascular in origin; global, Wernicke's, Broca's, amnesic, and nonclassifiable	1 early group received early therapy 1–4 mo postonset; 1 late group received therapy 4–12 mo postonset; 1 chronic group received therapy 12 or more mo postonset; each therapy period lasted 6–8 weeks with 9 60-min sessions/week; LOT therapy provided	Improvements observed in over 75% of early group, nearly 50% of late group, and 68% of chronic group compared to controls from other centers showing less improvement in early periods
Mazzoni et al.[49]	26	All vascular; strict selection criteria; moderate and severe Wernicke's, Broca's, conduction, global	13 subjects assigned to structured systematic language therapy for 45-min sessions 6 times/week for 3 months then reduced to 3–4 sessions/week at 4 mo for one third of subjects with great improvements for total of 7 mo; 13 self-selected no therapy	Therapy group significantly better than no therapy group for expressive and receptive language at 7 mo; fluent subjects who received therapy significantly more improved for expressive language at 7 mo than fluent subjects who did not receive therapy; significantly greater percentage of moderate subjects improved expressive language at 7 mo versus no therapy group

SLP = speech-language pathologist; LOT = language-oriented therapy
Adapted from Holland AL, Fromm DS, DeRuyter F, Stein M: Treatment efficacy: Aphasia. J Speech Hearing Res 39:S27–S36, 1996.

methodologies, and findings but do not represent an exhaustive survey of all published efficacy studies.

The overall finding from the efficacy group studies is that language therapy is more efficacious than no language therapy. Findings show that improvements in language performance are greater in individuals who receive treatment immediately following onset versus those whose treatment is delayed until after the spontaneous recovery period; however, individuals in the delayed treatment group can catch up if therapy is delivered over a longer time. The collective evidence indicates that individuals who suffer a single occlusive stroke, who are rated with mild to moderate impairment, and who are less than 6 months postonset are excellent candidates for language therapy.[7,62,73,89,90] Individuals who receive therapy at least 3 hours per week for 5 months[7] or 6 months,[67] 3 hours per week for 12 months,[73] 8 hours per week for 11 months,[89] or 18 hours per week for 12 months[25] will benefit more from language therapy than those who do not receive therapy.

The efficacy group studies are not unequivocally supportive of the positive effects of language therapy for aphasia. The only study using randomized controls, by Lincoln et al., found no significant differences in language between 104 randomly treated and 87 untreated individuals with aphasia of mixed etiologies (unilateral and bilateral, single and multiple strokes, brain tumors, dementia).[44] One of the major criticisms of Lincoln's[44] study, however, is that the subjects in the treated group received only 48 hours of general language stimulation—not language therapy—over 24 weeks. The limited amount of therapy, the ill-defined nature of the therapy, and the mixed etiologies and severity levels are often-cited design weaknesses. Sarno, Silverman, and Sands also found that chronic, severely aphasic individuals who receive language therapy from 7–46 hours over 4–36 weeks do not differ from control subjects who do not receive treatment, although their subjects were not randomly assigned.[68] On the other hand, Wertz et al. clearly showed the efficacy of the treatment over the randomized control group; the therapy for this randomized control group was deferred for 12 weeks, and the group caught up with the initially treated group at 24 weeks.[90]

Robey's meta-analysis of 21 studies on the efficacy of language therapy for aphasia revealed four important findings: (1) the performance of individuals who receive language therapy in the acute stage of recovery is nearly twice as large as the effect of spontaneous recovery alone; (2) language therapy initiated after spontaneous recovery has a positive, albeit small, effect on language performance; (3) a medium to large effect is present in comparisons of treated versus untreated individuals when therapy is begun in the acute phase; and (4) a small to medium effect is present in treated versus untreated groups when therapy is begun in the chronic stage of recovery (i.e., 6–12 months postonset).[65] Robey's more comprehensive meta-analysis of 55 studies confirmed the findings from his earlier work.[66] In addition, he observed that outcomes for treated versus untreated individuals are superior to those for untreated individuals at all severity levels. He also noted that more than 2 hours of language therapy per week achieves significantly greater gains than shorter amounts of therapy. Finally, he stated that large gains in performance are achieved by individuals with severe aphasia who are treated by speech-language pathologists. The findings of Robey and other recent investigators confirm that Darley's statement that "any all-conclusive statement about the efficacy of aphasia therapy would be ill-advised"[18] remains as true today as it did more than 25 years ago.

Effectiveness and Efficiency Studies

The past decade has seen such an exponential rise in the number of small group studies, case presentations, and single-subject trials showing the effectiveness and efficiency of language therapy for aphasia that they now vastly outnumber large and moderate-size group studies. The design of small group studies, case studies, and

TABLE 3. Summary of Selected Effectiveness and Efficiency Studies of Language Therapy and Aphasia

Study	Sample Size	Aphasia Types	Treatment Type	Outcome
Butfield and Zangwill[13]	70	14 head injury, 19 stroke, 37 tumors	Type not reported, range of sessions from 5–290	Language improved in half of group who received therapy within 6 mo post-onset; language improved in one third of group who received therapy after 6 mo postonset
Meikle et al.[53]	31 enrolled but results only from 29	Several types	16 subjects treated by SLPs using traditional stimulation and stimulus-response method; 15 subjects treated by teams of volunteers	No significant differences between SLP- versus volunteer-treated groups
Wertz et al.[89]	64	Several types; well-controlled-selection criteria with single occlusive infarct	Random assignment to individual treatment by SLPs for 8 hr/week for 44 weeks using stimulus-response or group therapy by SLP for 8 hr/week using	No significant differences between groups; both groups made significant improvements, with individual treatment group showing more improvements in selected areas
David et al.[20]	155 enrolled but only 96 completed full span of treatments	Several different types with multiple and heterogeneous etiologies	Random assignment of half of subjects to group treated by SLPs for about 30 hours in total; other half assigned randomly to group treated by untrained volunteers; treatments began 4–5 weeks postonset	Both groups improved but no significant differences between groups; indication that SLPs had better effect on subjects with severe aphasia than untrained volunteers

SLP = speech-language pathologist
Adapted from Holland AL, Fromm DS, DeRuyter F, Stein M: Treatment efficacy: Aphasia. J Speech Hearing Res 39:S27–S36, 1996.

single-subject trials limits, to some degree, the generalizability of their findings. Nonetheless, they form a sound body of work supporting the position that language interventions that target specific types of aphasia, particular severity levels, or single domains of language (e.g., word-finding problems in semantic domain, agrammatism in grammar domain) and functional communication (i.e., conversational performance in pragmatics domain) are more effective and efficient than no therapy. Moreover, they provide valuable information about the effects of specific types and qualities of therapies for subjects with certain types of aphasia. Tables 3 and 4 summarize selected effectiveness and efficiency studies, which represent examples of different designs, methodologies, and findings.

Several recent studies have documented the effects of different therapy approaches and different aphasia types on changes in functional communication.

TABLE 4.   Selected Citations of Recent Studies of the Effectiveness and
Efficiency of Language Therapy

Therapies for anomia	Therapies for computer use (cont.)
McNeil et al.[52]	Katz et al.[34]
Nickles and Best[56,57]	Petheram[61]
Thompson, Raymer, and le Grand[77]	Therapies for severe aphasia
Therapies for reading	Alexander and Loverso[1]
Bachy-Langedock and De Partz[5]	Colon and McNeil[15]
Kendall, McNeil, and Small[37]	Denes et al.[21]
Therapies for agrammatism	Therapies for mild aphasia
LeDorze, Jacob, and Coderre[43]	Marshall[47]
Thompson, Shapiro, and Roberts[78]	Penn, Jones and Joffe[60]
Thompson et al.[79]	Whitney and Goldstein[91]
Van De Sandt-Koenderman et al.[82]	Therapies for families
Therapies for groups	Hoen, Thelander and Worsley[27]
Avent[3]	Lyon et al.[46]
Bollinger, Musson and Holland[10]	Comparisons of different therapies
Brumfitt and Sheeran[12]	Carlomagno et al.[14]
Therapies for computer use	Hartman and Landau[26]
Crerar, Ellis and Dean[16]	Kearns and Yedor[36]
Katz and Wertz[33]	McNeil et al.[51]

Adapted from Holland AL, Fromm DS, DeRuyter F, Stein M: Treatment efficacy: Aphasia. J Speech
Hearing Res 39:S27–S36, 1996.

Springer and Willmes built on the findings of their earlier work to examine the differential effects of two different approaches for learning specific language structures.[75,76] Individuals with aphasia were taught the proper use of *wh-* questions and prepositions using a structured learning approach (i.e., traditional stimulus-response learning paradigm) and a stimulation approach (i.e., using auditory and prosodic cues such as intonation, hand tapping, and inflectional patterns in phrases). Twelve subjects with chronic Broca's and Wernicke's aphasia participated in a two-period cross-over design. The findings showed overall improvement in language performance irrespective of treatment method. In addition, the structured linguistic approach was more effective than the stimulation approach. However, the structured linguistic approach was more effective when preceded by the stimulation approach. Springer and Willmes observed that providing therapy tasks that stress the use of language structures in everyday situations before traditional language therapy helps to optimize learning and helps the use of specific language structures in individuals with chronic aphasia.[76]

Avent and Wertz investigated whether fluent or nonfluent aphasia and group or individual therapy influenced functional communication using data from Wertz et al.[4,89] Avent and Wertz studied the video recorded conversational performance of 10 fluent and 10 nonfluent individuals who were 48 weeks postonset. Subjects were assigned randomly to group treatment or individualized therapy. Group treatment (seven fluent and three nonfluent) and individualized therapy (three fluent and seven nonfluent) were provided by a speech-language pathologist for 6–8 hours per week for 44 weeks. All pre- and posttreatment evaluations were completed by speech-language pathologists who were blind to the treatment group assignment. Total improvement in functional communication was similar in the fluent and nonfluent groups at the end of the 44 weeks of therapy. No overall significant differences in functional communication were observed based on whether subjects received group or individual therapy. The only significant improvement occurred between weeks 4 and 15 of therapy, wherein the subjects who received group therapy made significantly more improvement than those who received individual therapy. This finding is not entirely surprising considering that group therapy focused on functional communication skills but individual therapy did not.

Recent work on the efficiency of language therapy has focused on determining the effects of different therapies for aphasia. For example, Murray and Holland compared the effects of conversational therapy to conversational therapy plus traditional didactic treatment on the expressive language and pragmatic skills of two pairs of subjects with acute aphasia (one pair with global aphasia and one pair with conduction aphasia).[55] Conversation therapy consisted of reinforcing any form of conversational interaction, such as taking turns, naming, and correcting misunderstandings in 15-minute daily sessions over an average of 14.5 days within the acute phase (the first 3 months). The traditional approach consisted of language stimulation approaches and stimulus-response tasks (e.g., picture naming) for at least 30 minutes each day over an average of 19.5 days. One subject in each pair received the conversational therapy only, and the other subject in the pair received the conversational therapy and the traditional approach. All subjects, regardless of therapy approach, showed improvement in language and pragmatic skills. During the acute phase of recovery after stroke, daily 15-minute conversation therapy sessions were found to be just as productive as daily 30-minute traditional language sessions plus 15 minutes of conversational therapy.

A long-standing controversial issue regarding the efficiency of language therapy for individuals with aphasia is whether therapy provided by speech-language pathologists is more efficient than therapy provided by volunteers. Several studies have compared the results of treatment by speech-language pathologists to the results of treatment by volunteers.[20,53,64,73] While all subjects who completed these trials showed significant improvements, no significant differences were observed according to whether a speech-language pathologist or volunteer provided the treatment. One of the negative outcomes from these studies, plus the influence of the findings of Lincoln et al.,[44] was a marked decrease in the provision of language therapy in Great Britain by speech-language pathologists for individuals with aphasia during the 1980s and early 1990s.[21a] These comparative studies also suffer from small sample sizes, lack of control groups, and concerns regarding statistical validity.[22] The large, well-controlled multicenter study by Marshall et al. also revealed no significant difference in improvement between individuals with aphasia treated by speech-language pathologists or by trained home volunteers.[48] They did observe that individuals treated by speech-language pathologists improved significantly more than individuals who did not receive treatment. However, like Wertz et al. and Shewan and Kertesz, Marshall et al. found no significant difference in performance in individuals who did not receive treatment and those whose treatment was provided by volunteers.[48,73,90]

Prognosis for Recovery

The equivocal and controversial findings from efficacy, effectiveness, and efficiency studies of aphasia continue to perplex researchers, clinicians, and patients and their families alike. Greater opportunities for large, multicenter trials, the emergence of robust single-subject study designs, and the recent development of standardized outcome measures of functional language and communication bode well for future studies. What remains problematic is determining the relative effects of combinations of factors that contribute to a positive recovery profile for individuals with

TABLE 5. Prognostic Factors and Recovery in Aphasia

Factor	Effect on Recovery
Size of lesion	Primary predictor of recovery; the larger the lesion, the poorer the recovery; interacts with site of lesion factor
Site of lesion	Primary predictor; poor recovery if cortical (e.g., Broca's and Wernicke's) and subcortical (e.g., thalamus, putamen, caudate nucleus) language areas infarcted
Initial severity	Primary factor of recovery
Etiology	Traumatic induced aphasia has better prognosis than vascular-based aphasia; occlusive stroke may have better prognosis than hemorrhagic stroke but opposite also possible; interaction with other factors such as size and site of lesion confound effects
Time postonset	Important factor; the earlier the intervention the greater potential for recovery; does interact with other factors such as size and site of lesion and initial severity
Aphasia type	Linked closely with initial severity; globals show poor recovery; Wernicke's and Broca's vary from fair to good recovery; anomic, conduction, and transcorticals generally have a good prognosis
Language domain	Mixed evidence for differential recovery of expressive (e.g., naming, grammar, writing) and receptive language skills; strong interaction with initial severity, type of aphasia, and size and site of lesion
Age	Conflicting evidence; not strong or important factor in recovery
Sex	Conflicting evidence; females may improve more than males on oral expression and auditory comprehension but evidence not firm
Handedness and hemispheric lateralization of language	Some evidence that left-handed and ambidextrous individuals may have better prognosis but not universally confirmed
Language therapy	Conflicting evidence but earlier intervention by speech-language pathologists in the acute postonset phase lasting through the chronic phase (6–18 mo postonset) results in better recovery than no language therapy
Other factors	Few effects on recovery of health status, premorbid intelligence, social support, level of education, occupational status, premorbid language proficiency

aphasia.[6,30,40,81] Table 5 summarizes selected prognostic factors that influence the recovery of individuals with aphasia. These factors can be used to help clinicians determine the prognosis for recovery and the suitability of referring individuals with aphasia to speech-language pathologists for language assessment and therapy. However, while we have some knowledge about the relative influence of single factors on recovery profiles, we know much less about how combinations of factors influence recovery. For example, the influence of size and site of lesion on recovery is well documented,[40] but less is known about how factors such as age, etiology, and time following onset interact with size and site of lesion to influence recovery. Further research aimed at uncovering the interactive effects of these factors is warranted.

CONCLUSIONS AND FUTURE CONSIDERATIONS

The literature on the efficacy, effectiveness, and efficiency of language therapy for aphasia has evolved over the past half century and has blossomed over the last quarter century. A definitive all-encompassing declaration that language therapy is efficacious for individuals with aphasia continues to elude researchers and clinicians,[18] but more recent work allows for carefully crafted, conditional statements. It is now agreed, although not without some controversy, that language therapy for individuals with aphasia is more efficacious than no therapy, especially when therapy begins in the acute phase of recovery. Additional empirically supported positions can be posited with some confidence about the effectiveness and efficiency of some types of therapy, when it is best to initiate therapy, and the types and severity levels of aphasia that may be more responsive to therapies. However, more needs to be learned about which types of therapy are best for particular profiles of language impairments and what aspects of therapy achieve the best outcomes.[31] Also less clear is the difference between the effects of language therapy provided by speech-language pathologists and the communication and socialization treatments provided by trained and untrained volunteers. The literature in this area is rife with serious design and methodologic flaws, making interpretations of findings difficult. Moreover, we still do not know which type of therapy is most efficient in acute aphasia and whether intervention in the acute phase is the most cost-effective use of resources, as suggested by Murray and Holland and by Wertz.[55,86] Therefore, where do aphasiologists and stroke rehabilitation specialists proceed based on current knowledge? One of the first steps is to ask questions about what constitutes efficacy, effectiveness, and efficiency from research and clinical perspectives. The terms *efficacy*, *effectiveness*, and *efficiency* have not been applied consistently and universally in the literature by aphasiologists. Clearer conceptualizations of what constitutes a positive meaningful outcome for patients, their caregivers, and their families will help advance our understanding of the effects of therapy on recovery.

Similarly, aphasiologists and stroke rehabilitation specialists need to reconceptualize their theoretical perspectives of how recovery may be occurring generally (e.g., reorganization of mental and linguistic processess versus relearning). Aphasiologists also need to develop new models of language recovery that can help answer questions about how language therapy may be remediating disordered language processes, facilitating their reorganization, or merely compensating for lost language skills. Models of language processing that have emerged over the past decade from the fields of cognitive psychology and cognitive neuropsychology provide a newer, different perspective on disorders of language and offer a framework within which to develop and test therapies that target specific language operations. The cognitive rehabilitation literature is replete with unique approaches on remediating reading disorders and naming problems for individuals with aphasia. The development of a new assessment tool, the Psycholinguistic Assessment of Language Processing in Aphasia (PALPA),[35] provides a hypothesis-driven test for assessing language and may aid in monitoring performance changes following targeted interventions. Despite its current lack of standardization, PALPA provides opportunities to help select treatment options and to help monitor their success rates.[85]

There also is a continuing need to pursue single-subject designs in effectiveness and efficiency studies of language therapy for aphasia.[67] Such studies provide a mechanism by which aphasiologists can observe detailed aspects of interventions that target specific language processes and language modalities. Although one cannot generalize findings from single-subject designs, these types of studies nonetheless offer opportunities to circumvent myriad confounding subject variables and control important factors that greatly influence recovery profiles. Most importantly, single-subject designs allow researchers and clinicians to monitor subtle performance changes over time and uncover nuances that might otherwise be lost in group studies where heterogeneity of performance and regression of data to the mean masks improvements.

The need to operationalize and describe in detail language therapies in future studies is paramount.[31] To date, there are large gaps in the descriptions of the therapies used in efficacy, effectiveness, and efficiency studies. Readers often come away with only a vague understanding of what was done in therapy, what stimulus materials were used, and when and how therapy was conducted. Future work must provide sufficient details about the nature of the therapy such that others can replicate the results.

Finally, there is a pressing need to develop clinically relevant and psychometrically valid outcome measures of the functional communication performance of individuals with aphasia. The lack of such measures at present hampers the evaluation of interventions that target everyday communication. Assessing the effectiveness and efficiency of therapies that target actual communication needs of individuals with aphasia is just as important a goal as validating a component of a model of language processing. Holland and Thompson stress the need for aphasiologists to develop measures that evaluate how the language problems of aphasia are reflected in an individual's ability to communicate functionally and, also, the nature and extent of how individuals with aphasia are able to participate fully in social and work-related activities.[31] Developing such measures would well serve individuals with aphasia, their families, an caregivers by offering greater opportunities to participate in meaningful therapy activities. Moreover, such measures would help advance our knowledge of the efficacy, effectiveness, and efficiency of functional communication interventions.

REFERENCES

1. Alexander MP, Loverso F: A specific treatment for global aphasia. Clin Aphasiol 21:277–289, 1993.
2. Au R, Albert MML, Obler LK: The relation of aphasia to dementia. Aphasiology 2:161–173, 1988.
3. Avent JR: Group treatment in aphasia using cooperative learning methods. J Med Speech Lang Pathol 5:9–26, 1997.
4. Avent JR, Wertz RT: Influence of type of aphasia and type of treatment on aphasic patients' pragmatic performance. Aphasiology 10:253–265, 1996.
5. Bachy-Langedock N, De Partz MP: Coordination of two reorganization therapies in a deep dyslexic patient with oral naming disorder. In Seron X, Deloche D (eds): Cognitive Approaches in Neuropsychological Rehabilitation. Hillsdale, NJ, Lawrence Erlbaum, 1989, pp 211–247.
6. Basso A: Prognostic factors in aphasia. Aphasiology 6:337–348, 1992.
7. Basso A, Capitani E, Vignolo L: Influence of rehabilitation of language skills in aphasic patients: A controlled study. Arch Neurol 36:190–196, 1979.
8. Bayles KA: Management of neurogenic communication disorders associated with dementia. In Chapey R (ed): Language Intervention Strategies in Adult Aphasia. Baltimore, Williams & Wilkins, 1994, pp 535–545.
9. Benson DF: Aphasia, Alexia, and Agraphia. New York, Churchill Livingstone, 1979.
10. Bollinger RL, Musson ND, Holland AL: A study of group communication intervention with chronically aphasic persons. Aphasiology 7:301–313, 1993.
11. Brookshire RH: Group studies of treatment for adults with aphasia: Efficacy, effectiveness, and believability. Div 2 Newsl Am Speech Lang Hear Assoc 4:5–13, 1994.
12. Brumfitt SM, Sheeran P: An evaluation of short-term group therapy for people with aphasia. Disabil Rehabil 19:221–230, 1997.
13. Butfield E, Zangwill O: Re-education in aphasia: A review of 70 cases. J Neurol Neurosurg Psychiatry 9:75–79, 1946.
14. Carlomagno S. Colombo A, Casadio P, et al: Cognitive approaches to writing rehabilitation in aphasics: Evaluation of two treatment strategies. Aphasiology 5:355–360, 1991.
15. Colon CP, McNeil MR: The efficacy of treatment for two globally aphasic adults using visual action therapy. Clin Aphasiol 19:185–195, 1991.
16. Crerar MA, Ellis AW, Dean EC: Remediation of sentence processing deficits in aphasia using a computer-based microworld. Brain Lang 52:229–275, 1996.

17. Cummings JL, Benson DF, Hill MA, Read S: Aphasia in dementia of the Alzheimer type. Neurology 35:394–397, 1985.
18. Darley FL: The efficacy of language rehabilitation in aphasia. J Speech Hear Disord 37:3–21, 1972.
19. Darley FL: Aphasia. Philadelphia, WB Saunders, 1982.
20. David RM, Enderby P, Bainton D: Progress report on an evaluation of speech therapy for aphasia. Br J Disord Commun 14:85–88, 1982.
21. Denes G, Perazzolo C, Piani A, Piccione F: Intensive versus regular speech-therapy in global aphasia: A controlled study. Aphasiology 10:385–394, 1996.
21a. Ebriham S: [personal communication], 1997.
22. Enderby P, Emerson J: Does Speech and Language Therapy Work?: A Review of the Literature. San Diego, Singular Publishing Group, 1995.
23. Frattali C, Thompson C, Holland A, et al: American Speech-Language-Hearing Association Functional Assessment of Communication Skills for Adults. Rockville, MD, American Speech-Language Hearing Association, 1995.
24. Goodglass H, Kaplan E: Boston Diagnostic Examination for Aphasia. 2nd ed. Philadelphia, Lea & Febiger, 1983.
25. Hagen C: Communication abilities in hemiplegia: Effect of speech therapy. Arch Phys Med Rehabil 54:454–463, 1973.
26. Hartman J, Landau WM: Comparison of formal language therapy with supportive counseling for aphasia due to acute vascular accident. Arch Neurol 44:646–649, 1987.
27. Hoen B, Thelander M, Worsely J: Improvement in psychological well-being of people with aphasia and their families: Evaluation of a community-based programme. Aphasiology 11:681–691, 1997.
28. Holland AL: Communicative Activities of Daily Living. Austin, TX, ProEd, 1980.
29. Holland AL, Fromm DS, DeRuyter F, Stein M: Treatment efficacy: Aphasia. J Speech Hearing Res 39:S27–S36, 1996.
30. Holland AL, Greenhouse JB, Fromm D, Swindell CS: Predictors of language restitution following stroke: A multivariate analysis. J Speech Hear Res 32:232–238, 1989.
31. Holland AL, Thompson CK: Outcomes measurement in aphasia. In Frattali CM (ed): Measuring Outcomes in Speech-Language Pathology. New York, Thieme, 1998, pp 245–266.
32. Holland AL, Wertz RT: Measuring aphasia treatment effects: Large-group, small-group, and single-subject studies. In Plum F (ed): Language, Communication, and the Brain. New York, Raven Press, 1988.
33. Katz RC, Wertz RT: The efficacy of computer-provided reading treatment for chronic aphasia adults. J Speech Lang Hear Res 40:493–507, 1997.
34. Katz RC, Wertz RT, Lewis SM, et al: A comparison of reading treatment, computer stimulation, and no treatment for aphasia. Clin Aphasiol 19:243–254, 1991.
35. Kay J, Lesser R, Coltheart M: PALPA: Psycholinguistic Assessments of Language Processing in Aphasia. Hove, Lawrence Erlbaum, 1992.
36. Kearns KP, Yedor K: An alternating treatments comparison of lose training and a convergent treatment strategy. Clin Aphasiol 20:223–238, 1991.
37. Kendall DL, McNeil MR, Small SL: Rule-based treatment for acquired phonological dyslexia. Aphasiology 12:587–600, 1998.
38. Kertesz A: Aphasia and Associated Disorders: Taxonomy, Localization, and Recovery. New York, Grune & Stratton, 1979.
39. Kertesz A: Western Aphasia Battery. New York, Grune & Stratton, 1982.
40. Kertesz A: Prognostic factors and recovery in aphasia. Ann Readapt Med Phys 35:81–88, 1992.
41. Kertesz A, McCabe P: Recovery patterns and prognosis in aphasia. Brain 100:1–18, 1977.
42. Last JM: A Dictionary of Epidemiology. 3rd ed. New York, Oxford University Press, 1995.
43. LeDorze G, Jacob A, Coderre L: Aphasia rehabilitation with a case of agrammatism: A partial replication. Aphasiology 5:63–85, 1991.
44. Lincoln N, McGuirk E, Mulley G, et al: Effectiveness of speech therapy for aphasic stroke patients: A radomised controlled trial. Lancet 1:1197–1200, 1984.
45. Lomas J, Pickard L, Bester S, et al: The communicative effectiveness index: Development and psychometric evaluation of a functional communication measure for adult aphasia. J Speech Hear Disord 54:113–124, 1989.
46. Lyon JG, Carisk D, Keisler L, et al: Communication partners: Enhancing participation in life and communication for adults with aphasia in natural settings. Aphasiology 11:693–708, 1997.
47. Marshall RC: Problem-focused group treatment for clients with mild aphasia. Am J Speech Lang Pathol 2:31–37, 1993.
48. Marshall RC, Wertz TR, Weiss DG, et al: Home treatment for aphasic patients by trained professionals. J Speech Hear Disord 54:462–470, 1989.

49. Mazzoni M, Vista M, Geri E, et al: Comparison of language recovery in rehabilitated and matched, non-rehabilitated aphasic patients. Aphasiology 9:553–563, 1995.

50. McNeil MR: The nature of aphasia in adults. In Lass NJ, McReynolds LV, Northern JL, Yoder DE (eds): Speech, Language, and Hearing. Vol 2. Philadelphia, WB Saunders, 1982, pp 692–740.

51. McNeil MR, Doyle PJ, Spencer KA, et al: A double-blind, placebo-controlled study of pharmacological and behavioural treatment of lexical-semantic deficits in aphasia. Aphasiology 11:385–400, 1997.

52. McNeil MR, Doyle PJ, Spencer K, et al: Effects of training multiple form classes on acquisition, generalization, and maintenance of word retrieval in a single subject. Aphasiology 12:575–585, 1998.

53. Meikle M, Wechsler E, Tupper A, et al: Comparative trial of volunteer and professional treatment of aphasia after stroke. BMJ 2:87–89, 1979.

54. Murdoch BE: Language disorders in dementia as aphasia syndromes. Aphasiology 2:181–185, 1988.

55. Murray LL, Holland AL: The language recovery of acutely aphasic patients receiving different therapy regimens. Aphasiology 9:397–405, 1995.

56. Nickles L, Best W: Therapy for naming disorders (Part I): Principles, puzzles and progress. Aphasiology 10:21–47, 1996.

57. Nickles L, Best W: Therapy for naming disorders (Part II): Specifics, surprises and suggestions. Aphasiology 10:109–136, 1996.

58. Olswang LB: Treatment efficacy: The breadth of research. In Olswang LB, Thompson CK, Warren SF, Minghetti NJ (eds): Treatment Efficacy Research in Communication Disorders. Rockville, MD, American Speech-Language-Hearing Association, 1990, pp 99–104.

59. Penn C: The profiling of syntax and pragmatics in aphasia. Clin Linguist Phonet 2:179–207, 1988.

60. Penn C, Jones D, Joffe V: Hierarchical discourse therapy: A method for the mild patient. Aphasiology 11:601–632, 1997.

61. Petheram B: Exploring the home-based use of microcomputers in aphasia therapy. Aphasiology 10:267–282, 1996.

62. Poeck K, Huber W, Willmes K: Outcome of intensive language treatment in aphasia. J Speech Hear Disord 54:471–479, 1989.

63. Prutting CA, Kirchner DM: A clinical appraisal of the pragmatic aspects of language. J Speech Hear Disord 52:105–119, 1987.

64. Quinteros B, Williams DR, White CA, Pickering M: The costs of using trained and supervised volunteers as part of a speech therapy service for dysphasic patients. Br J Disord Commun 19:205–212, 1984.

65. Robey RR: The efficacy of treatment for aphasic persons: A meta-analysis. Brain Lang 47:582–608, 1994.

66. Robey RR: A meta-analysis of clinical outcomes in the treatment of aphasia. J Speech Lang Hear Res 41:172–187, 1998.

67. Rosenbek JC, LaPointe LL, Wertz RT: Aphasia: A Clinical Approach. Austin, TX, ProEd, 1989.

68. Sarno M, Silverman M, Sands E: Speech therapy and language recovery in severe aphasia. J Speech Hear Res 13:607–623, 1970.

69. Sarno MT: The Functional Communication Profile: Manual of Direction. New York, Institute of Rehabilitative Medicine, New York University Medical Center, 1969.

70. Schuel H, Jenkins JJ, Jimnez-Pabn E: Aphasia in Adults. New York, Harper & Row, 1964.

71. Shewan CM: The history and efficacy of aphasia treatment. In Chapey R (ed): Language Intervention Strategies in Adult Aphasia. Baltimore, Williams & Wilkins, 1986, pp 28–43.

72. Shewan CM, Bandur DL: Treatment of Aphasia: A Language-Oriented Approach. Austin, TX, ProEd, 1986.

73. Shewan CM, Kertesz A: Effects of speech and language treatment on recovery from aphasia. Brain Lang 23:272–299, 1984.

74. Sparks R, Helm N, Albert M: Aphasia rehabilitation resulting from melodic intonation therapy. Cortex 10:303–316, 1974.

75. Springer L, Glindemann R, Huber W, Willmes K: How efficacious is PACE-therapy when "Language Systematic Training" is incorporated? Aphasiology 5:391–401, 1991.

76. Springer L, Willmes K: Efficacy of language systematic learning approaches to treatment. In Paradis M (ed): Foundations of Aphasia Rehabilitation. Oxford, England, Pergamon Press, 1993, pp 77–98.

77. Thompson CK, Raymer A, le Grand H: Effects of phonologically based treatment on aphasic naming deficits: A model-drive approach. Clin Aphasiol 20:239–259, 1992.

78. Thompson CK, Shapiro LP, Roberts MM: Treatment of sentence production deficits in aphasia: A linguistic-specific approach to Wh-interrogative training and generalization. Aphasiology 7:111–133, 1993.

79. Thompson CK, Shapiro LP, Tait ME, et al: Training Wh-question production in agrammatic aphasia: Analysis of argument and adjunct movement. Brain Lang 52:175–228, 1996.

80. Tompkins CA: Right Hemisphere Communication Disorders: Theory and Management. San Diego, Singular Publishing Group, 1995.

81. Tompkins CA, Jackson ST, Schulz R: On prognostic research in adult neurologic disorders. J Speech Hear Res 33:398–401, 1990.

82. Van De Sandt-Koenderman WME, Bonta E, Wielaert SM, Visch-Brink EG: Stimulating sentence production in agrammatic patients: The effect of the visual cue programme on spontaneous speech. Aphasiology 11:735–759, 1997.

83. Vignolo L: Evolution of aphasia and language rehabilitation: A retrospective exploratory study. Cortex 1:344–367, 1964.

84. Ylvisaker M, Szekeres SF: Communication disorders associated with closed head injury. In Chapey R (ed): Language Intervention Strategies in Adult Aphasia. Baltimore, Williams & Wilkins, 1994, pp 546–568.

85. Wertz RT: The PALPA's proof is in the predicting. Aphasiology 10:180–190, 1996.

86. Wertz RT: Comments on "Aphasia treatment in the early postonset period: Managing our resources effectively." Am J Speech Lang Pathol 6:12–18, 1997.

87. Wertz RT: Language treatment for aphasia is efficacious, but for whom? Top Lang Disord 8:1–10, 1987.

88. Wertz RT: Efficacy of various methods. In Paradis M (ed): Foundations of Aphasia Rehabilitation. Oxford, England, Pergamon Press, 1993, pp 61–75.

89. Wertz RT, Collins MJ, Weiss D, et al: Veterans Administration cooperative study on aphasia: A comparison of individual and group treatment. J Speech Hear Res 24:580–594, 1981.

90. Wertz RT, Weiss DG, Aten JL, et al: Comparison of clinic, home and deferred language treatment for aphasia: A Veterans Administration cooperative study. Arch Neurol 43:653–658, 1986.

91. Whitney J, Goldstein H: Using self-monitoring to reduce disfluencies in speakers with mild aphasia. J Speech Hear Disord 54:576–586, 1989.

92. Whur R, Lorch MP, Nye C: A meta-analysis of studies carried out between 1946 and 1988 concerned with the efficacy of speech and language therapy treatment for aphasic patients. Eur J Disord Commun 27:1–17, 1992.

93. World Health Organization: International Classification of Impairments, Disabilities and Handicaps. Geneva, WHO, 1980.

LEORA C. SWARTZMAN, PhD, CPsych
MARGARET C. GIBSON, PhD, CPsych
TAMARA L. ARMSTRONG, MA

PSYCHOSOCIAL CONSIDERATIONS IN ADJUSTMENT TO STROKE

From the Department of
    Psychology
University of Western Ontario
    and
Veteran's Care Program (LCS,
    TLA)
St. Joseph's Health Centre
London, Ontario
Canada

Reprint requests to:
Leora C. Swartzman, PhD, CPsych
Associate Professor
Department of Psychology
The University of Western Ontario
London, Ontario N6A 5C2
Canada

This chapter addresses psychosocial considerations in adjustment to stroke. We review the literature indicating how the common neurobehavioral sequelae of a stroke can compromise the rehabilitation process and affect long-term adjustment. This chapter, which builds on an earlier review on psychological consequences of stroke,[153] strives to update information on current treatments, with an emphasis on those whose efficacy has been demonstrated via randomized controlled trials, and to increase the practical utility by providing information on instruments for screening and tracking the neurobehavioral consequences of stroke. A section on social support, an acknowledged important psychosocial resource in adjustment and recovery from stroke, has been added. We distinguish between the prevalence of psychosocial sequelae and treatment strategies implemented during the subacute (1–6 months poststroke) and chronic (at least 6 months poststroke) stages, when such a distinction is made in the literature.

Moreover, our conceptual framework is of stroke as a biopsychosocial, as opposed to a biomedical, event. This has implications for models of etiology, disability and rehabilitation, and relevant health outcome measures.

Hafsteindottir et al. note that, whereas health care providers and researchers working with stroke patients tend to measure recovery in terms of "isolated and discrete return of movement" (i.e., a focus on motor function and functional disability), their review of qualitative studies on

TABLE 1. Factors Contributing to Poststroke Behavior

Prestroke (premorbid) behavior
Psychological reaction to the stroke and subsequent disability
Neurobehavioral deficits such as aphasia, apraxia, and perceptual problems
Organic cerebral changes
Environmental situation
Social supports

Adapted from Anderson TP: Rehabilitation of patients with completed stroke. In Kottke EJ, Stillwell GK, Lehmann JF (eds): Krusen's Handbook of Physical Medicine and Rehabilitation. Philadelphia, WB Saunders, 1982, pp 583–603.

patients' experience of stroke suggests that, for patients, recovery is a return to previously valued activities, which are more tied to psychosocial functioning and social support.[58] Accordingly, this chapter also includes a section on the measurement of health-related quality of life.

STROKE: A BIOPSYCHOSOCIAL APPROACH

Physicians who treat and manage stroke patients have described their role as being more than strictly biomedical—as involving the combination of good medicine with an awareness of the social problems and circumstances of their patients.[79] This perspective is consistent with the biopsychosocial model,[38] which postulates that health and illness are determined and maintained by the interplay between organismic, behavioral, and environmental factors, including social support. James and Minichiello argue that the multifactorial biopsychosocial perspective is particularly applicable to disability and rehabilitation in the elderly.[73]

The biopsychosocial model is quite applicable to stroke. As Anderson argues, the reaction of each stroke patient is likely to be shaped by his or her premorbid personality, the individual's characteristic manner of coping with stress, support of family and friends, and the cognitive/perceptual deficits created by the stroke itself[9] (Table 1).

The biopsychosocial model largely has been applied to investigate causes of illness and disability, and less attention has been paid to the determinants of behavioral health outcomes. It has been argued, however, that because behavioral outcomes including health-related quality of life and symptomatic complaints are major concerns of patients, they also should be a major concern of health care practitioners and researchers.[78] The literature regarding stroke is beginning to shift attention from survival and functional outcomes to psychological factors that influence poststroke quality of life and subjective well being.[164]

The following sections review psychological and behavioral problems that commonly appear poststroke. Readers also are referred to other recent reviews to supplement this materal.[52,58,68,81,86,87,126]

DEPRESSION

Etiology

Depression is generally considered a common sequela of stroke and has received the greatest share of research attention. Whether depression poststroke is better understood as a reaction to the functional and cognitive losses faced by the stroke patient, or is intrinsically related to the brain damage itself, has been debated for 20 years without resolution.[64] Debate also exists as to whether depression following a stroke is a disease-specific syndrome or a generic condition that encompasses a variety of syndromes, each with its distinct prevalence rate and prognosis.[106]

The complex association between lesion location and susceptibility to poststroke depression is not well understood.[52] While some studies have shown depression to be more prevalent in patients with lesions affecting the frontal brain regions,[43,48,93,130,132] others have not confirmed this result.[4,36,37,45,64,85,129] Temporal factors may moderate this relationship.[115] Astrom and colleagues found that left anterior lesions were associated with depression in the acute stage but not at 3, 12, 24, or 36 months poststroke.[11] In contrast, Parikh et al. found an association at 12 months but not at 2 years.[116] This pattern of results has led Astrom and colleagues to hypothesize that depression that develops shortly after stroke may have a neuroanatomic and neurophysiological basis, but depression observed later in recovery may, in part, be a reaction to psychosocial factors including situational stresses.[10,11]

The situational stresses encountered poststroke typically involve losses[17,22,101] in finances, family status, personal appearance, leizure, and social activities,[101] which results in a reduction of positive reinforcement in the individual's environment. Reduced access to positive reinforcement has been implicated in depression.[90] Moreover, exposure to uncontrollable, aversive events (i.e., learned helplessness) can lead to depression,[1,136] as can seeing one's disability or chronic illness as beyond one's control.[2,22,134] Arguably, stroke survivors are exposed to many unpredictable and uncontrollable events, including the stroke itself and its social sequelae.[31]

The precise etiologic relationships between psychosocial factors and poststroke depression await further study. Preliminary evidence suggests that psychosocial risk factors that may be associated with poststroke depression include premorbid personal and social characteristics.[84]

Assessment

Some researchers have adhered to the criteria for major depression found in the *Diagnostic and Statistical Manual of Mental Disorders* (DSM).[5,11] Others have used modified DSM criteria[4,138] or have relied on standardized questionnaires[37,64,85] or nonstandardized observational data.[42]

The validity of using DSM criteria to diagnose depression in stroke patients has been criticized because some of the criteria rely on patients' verbal reports.[119,131] Thus, depression may be particularly difficult to establish in stroke survivors who have aphasia or dementia. Another concern is that the diagnostic criteria for depression include vegetative symptoms of depression (i.e., sleep and appetite disturbance, fatigue, and psychomotor retardation) that may be consequences of the stroke itself[41] or other medical conditions.[118] However, in a recent study, depression was not shown to be overdiagnosed using DSM criteria.[115]

Standardized self-report questionnaires are also compromised by reliance on self-report and intact verbal abilities.[119] They, however, are more practical and may better capture patterns of depressive symptomatology that may be missed when looking for depressive syndromes using DSM criteria alone.[4,75] Moreover, scales have the added advantage of enabling clinicians to chart changes in depressive symptomatology in response to treatment; however, their sensitivity in this regard has not been fully explored. Table 2 describes some depression measures that have been used with stroke patients.

If the goal of assessing depression is, in part, to identify which patients might benefit from antidepressant therapy, the dexamethasone suppression test (DST) may

TABLE 2. Selection of Depression Measures Used with Stroke Patients

Instrument	Scales/Description	No. Items	Reliability: Internal	Reliability: Test-Retest	Comments
Beck Depression Inventory (BDI)[15]	Self-administered. Items refer to specific behavioral manifestations of depression	21	0.88[15] 0.91[50]	0.90 (6–21 days)[50]	Sensitive to antidepressant treatment effects in a stroke population[142] and an outpatient rehabilitation program[85]
Hamilton Depression Rating Scale (HRS-D)[59]	Interviewer-administered. Recently-developed self-report version[123]	Original: 17 items. Newer 6-item version[113]	0.90 (in a geriatric population)[165]. Self-report version: 0.91[123]	Self-report version 0.95[123]	Original scale is sensitive to antidepressant treatment effects in a stroke population.[7,88,89,94,142] 6-item version as sensitive as longer versions to anti-depressive treatment effects[113]
Zung Self-Rating Depression Scale (SDS)[167]	Self-rating scale that includes symptoms tapping depressed affect and its physiologic and psychological concomitants	20	0.83 (in a stroke population)[3] 0.87 (in a stroke population)[165]	N/A	Sensitivity of 0.76 and specificity of 0.96 (cut-off of 45).[3] Sensitive to treatment effects[167]
Hospital Anxiety and Depression Scale (HADS)[166]	Self-administered. Two scales: anxiety (A) and depression (D). Developed for use in nonpsychiatric hospital patients and thus excludes questions about physical complaints	Depression scale: 7	0.81[63]	0.85 < 2 wk; 0.76 2–4 wk; 0.7 > 6 wk[63]	Correlation with psychiatric rating of depression severity = 0.70.[166] Sensitivity of 0.83[75] and 0.80.[111] Specificity of 0.44[75] and 0.79[111] for detecting clinically diagnosed depression
Geriatric Depression Scale (GDS)[165]	Self-administered. Yes/no response format, which is assumed to be easier for elderly than the 3–5 point rating scales typical of most other self-report depression inventories	30. Shorter form available[139]	0.94 (in a geriatric population)[165]. 0.90 (in a geriatric stroke population)[3]	0.85 (1-wk)[165]	Sensitivity of 0.84, specificity of 0.66 for detecting clinically diagnosed depression.[75] Sensitivity of 0.88 and specificity of 0.64[3]
General Health Questionnaire (GHQ)[55]	Self administered psychiatric screening test. Comprises 4 subscales: somatic symptoms, anxiety and insomnia, social dysfunction, severe depression	28 in original version. Later versions have more (30) or fewer (12, 20, 25) items	0.78 (GHQ-12): 0.84 (GHQ-28)[82]	Reported to be high[61]	Sensitivity of 0.89[75] and 0.80.[111] Specificity of 0.75[75] and 0.76[111] (cut-off score of 4/5) for detecting clinically diagnosed depression

N/A = not applicable or not available from published literature

serve as a suitable alternative to self-report inventories and diagnostic interviews. The DST has been shown to predict response to tricyclic antidepressant medications,[43,94,121] but its specificity for the diagnosis of poststroke depression is reportedly low.[95,121] However, in a longitudinal study of a population-based stroke survivor cohort, Astrom et al. found that the predictive value of the DST, 91%, was acceptably high.[12] The DST is advantageous because it does not rely on patients' intact verbal abilities; however, biochemical testing-based tool may not be practical economically, particularly in large-scale population studies.[159]

Prevalence

Given the diversity of measurement approaches, study populations, and sampling times used in different studies, it is not surprising that estimates of the prevalence of depression poststroke can vary from 18–60%.[37,41,42,64,83,85,93,121] It has even been argued that, once methodologic variations are considered, the prevalence of depression among stroke patients may not be any higher than among other groups of patients;[69] however, there are data to the contrary.[45,144]

Recent reviewers[6] concluded that the prevalence of depression in the acute stage was about 40%, with equivalent proportions of major and minor depression.[52] In general, depression rates during the subacute stage are higher. Rates of 40–60% have been found in patient samples drawn from rehabilitation settings.[96,128] Rates during the chronic stage are lowest, ranging from 16–23% in population-based samples.[23,63,85]

Prognosis and Implications for Adjustment

The natural course of poststroke depression is unclear. Symptom remission tends to occur,[69] as evidenced by the fact that the difference in prevalence of depression between stroke survivors and age-matched peers tends to decrease as time after stroke increases.[69,138]

However, poststroke depression has implications for recovery. In longitudinal studies, poststroke depression has been shown to predict recovery at both the subacute and chronic stages. For example, depression has been shown to predict functional outcome 2½ months after discharge[84] and activities of daily living 2 years poststroke.[144] Depression even has been shown to predict mortality 10 years poststroke.[103] Morris et al found that stroke patients with diagnoses of major or minor depression diagnosed about 2 weeks poststroke were 3.4 times more likely to have died during the 10-year follow-up period than were nondepressed stroke patients.[103] These differences were not attributable to differences on other measured risk factors, including age, sex, social class, type and location of lesions, level of social functioning, and prestroke depression.[106] Given its demonstrated impact on rehabilitation outcome, long-term functional status, and even mortality, we concur with Koivisto et al. that the "diagnosis and treatment of poststroke depression is essential in clinical practice."[84]

Treatment

Pharmacologic treatment may be the most viable treatment option for poststroke depression. Treatment of depression in stroke patients can be as effective as in any other patient group experiencing clinical depression.[81] There are several approaches to the treatment of poststroke depression, including electroconvulsive therapy (ECT), psychosocial interventions, and pharmacologic approaches with tricyclics, selective serotoninergic reuptake inhibitors (SSRIs), and psychostimulants.

PHARMACOLOGIC APPROACHES

Tricyclics.   Lipsey et al. found that nortriptyline (25 mg initially, raised to up to 100 mg daily) significantly improved depression in stroke patients over an untreated matched control group.[94] However, the sample size was small and the dropout rate high (6 of 17) due to side effects. Reding examined the effect of trazodone (target dose 200 mg/day) in the treatment of depressed and nondepressed stroke patients.[121] Depressed patients showed a trend toward greater improvement in ADLs with trazodone than with placebo. Moreover, an abnormal DST test was more predictive of a positive response to trazodone than to placebo. Although the treatment was deemed effective, a quarter of the patients were withdrawn from the study because of side effects. Virtually identical results are reported by Rafaelle et al. in a randomized control trial of trazodone (300 mg/day) in 22 stroke patients.[120]

In a sample of 20 inpatients identified as depressed as per the Hamilton Scale, Lauritzen et al. found that imipramine (mean dose 75 mg/day) plus mianserin (mean dose 25 mg/day) was superior to desipramine (66 mg/day) plus mianserin (27 mg/day).[88] Both regimens were well tolerated. The superiority of imipramine (which affects both noradrenergic and serotonergic receptors) over desipramine (which affects only the noradrenergic receptors) led the authors to predict that SSRIs might be of clinical utility.

SSRIs.   Because SSRIs have fewer adverse effects than the older tricyclic antidepressants and because the side effects tend to subside after a few weeks of treatment, SSRIs may be promising treatment approaches. Andersen et al. have reported the only published controlled clinical trial on the effectiveness of this class of drugs on poststroke depression.[7] In their 6-week double-blind placebo-controlled trial of citalopram (10–40 mg/day) involving 66 depressed stroke patients, a significant improvement in Hamilton depression scores was observed for patients receiving treatment versus placebo. The treatment effect was more pronounced in patients who became depressed in the subacute stage than in those entering the trial 2–6 weeks after stroke. The authors note that this is, in part, a function of the high degree of spontaneous recovery of depression in the early stage of stroke. Side effects were mild and usually transient.

In a small, uncontrolled study of five stroke patients with major depression[142] fluoxetine (20 mg in the morning for 8 weeks), another SSRI, statistically reduced depression scores and increased functionality. Marked improvement occurred within 14 days of treatment, and no patient discontinued treatment due to side effects.

Psychostimulants.   Although psychostimulants have a role in the treatment of poststroke depression, the literature consists mostly of uncontrolled case studies.[86] For example, retrospective studies involving hospital chart reviews suggest that psychostimulants are a safe and effective treatment alternative to tricyclics for stroke patients.[92,100] About 80% of patients showed full or partial improvement of symptoms of depression within 1–2 weeks of onset of treatment. Side effects were not marked. In a subsequent 3-week uncontrolled efficacy and side effect trial[89] of methylphenidate, 80% of 10 treated patients evidenced complete or partial alleviation of their depression within 1–2 weeks of treatment. (Treatment was started at 2.5 mg or 5 mg orally in the morning and at noon and slowly increased to as much as 40 mg/day; the mean final dosage was 17.0 mg/day.) No significant electrocardiographic changes were observed for any of the 10. None had to leave the study because of side effects, but the patients were only followed for 3 weeks. The impact of longer administration of psychostimulants on cardiac functioning in these patients has not been assessed. This, paired with the fact that methylphenidate can be highly additive and can suppress appetite, has led to the recommendation that it be used cautiously poststroke.[153]

Electroconvulsive Therapy. ECT has been regarded as a suitable alternative for patients who fail to respond to antidepressants, who are considered at high risk for suicide, or who have marked neurovegetative or psychotic symptoms.[119] ECT appears relatively safe and generally efficacious in the treatment of poststroke depression[108] but should not be administered within 3 months of a stroke.[153]

Psychosocial Interventions. Cognitive behavior therapy is an active, directive, time-limited approach to a variety of psychological disorders, including depression. However, the results of a pilot study evaluating cognitive behavioral treatment for depression in poststroke patients are disappointing.[91] Only 19 of the 111 (17%) patients who were eligible for and offered the cognitive behavior therapy (an average of 8.4 ± 3 sessions over 3 months) agreed to participate. Moreover, the efficacy of the intervention for patients who did participate was low; only eight of the 19 benefitted from therapy, as shown by scores on the Beck Depression Inventory.[11]

In the Finnstroke study, the prevalence of depression, as measured by the BDI, in patients discharged from hospitals with an after-hospital discharge program was significantly lower than in those discharged without such programs; the differences were maintained at 12 months.[85] There were no differences in the rate of pharmacotherapy for depression across districts. Although the authors suggest the programs worked because they facilitated the establishment of social ties, they provide no data to support this assumption.

ANXIETY

Etiology

Comorbidity between poststroke generalized anxiety disorder (GAD) and depression is high.[10,24–26,135,144] The comorbidity is particularly marked in the acute stage but diminishes by 2 years after stroke.[135] Whether poststroke anxiety, depression, and anxious-depression are manifestations of the same condition or discrete clinical entities is unknown.[26]

Both neurologic and psychosocial factors have been implicated in the etiology of anxiety disorders poststroke. Comorbid depression and GAD have been associated with left hemispheric lesions, but GAD alone has been associated with right hemispheric lesions.[10,26]

Other risk factors for poststroke anxiety may include personal and family history of psychiatric illness. Although Castillo and colleagues initially found no evidence for this association in acute poststroke patients,[26] they observed an association in a subsequent study;[25] stroke survivors with early-onset GAD were more likely to have had a psychiatric history than those with late-onset GAD. Finally, poststroke GAD is more prevalent in women and in persons who have their strokes at a younger age.[135]

Measurement

The factors that complicate measurement of depression—standardization of diagnostic criteria and reliance on self-report tools that require verbal ability—also hold for the assessment of poststroke anxiety. GAD is the DSM diagnostic category of choice for some researchers. Even so, when applying DSM diagnostic criteria for GAD to stroke patients, one should deemphasize autonomic symptoms and relax the temporal criteria.[135] Other anxiety disorders, such as agoraphobia and panic disorder, seldom have been addressed poststroke.[24,69]

The results of apparently the only study evaluating the utility of self-report measures of anxiety for use with stroke patients were disappointing.[24] The researchers found that standardized scales such as the Hospital Anxiety and Depression Scale[166] and the General Health Questionnaire[55] had low specificity and poor predictive value for screening poststroke anxiety disorders.

Prevalence

The reported prevalence of GAD poststroke has ranged from 3–31%.[10,25,26,53,69,137,144] Astrom found the prevalence of GAD to be 28% in the acute stage, with no appreciable decrease in prevalence over 3 years of follow-up.[10]

Prognosis and Implications for Adjustment

Given that the prevalence of GAD is similar at the acute and chronic stages, it is not surprising that Astrom found that only one in four stroke survivors diagnosed with GAD in the first 3 months poststroke had recovered 1 year after stroke.[10] Moreover, at 3-year follow-up, 62% still had not recovered. Thus, GAD does not tend to spontaneously remit. Some data suggest that poststroke anxiety, but not necessarily GAD, is associated with more frequent use of avoidant coping strategies, which arguably can interfere with the rehabilitative process.[53] Some evidence exists, however, that the impact of anxiety on functional outcome is manifested at the acute rather than chronic phase.[135] Consistent with this finding, Castillo et al. report that stroke survivors who had developed either early- or late-onset anxiety were no more impaired socially, cognitively, or physically at follow-up than those who had not.[25]

Treatment

There appear to be no published treatment outcomes studies for poststroke anxiety.[126] Robinson notes that, although benzodiazepines are used to treat GAD in the general population, their use poststroke must be tempered by the recognition that stroke patients may be particularly vulnerable to the side effects of benzodiazepines, including sedation, ataxia, disinhibition, and confusion. Given the comorbidity of depression and anxiety in stroke patients, Robinson also suggests that antidepressants might be of benefit, but their efficacy for poststroke anxiety has not been formally assessed.[126]

OTHER NEUROBEHAVIORAL DISORDERS

Emotional Lability and Disinhibition

ETIOLOGY

Stroke patients can develop some combination of disinhibition syndromes, including motor disinhibition (e.g., hyperactivity, pressured speech), behavioral disinhibition (resulting in socially inappropriate behavior), and emotional disinhibition (e.g., emotional lability, anger). Starkstein and Robinson recently provided an excellent review of behavioral and motor disinhibition syndromes.[150] Accordingly, this section focuses on emotional lability. The next section discusses a second manifestation of emotional disinhibition: catastrophic reactions and aggression.

Emotional lability and its most dramatic manifestation, pathologic laughing and crying, refer to the display of affect that is situationally inappropriate or does not correspond with the underlying emotional state. Although it is observed in a variety of central nervous system disorders,[104] its neurophysiologic basis has not been elucidated.

Emotional lability, also referred to as emotional incontinence and pathologic emotionalism, presents as a part of the syndrome of pseudobulbar palsy, which occurs in patients who have had bilateral subcortical infarcts and is not uncommon after right hemispheric lesions.[29,37,70,144] That antidepressants have been effective in treating emotional lability[8,107,127] suggests that its underlying mechanism may involve serotonin or other biogenic amine systems.[127] Furthermore, findings that stroke patients with more anterior lesions are at greater risk for emotional lability[104] suggest that anterior lesions may produce disinhibition of emotional control,[109,148] similar to the way frontal lobe damage produces irritability and disinhibition of social behavior.[70]

The observed comorbidity of depression and emotional lability has led Jorge et al. to question the independence of these two emotional disturbances, but their data indicate no association between pathologic crying and depression in stroke patients.[76] Data from Morris, Robinson, and Rafaelle similarly suggest that depression and pathologic laughing and crying are distinct enough to be considered separate entities.[104]

MEASUREMENT

The only measure of emotional lability of which we are aware is the Pathological Laughter and Crying Scale (PLACS), developed by Robinson et al. to assess symptoms of extreme emotional lability in stroke patients.[127] PLACS has been demonstrated to be reliable and valid and has proven useful in the quantification of emotional lability (Table 3).

PREVALENCE

Morris, Robinson, and Rafaelle found that 18% of their sample experienced repeated episodes of emotional lability poststroke.[104] House observed prevalence rates of 15% at 1 month and 12% at 1 year poststroke.[70]

PROGNOSIS AND IMPLICATIONS FOR ADJUSTMENT

Little is known about the natural course of emotional lability poststroke. The clinical presentation usually occurs 4–6 weeks after a stroke and is almost always triggered by minor stimuli.[107] In some cases, the emotional lability is so severe and persistent that it leads to prolonged distress and social embarrassment and interferes with the patient's rehabilitation.[127] Firsthand accounts by patients reveal that, when insight is intact, stroke survivors are often embarrassed by their emotional outbursts.[77,117] In the absence of insight, disinhibited behavior and emotional lability will not disturb the patient but are likely to distress others.[19]

TREATMENT

In one study, stroke patients treated with the tricyclic antidepressant nortriptyline (50 mg/day gradually increased to 100 mg/day) showed significantly greater improvement in emotional lability after 4 and 6 weeks of treatment than placebo-treated controls.[127] Although about half of the patients also had major or minor depression, nortriptyline-related improvements in PLACS scores were observed for both the depressed and nondepressed patients. Moreover, nondepressed patients tended to improve more on PLACS than the depressed patients, suggesting that the observed effect was not mediated by the amelioration of depression.[125]

TABLE 3. Emotional Lability Measures Used with Stroke Patients

Instrument	Scales/ Description	No. Items	Reliability: Internal	Reliability: Test-Retest	Comments
Pathological Laughter and Crying Scale (PLACS)[127]	Semistructured patient interview that requires the rating of the frequency of unexplained or inappropriate emotion	18	N/A	0.85 (2 wk)[127]	Sensitivity of the PLACS for detecting clinically diagnosed emotional lability is 0.88; scale specificity is 0.96, sensitive to treatment effects[127]
Catastrophic Reaction Scale (CRS)[145]	Brief, quantitative measure of patients' behavior poststroke. Assesses the frequency of behaviors typical of a catastrophic reaction (e.g., "patient became tearful")	11	0.85[145]	N/A	Interrater agreement: 91%[145]

N/A = not applicable or not available from published literature

In a double-blind placebo-controlled crossover study, 73% of 16 patients treated with the SSRI citalopram (20 mg/day before bed for patients younger than 66 and 10 mg/day for older patients) evidenced significant decreases in crying frequency, as determined by semistructured interviews and diaries.[8] Finally, significant decreases in PLACS scores and increases in functional independence were observed in two poststroke patients treated with sertraline (daily dosages of 50 and 75 mg), a short-acting SSRI.[107]

Catastrophic Reactions and Aggression

ETIOLOGY

Catastrophic reactions, first described by Goldstein,[56] involve extremely disruptive emotional outbursts characterized by physically aggressive behavior toward family and staff, refusal to comply with directions, difficulty settling down, swearing or other verbal abuse, and an inability to be reasoned with. Although catastrophic reactions have been shown to be more prevalent in patients with basal ganglia lesions,[145] left anterior lesions,[114] and expressive or Broca's aphasia,[48] the neurophysiologic basis of catastrophic reactions has not been determined.[143]

From a psychological standpoint, catastrophic reactions can be conceptualized as an understandable response to a frustrating situation. The concept of "rehabilitation as punishment"[46] is germane here, in that stroke survivors enter into disability and consequent rehabilitation involuntarily and are required to perform laborious rehabilitation exercises that they may find extremely aversive. At the same time, many of the patient's positive reinforcers, such as social contacts, material comforts, family contacts, sexual activity, and work, are not available during the recovery period. Accordingly, catastrophic reactions and less extreme acts of aggression can be understood as a natural response to frustration and perceived punishment.[46] As one physician said: "I encourage the expression of anger and depression because I think it is realistic. If it were me, I'd be in a blind rage if I had a stroke."[79]

In support of the view that catastrophic reactions are, in part, a response to an actual or perceived external threat, it has been observed that they are often triggered by stressors[44,48] such as a demanding language task.[17]

Risk factors for catastrophic reactions include younger age, cognitive and functional impairment, and depression.[114] Some researchers have suggested that catastrophic reactions are best understood as a symptom of major depressive syndrome in stroke patients.[49,149]

MEASUREMENT

The Catastrophic Reaction Scale has been shown to be a reliable instrument for the assessment of catastrophic reaction symptoms poststroke[145] (see Table 3).

PREVALENCE

Catastrophic reactions are not an infrequent sequelae of stroke. Starkstein et al. identified catastrophic reactions in 19% of patients in the acute phase, and 9–29% demonstrate irritability and agitation of sufficient magnitude to interfere with the rehabilitation process.[71,145] Aggression ranks third, behind depression and memory loss, among changes causing concern to caregivers of stroke patients.[60]

PROGNOSIS AND IMPLICATIONS FOR ADJUSTMENT

Empiric studies on the natural course of catastrophic reactions and aggressive behaviors poststroke are lacking. This issue is important, however, because aggressive behaviors can compromise rehabilitation efforts and the maintenance of gains once rehabilitation is completed.[19] Aggressive outbursts may impair adjustment because they lead to a breakdown of caretaking and needed support relationships. Health care workers and family members may respond with negative sanctions, such as withholding privileges, in response to these behaviors, thereby increasing the patient's perception of rehabilitation as punishment.

TREATMENT

Antipsychotic medications are sometimes administered to agitated patients. On the basis of a meta-analysis of controlled clinical trials, Schneider et al. conclude that hostility and combativeness in stroke patients can be reduced with antipsychotic medications.[133] Moreover, a more recent case report showed that the SSRI fluoxetine was effective in reducing anger and hostility in a patient with poststroke depression accompanied by anger attacks.[162]

Behavioral considerations are also important for preventing outbursts or for mitigating their impact. Thus, the decision about where a patient can best be managed is important. Behaviors that may be dangerous on a medical unit may be more easily managed on a psychiatric ward or in a long-term care facility. Responding to the outbursts by restraining patients or threatening to punish them only aggravates the situation; patients should be given plenty of space and preferably housed in a single room, to avoid the threat of danger to roommates.[19]

Indifference Reactions

ETIOLOGY

Indifference reactions encompass a host of psychological phenomena that can occur poststroke, including lack of appropriate concern or anxiety, denial of obvious disabilities, apathy, and unmotivated behavior.[163] Although some research suggests

TABLE 4. Denial and Apathy Measures Used with Stroke Patients

Instrument	Scales/ Description	No. Items	Reliability: Internal	Reliability Test-Retest	Comments
Apathy Evaluation Scale (AES)[98]	Three versions are available; clinician, informant, and self-rated (AES-C, AES-I, AES-S)	18	0.86–0.94[98]	0.76–0.94 (Mean 25.4 days)	Convergent and discriminant validity have been shown using the multitrait-multimethod matrix procedure[98]
Apathy Scale[147]	Brief, structured interview assessing patient's level of interest and general affect. Abridged version of AES	14	0.76[147]	0.90 (1 wk)[147]	Interrater reliability: 0.81[147]
Anosognosia Questionnaire[146]	Semistructured clinician interview assessing patient's level of awareness of physical limitations	6–11 (depends on presence of denial)	N/A	N/A	

N/A = not applicable or not available from published literature

that indifference reactions are related to specific anatomic lesions, particularly in the anterior temporal regions,[112] other studies[65,140,163] have failed to show such associations. Indifference also can arise from nonneurologic proximal causes, such as fatigue, depression, concurrent medical and mental conditions, and social factors fostering dependency.[19]

MEASUREMENT

Table 4 summarizes several tools to measure indifference reactions.

PREVALENCE

Reding and colleagues observed neglect or denial of deficit in 43% of stroke survivors and a combination of depression, apathy, lack of motivation, inappropriate fatigue, withdrawal, and crying in 25% of survivors.[122] These behaviors were sufficient to interfere with the rehabilitation process. Hibbard et al. report that although only three of 82 of their stroke patients denied their illness, about half minimized its impact.

PROGNOSIS AND IMPLICATIONS FOR ADJUSTMENT

Indifference reactions interfere with engagement in rehabilitation and are one of the primary reasons patients leave the hospital against medical advice.[122] Little is known about their natural course poststroke.

TREATMENT

There appear to be no studies on the treatment of indifference reactions. Swartzman and Teasell suggest that confrontation of denial is only warranted when the denial interferes with the rehabilitation process, and it is best accomplished by discussing the disability and its possible permanence in a hopeful, optimistic, and gradual fashion.[153]

TABLE 5. Social Support Measures Used with Stroke Patients

Instrument	Scales/Description	No. Items	Reliability: Internal	Reliability: Test-Retest	Comments
Social Ties Checklist[153]	Brief, quantitative measure of patient's social connectedness. Assesses whether a specific social activity (e.g., having lunch with someone) is part of a patient's life. It does not assess satisfaction with social functioning.	10	N/A	N/A	Behavioral specificity of scale requires less interpretation and thus may be well suited for proxy respondents. Predicts 10-year poststroke mortality[103]
Social Support Inventory for Stroke Survivors: SSISS[102]	Assesses quality, quantity, and satisfaction with five sources of social support: family, friend, community, group, and professional. By interview or self-administered	75 (15 for each of 5 sources).	0.85[102]	0.95 (1 wk)[102]	Not sensitive to change in response to a social support intervention[47]
Interpersonal Support Evaluation List: ISEL 5	Availability of support in 4 domains: appraisal, belonging, tangibility, self-esteem	40	0.77–0.90[28]	0.87 (2 day); 0.70 (6 wk)[28]	Not sensitive to change in response to a social support intervention[47]
Older American Resources and Services (OARS) Social Service Scale[35]	Structured interview	Overall rating. 1 = excellent 4 = poor	N/A	N/A	Predicts postrehabilitation discharge status[21]
Inventory of Socially Supportive Behaviors[13,14]	Frequency of available social support in 3 domains: emotional, instrumental, informational	40	0.93[62]	0.88 (2 day)[62]	Behavioral specificity of scale requires less interpretation and thus may be suited for proxy respondents

N/A = not applicable or not available from published literature

SOCIAL SUPPORT

In the last two decades, social support has been studied to a greater extent than any other psychosocial variable and variously has been "heralded as a magic bullet" and "attacked as a myth."[54] Glass and Maddox discuss the mechanisms by which social support might exert its effect on stroke patients.[54]

In the literature, a distinction is often made between instrumental (i.e., practical) support (e.g., assistance with daily chores in and around the house), emotional support (talking about feelings and emotions), and informational social support. This distinction fits well with research by Evans and Northwood, who argue that social interaction for stroke patients is supportive when it meets the patients' emotional needs, provides patients with access to information about available services and resources, and gives patients practical help with the tasks of daily living.[40]

Measurement

Heitzmann and Kaplan comprehensively review measures available for assessing social support.[63] Table 5 presents information about social support measures that have been used in stroke patients.

Prognosis and Implications for Adjustment

Several longitudinal studies clearly indicate that social support has an impact on adjustment to stroke at both the subacute and chronic stages. In a study of 152 stroke patients enrolled in a stroke rehabilitation program in a general hospital, Brosseau et al. found that stroke survivors with poor social support were 2.6 times more likely to be referred to a long-term care facility and 1.8 times more likely to go to a rehabilitation facility, as opposed to home, than those with adequate support.[21] Similarly, in a prospective study of stroke outcome in a sample of 536 consecutive admissions to a rehabilitation unit in a general hospital, Ween et al. found that the absence of a committed caregiver significantly reduced the rate of home discharge, from 77% to 65%.[161] These results suggest that social support indices can be useful for the rational planning of discharge dispositions.

Social support has an even stronger impact on adjustment in the chronic stage. The Framingham study showed that, for stroke patients, social factors were as much a determinant of independent functioning in the chronic phase as disability.[80] Moreover, in a longitudinal study aimed at examining the impact of emotional, instrumental, and informational social support on functional capacity at different stages of the recovery process, Glass and Maddox followed 44 stroke patients 6 months poststroke.[54] The impact of social support did not appear during the first month of rehabilitation. Patients reporting high levels of emotional support showed dramatic improvement despite having the lowest functional status. Instrumental support was related to positive outcomes only when provided in moderate amounts. Finally, informational support was beneficial but not for patients who had had more severe strokes; it is likely that cognitive impairment prevented patients in this subgroup from using this resource.

Finally, the lack of social support has been shown to increase the risk of depression on mortality 10 years poststroke.[103] That is, patients who were depressed *and* had few social ties 1–3 weeks poststroke had a much higher mortality rate (92%) than those who were depressed but had adequate social ties (58%).

Although social support networks typically are considered assets, they also can be liabilities.[110,152,155] Well-meant, yet oversolicitous care by family members and friends that stifles patients' autonomy may be more hindrance than help. For example, stroke patients whose primary caregivers were overprotective of them felt that they had less control over their recovery and were more depressed 9 months poststroke than those whose caregivers were not overprotective.[155] Moreover, the finding by Glass and Maddox that moderate but not high levels of instrumental support were related to positive outcomes suggests that too much instrumental support may have engendered dependency and lack of motivation in achieving rehabilitative goals.[54] Horgas et al. comprehensively discuss dependency in later life,[67] and Evans et al. provide a thoughtful discussion of the crucial role of the family in poststroke rehabilitation.[39]

Taken together, these findings suggest that social support is an important predictor of recovery from stroke. Moreover, they indicate that it is important to take the timing, type, and amount of support into account. Failure to do so may lead to an underestimate of the impact of social support and may weaken the observed effect of treatment aimed at increasing social support.

Treatment

Geddes and Chamberlain evaluated the impact of the Volunteer Stroke Scheme, a community service offering support to stroke patients in the form of attendance at a weekly club and regular home visits by volunteers.[51] Thirty-four patients receiving support were compared to a matched sample of 10 control patients and were assessed both before and a year after entry into the program. Marshall and Sacchett note that the results are modest at best.[99] The intervention did not have an impact on functionality. However, a significant increase in social and home-based activities was observed in the treatment but not the control group.

Friedland and McColl conducted a randomized trial of a social support intervention for stroke survivors at the chronic stage (an average 11.4 months poststroke), which was aimed at working with members of the patients' existing support system to improve social support and to establish new supports.[47] Although the 48 patients in the treatment group improved with respect to their perceived quality of relationships relative to the 40 patients who received no treatment, there were no treatment effects on psychosocial adjustment and adjustment to disability, and there was no impact on broad social support networks or community integration.

The authors hypothesize that this weak treatment effect may have occurred because the timing of the intervention (9.7 months after discharge from the hospital) was too late. They suggest that, to be effective, social support interventions may have to begin earlier, before previously existing supports begin to fall away. They hypothesize that the critical period for social support interventions might be during hospitalization, when patients are in crisis and thus may be particularly open to intervention. They also note, however, that if intervention begins too soon, recipients may not be able to benefit because they have yet to come to terms with the permanence of their disability.

These findings suggest that the timing of social support interventions merits further examination. Moreover, to be effective, interventions should be guided by what is known about helpful versus unhelpful support[54,152,155] in the natural environment.

Finally, one cannot rule out the possibility that the modest effects of treatment outcome studies may reflect the fact that social support is a powerful resource that is embedded in one's longstanding social network and, thus, may not be modified easily. However, given that social support has been demonstrated to be a strong predictor of outcome in stroke patients, and given the availability of good, sensitive

TABLE 6.   Activities of Daily Living Measures Used with Stroke Patients

Instrument	Scales/ Description	No. Items	Reliability: Internal	Reliability: Test-Retest	Comments
Frenchay Activities Index[158]	Activities (both inside and outside the home) that require some decision making and organization on the part of the patient (e.g., housework, shopping, social activities, pursuit of hobbies, travel)	15	High communality for the items (mean = 60, range = 0.44–0.77).[158]	N/A	Scoring is based on the frequency rather than quality of activities, which minimizes subjectivity. Demonstrated content validity. Interrater reliability: 80. Sensitive to recovery[158]
Activities Index for Stroke patients[66]	Designed to assess patient's "lifestyle," prestroke (assessed retrospectively) and poststroke in 3 domains: domestic chores, leisure/work, and outdoor activities	15	N/A	N/A	Prestrokes scores (obtained retropsectively) were higher than those obtained 12 months poststroke, indicating scale sensitivity[66]

N/A = not applicable or not available from published literature

measurement instruments, social support routinely should be assessed at various stages in the rehabilitation process to identify high-risk patients who might benefit from additional support upon discharge.

ACTIVITIES OF DAILY LIVING AND QUALITY OF LIFE MEASURES

Health care providers and researchers working with stroke patients typically measure recovery in terms of motor function and broader functional abilities. This focus has resulted in the development of well-validated instruments sensitive enough to detect changes associated with functional recovery in stroke patients, including the Barthel Index[72,97] and the Functional Independence Measure.[57] Other recent reviews appraise other common scales used to measure deficits and disability in stroke patients during the acute/subacute[124] and chronic[30] stages.

However, whereas researchers tend to measure recovery in terms of physical functioning, Hafsteinsdottir and Grypdonck found that, for patients, recovery is viewed as a return to previously valued activities. For example, despite being less functionally impaired, patients with higher education and income levels had a lower quality of life than those with less education because their leisure activities were more affected by the perceived social stigma associated with having had a stroke. Thus, it is important to tap the activities that are valued by patients themselves. Accordingly, extended activities of daily living measures (that go beyond basic self-care activities) and quality of life measures (some of which assess valued activities) have an important role to play in the ongoing assessment of stroke patients (Tables 6 and 7).

SUMMARY

There are a wide range of psychological sequelae of stroke, most of which affect recovery, that are readily measurable, and are themselves amenable to treatment. Social support is a measurable resource that also affects recovery, but its amenability to treatment is questionable.

TABLE 7. Quality of Life Measures Used with Stroke Patients

Instrument	Scales/Description	No. Items	Reliability: Internal	Reliability: Test-Retest	Comments
SF-36[160]	Assesses eight domains: limitations in physical, social and usual role activities due to health problems, bodily pain, general mental health, limitations in usual role activities due to emotional problems, vitality, and general health perceptions	36	Range: 0.80–0.96[32]	0.70 (3 wk) (average over 8 domains) Range: 0.30 (mental health) to 0.81 (general health and body pain)[32]	Can be self-administered or administered by a trained interviewer in person or by telephone[160]
EuroQol[154]	Short, simple, descriptive profile of health (subjectively rated) in 5 domains: mobility, self-care, social, pain, and psychological function. Designed as an instrument for describing and valuing health states.	5	N/A	Test-retest reliability adequate, with kappa ranging from 0.63–0.80 for the 6 domains[32]	Discriminated among patients with different stroke syndromes and severities.[33] Proxy ratings are reasonably accurate for observable domains (self-care, mobility, social functioning) but less accurate for more subjective domains (pain and psychological functioning)[34]
Sickness Impact Profile (SIP)[18]	Items describe behavior in 12 categories: household management, ambulation, mobility, body care and movement, social interaction, alertness, emotional behavior, communication, sleep and rest, eating, work, and recreation and pastimes	136	0.94[18,156]	Total score: 0.92 Category subscale scores: 0.82 (mean). (1 day)[18]	Consistency between self- and interviewer-administration: 0.87.[18] Can effectively be completed by proxy. Proxy ratings are sensitive to differences in patients' functional health[141]
Stroke Adapted version of the SIP (SA-SIP30)[156]	Eight categories: household management, ambulation, mobility, body care and movement, social interaction, alertness, emotional behavior, and communication	30	N/A	0.85[156]	Correlation with SIP (136) scores: 0.96 (i.e., 92% shared variance)[156]

N/A = not applicable or not available from published literature

The literature focuses predominantly on depression and less on the other seque-lae.[74] Johnson postulates that this emphasis on depression stems, in part, from the fact that depression may tend to elicit the concern of others.[74] Accordingly, health care professionals may be moved to alleviate the suffering of depressed patients and thus might be more likely to request psychiatric referrals on the basis of depressive symptoms than anxiety symptoms. Johnson suggests that this concept, paired with the availability of effective treatments for depression in younger patients, has fueled the interest in depression.

In our view, the focus on depression is not misguided, given that it clearly has been shown to predict recovery and can be treated effectively in stroke patients. However, other sequelae—anxiety, apathy, emotional lability, anger, and hostility—merit more research attention.

ACKNOWLEDGMENTS

Preparation of this chapter was facilitated by a University of Western Ontario Vice-President Research Grant and a grant from the Agnes Cole Dark Fund (Faculty of Social Science, The University of Western Ontario) to LCS.

REFERENCES

1. Abramson LY, Seligman MEP, Teasdale JD: Learned helplessness in humans: Critique and reformulation. J Abnorm Psychol 87:49–74, 1978.
2. Affleck G, Tennen H, Pfeiffer C, Fifield J: Appraisals of control and predictability in adapting to a chronic disease. J Pers Soc Psychol 53:273–279, 1987.
3. Agrell B, Dehlin O: Comparison of six depression rating scales in geriatric stroke patients. Stroke 20:1190–1194, 1989.
4. Agrell B, Dehlin O: Depression in stroke patients with left and right hemisphere lesions. A study in geriatric rehabilitation in-patients. Aging Clin Exp Res 6:49–56, 1994.
5. American Psychiatric Association: Diagnostic and Statistical Manual of Mental Disorders. 4th ed. Washington, DC, American Psychiatric Association, 1994.
6. Andersen G, Vestergaard K, Ingemann-Nielsen M, Lauritzen L: Risk factors for poststroke depression. Acta Psychiatr Scand 92:193–198, 1995.
7. Andersen G, Vestergaard K, Lauritzen L: Effective treatment of poststroke depression with the selective serotonin reuptake inhibitor citalopram. Stroke 25:1099–1104, 1994.
8. Andersen G, Vestergaard K, Riis JO: Citalopram for post-stroke pathological crying. Lancet 342:837–839, 1993.
9. Anderson TP: Rehabilitation of patients with completed stroke. In Kottke EJ, Stillwell GK, Lehmann JF (eds): Krusen's Handbook of Physical Medicine and Rehabilitation. Philadelphia, WB Saunders, 1982, pp 583–603.
10. Astrom M: Generalized anxiety disorder in stroke patients. A 3-year longitudinal study. Stroke 27:270–275, 1996.
11. Astrom M, Adolfsson R, Asplund K: Major depression in stroke patients. A 3-year longitudinal study. Stroke 24:976–982, 1993.
12. Astrom M, Olsson T, Asplund K: Different linkage of depression to hypercortisolism early versus late after stroke. A 3-year longitudinal study. Stroke 24:52–57, 1993.
13. Barrera MA: A method for the assessment of social support networks in community survey research. Connections 3:8–13, 1980.
14. Barrera M, Sandler IN, Ramsey TB: Preliminary development of a scale of social support: Studies on college students. Am J Community Psychol 9:435–447, 1981.
15. Beck AT, Steer RA: Internal consistencies of the original and revised Beck Depression Inventory. J Clin Psychol 40:1365–1367, 1984.
16. Beck AT, Ward CH, Mendelson M, et al: An inventory for measuring depression. Arch Gen Psychiatry 4:561–571, 1961.
17. Benson DF: Psychiatric aspects of aphasia. Fr J Psychiatry 123:555–556, 1973.
18. Bergner M, Bobbit RA, Carter WB, et al: The sickness impact profile: Development and final revision of a health status measure. Med Care 19:787–805, 1981.
19. Birkett DP: The Psychiatry of Stroke. Washington, DC, American Psychiatric Press, 1996.
20. Brink TA, Yesevage JA, Lum O: Screening tests for geriatric depression. Clin Gerontol 1:37–44, 1982.

21. Brosseau L, Potvin L, Philippe P, et al: Post-stroke inpatient rehabilitation: II. Predicting discharge disposition. Am J Phys Med Rehabil 75:431–436, 1996.
22. Bulman R, Wortman C: Attributions of blame and coping in the "real world": Severe accident victims react to their lot. Pers Soc Psychol 35:351–363, 1977.
23. Burvill PW, Johnson GA, Jamrozik KD, et al: Prevalence of depression after stroke: The Perth Community Stroke Study. Br J Psychiatry 166:320–327, 1995.
24. Burvill PW, Johnson GA, Jamrozik KD, et al: Anxiety disorders after stroke: Results from the Perth Community Stroke Study. Br J Psychiatry 166:328–332, 1995.
25. Castillo CS, Schultz SK, Robinson RG: Clinical correlates of early-onset and late-onset poststroke generalized anxiety. Am J Pyschiatry 152:1174–1179, 1995.
26. Castillo CS, Starkstein SE, Fedoroff JP, et al: Generalized anxiety disorder after stroke. J Nerv Ment Dis 181:100–106, 1993.
27. Charaton FB, Fisk A: Th emental and emotional results of strokes. N Y State J Med 78:1403–1405, 1978.
28. Cohen S, Mermelstein R, Kamarck T, et al: Measuring the functional components of social support. In Sarason IG, Sarason BR (eds): Social Support: Theory, Research and Applications. Boston, Martinus Nijhoff, 1985, pp 75–94.
29. Cutting I: Memory in functional psychosis. J Neurol Neurosurg Psychiatry 42:1031–1037, 1979.
30. D'Olhaberriague L, Litvan I, Mitsias P, et al: A reappraisal of reliability and validity studies in stroke. Stroke 27:2331–2336, 1996.
31. Doolittle N: Clinical ethnography of lacunar stroke: Implications for acute care. J Neurosci Nurs 23:235–240, 1991.
32. Dorman P, Slattery J, Farrell B, et al: Qualitative comparison of the reliability of health status assessments with the EuroQol and SF-36 questionnaires after stroke. Stroke 29:63–68, 1988.
33. Dorman PJ, Waddell F, Slattery J, et al: Is the EuroQol a valid measure of health-related quality of life after stroke? Stroke 28:1876–1882, 1997.
34. Dorman PJ, Waddell F, Slattery J, et al: Are proxy assessments of health status after stroke with the EuroQol questionnaire feasible, accurate, and unbiased? Stroke 28:1883–1887, 1997.
35. Duke University Center for the Study of Aging and Human Development: Multidimensional functional assessment: The OARS methodology. In Kanem RA, Kane RL (eds): Assessing the Elderly: A Practical Guide to Measurement. Lexington, MA, Lexington Books, 1984, pp 166–168.
36. Eastwood MR, Rifat SL, Nobbs H, et al: Mood disorder following cerebrovascular accident. Br J Psychiatry 154:195–200, 1989.
37. Ebrahim S, Barer D, Nouri F: Affective illness after stroke. Br J Psychiatry 151:52–56, 1987.
38. Engel GL: The need for a new biomedical model: A challenge for biomedicine. Science 196:129–136, 1977.
39. Evans R, Connis RT, Bishop RD, et al: Stroke: A family dilemma. Disabil Rehabil 3:110–118, 1994.
40. Evans RL, Northwood LK: Social support needs in adjustment to stroke. Arch Phys Med Rehabil 64:61–64, 1983.
41. Feibel JH, Berk SS, Joynt RJ: Unmet needs of stroke survivors. Neurology 29:592, 1979.
42. Feibel JH, Springer CJ: Depression and failure to resume social activities after stroke. Arch Phys Med Rehabil 63:276–278, 1982.
43. Finkelstein S, Benowitz LI, Baldessarian RJ, et al: Mood, vegetative disturbance and dexamethasone suppression test after stroke. Ann Neurol 12:463–468, 1982.
44. Fisher SH: Psychiatric considerations of cerebral vascular disease. Am J Cardiol 7:379–385, 1961.
45. Folstein MF, Mailberger R, McHugh PR: Mood disorder as a specific complication of stroke. J Neurol Neurosurg Psychiatry 40:1018–1022, 1977.
46. Fordyce WE: Behavioral methods in medical rehabilitation. Neurosci Biobehav Rev 5:391–396, 1981.
47. Friedland JF, McColl, M: Social support intervention after stroke: Results of a randomized trial. Arch Phys Med Rehabil 73:573–581, 1992.
48. Gainotti G: Emotional behavior and hemispheric side of the lesion. Cortex 8:41–55, 1972.
49. Gainotti G: Disorders of emotions and affect in patients with unilateral brain damage. In Boller F, Graffman J (eds): Handbook of Neuropsychology. Vol 3. Amsterdam, Elsevier, 1989, pp 345–361.
50. Gallagher D, Nies G, Thompson LW: Reliability of the Beck Depression Inventory with older adults. J Consult Clin Psychol 50:152–153, 1982.
51. Geddes JML, Chamberlain MA: Improving social outcome after stroke: An evaluation of the volunteer stroke scheme. Clin Rehabil 8:117–126, 1994.
52. Ghika-Schmid F, Bogousslavsky J: Affective disorders following stroke. Eur Neurol 38:75–81, 1997.

53. Gillespie DC: Poststroke anxiety and its relationship to coping and stage of recovery. Psychol Rep 80:1059–1064, 1997.
54. Glass TA, Maddox GL: The quality and quantity of social support: Stroke recovery as psycho-social transition. Soc Sci Med 34:1249–1261, 1992.
55. Goldberg DP, Hillier VF: A scaled version of the General Health Questionnaire. Psychol Med 9:139–145, 1979.
56. Goldstein K: Language and Language Disturbances. New York, Grune & Stratton, 1948.
57. Granger CV, Hamilton BB, Keith RA, et al: Advances in functional assessment for medical rehabilitation. Top Geriatr Rehabil 1:59–74, 1986.
58. Hafsteinsdottir TB, Grypdonck M: Being a stroke patient: A review of the literature. J Adv Nurs 26:580–588, 1997.
59. Hamilton M: Development of a rating scale for primary depressive illness. Br J Soc Clin Psychol 6:278–296, 1967.
60. Hanger HC, Mulley GP: Questions people ask about stroke. Stroke 24:536–538, 1993.
61. Havenaar JM, Rumyantzevam GM, Poelijoe NW, et al: The reliability and validity of two psychiatric screening questionnaires in the Russian Federation. Intl J Methods Psychiatric Res 9:237–242, 1996.
62. Heitzman CA, Kaplan RM: Assessment of methods for measuring social support. Health Psychol 7:75–109, 1988.
63. Herrmann C: International experience with the hospital anxiety and depression scale: A review of validation data and clinical results. J Psychosom Res 42:17–41, 1997.
64. Herrmann N, Black SE, Lawrence J, et al: The Sunnybrook Stroke Study. A prospective study of depressive symptoms and functional outcome. Stroke 29:618–624, 1998.
65. Hibbard MR, Gordon WA, Stein PN, et al: Awareness of disability in patients following stroke. Rehabil Psychol 37:103–120, 1992.
66. Holbrook ME, Skilbeck CE: An activities index for use with stroke patients. Age Ageing 12:166–170, 1983.
67. Horgas AL, Wahl HW, Baltes MM: Dependency in late life. In Carstensen LL, Edelstein BA, Dorbrand L (eds): The Practical Handbook of Clinical Gerontology. Thousand Oaks, CA, Sage, 1996, pp 54–75.
68. House A: Depression associated with stroke. Neuropsychiatr Pract Opin 4:453–457, 1996.
69. House A, Dennis M, Mogridge L, et al: Mood disorders in the year after first stroke. Br J Psychiatry 158:83–92, 1991.
70. House A, Dennis M, Molyneux A, et al: Emotionalism after stroke BMJ 298:991–994, 1989.
71. Isaacs B, Neville Y, Rushford I: The stricken: Social consequences of stroke. Age Ageing 5:188–192, 1976.
72. Jacelon CS: The Barthel Index and other indices of functionality. J Rehabil Nurs 11:9–11, 1986.
73. James JE, Minichiello V: Disability and rehabilitation in older persons: Biopsychosocial foundations [editorial]. Disabil Rehabil 16:95–97, 1994.
74. Johnson GA: Research into psychiatric disorder after stroke: The need for further studies. Aust N Z J Psychiatry 25:358–370, 1991.
75. Johnson G, Burvill PW, Anderson CD, et al: Screening instruments for depression and anxiety following stroke: Experience in the Perth Community Stroke Study. Acta Psychiatr Scand 91:252–257, 1995.
76. Jorge RE, Robinson RG, Starkstein SE, et al: Secondary mania following traumatic brain injury. Am J Psychiatry 150:916–921, 1993.
77. Josephs A: Stroke: An Owner's Manual. Long Beach, CA, Amadeus Press, 1992.
78. Kaplan RM: Behavior as the central outcome in health care. Am Psychol 45:1211–1220, 1990.
79. Kaufman SR, Becker G: Content and boundaries of medicine in long-term care: Physicians talk about stroke. Gerontologist 31:238–245, 1991.
80. Kelly-Hayes M, Wolf PA, Kannel WB: Factors influencing survival and need for institutionalization following stroke: The Framingham Study. Arch Phys Med Rehabil 69:415–418, 1988.
81. Kelly-Hayes M, Paige C: Assessment and psychologic factors in stroke rehabilitation. Neurology 45:S29–S32, 1995.
82. Kilic C, Rezaki M, Rezaki B, et al: General health questionnaire (GH12 & GH28): Psychometric properties and factor structure of the scales in a Turkish primary care sample. Soc Psychiatry Psychiatr Epidemiol 32:327–331, 1997.
83. King RB: Quality of life after stroke. Stroke 27:1467–1472, 1996.
84. Koivisto K, Viinamake H, Riekkinen P: Poststroke depression and rehabilitation outcome. Nord J Psychiatry 47:245–249, 1993.
85. Kotila M, Numminen H, Waltimo O, et al: Depression after stroke: Results of the FINNSTROKE study. Stroke 29:368–372, 1998.

86. Kraus MF: Neuropsychiatric sequelae of stroke and traumatic brain injury: The role of psychostimulants. Int J Psychiatry Med 25:39–51, 1995.

87. Kriegsman DM, Deeg DJ, Van Eijk JT, et al: Does family support buffer the impact of specific chronic diseases on mobility in community-dwelling elderly? Disabil Rehabil 19:71–83, 1997.

88. Lauritzen L, Bendsen BB, Vilar T, et al: Post-stroke depression: Combined treatment with imipramine or desipramine and mianserin. A controlled clinical study. Psychopharmacology 114:119–122, 1994.

89. Lazarus LW, Winemiller DR, Lingam VR, et al: Efficacy and side effects of methylphenidate for poststroke depression. J Clin Psychiatry 53:447–449, 1992.

90. Lewinsohn PM, Biglan A, Zeiss AM: Behavioral treatment of depression. In Davidson PO (ed): The Behavioral Management of Anxiety, Depression, and Pain. New York, Brunner/Mazel, 1976, pp 91–146.

91. Lincoln NB, Flannaghan T, Sutcliffe L: Evaluation of cognitive behavioural treatment for depression after stroke: A pilot study. Clin Rehabil 11:114–122, 1997.

92. Lingam VR, Lazarus LW, Groves L, et al: Methylphenidate in treating poststroke depression. J Clin Psychiatry 29:46–49, 1988.

93. Lipsey JR, Robinson RG, Pearlson GD, et al: Mood change following bilateral hemispheric brain injury. Br J Psychiatry 143:266–273, 1983.

94. Lipsey JR, Robinson RG, Pearlson GD, et al: Nortriptyline treatment in post-stroke depression: A double-blind study. Lancet 3372:297–300, 1984.

95. Lipsey JR, Robinson RG, Pearlson GD, et al: Dexamethasone suppression test and mood following strokes. Am J Psychiatry 142:318–323, 1985.

96. Loong CK, Ng Kwan Chung K, Paulin ST: Post-stroke depression: Outcome following rehabilitation. Aust N Z J Psychiatry 29:609–614, 1995.

97. Mahoney FI, Barthel DW: Functional evaluation: The Barthel index. Md State Med J 14:61–65, 1965.

98. Marin RS, Biedrzycki RC, Firinciogullari S: Reliability and validity of the apathy evaluation scale. Psychiatry Res 38:143–162, 1991.

99. Marshall J, Sacchett C: Does the Volunteer Stroke Scheme improve social outcome after stroke? A response to Geddes and Chamberlain. Clin Rehabil 10:104–111, 1996.

100. Masand PS: Psychostimulants, poststroke depression, and side effects [letter]. J Clin Psychiatry 54:356, 1993.

101. McCaffrey RJ, Fisher JM: Cognitive, behavioural and psychosocial sequelae of cerebrovascular accidents and closed head injuries in older adults. In Carstensen LL, Edelstein BA (eds): Handbook of Clinical Gerontology. New York, Pergammon Press, 1987, pp 277–288.

102. McColl MA, Friedland J: Development of a multidimensional index for assessing social support in rehabilitation. Occup Ther J Res 9:218–234, 1989.

103. Morris PLP, Robinson RG, Andrzejewski P, et al: Association of depression with 10-year poststroke mortality. Am J Psychiatry 150:124–129, 1993.

104. Morris PLP, Robinson RG, Raphaelle B: Emotional lability after stoke. Aust N Z J Psychiatry 27:601–605, 1993.

105. Morris PL, Shields RB, Hopwood MJ, et al: Are there two depressive syndromes after stroke? J Nerv Ment Dis 182:230–234, 1994.

106. Morris PLP, Robinson RG: Drs. Morris and Robinson reply to Cooney JA. Am J Psychiatry 151:152, 1994.

107. Mukand J, Kaplan M, Senno RG, et al: Pathological laughing and crying: Treatment with sertraline. Arch Phys Med Rehabil 77:1309–1311, 1996.

108. Murray GB, Shea V, Conn DK: Electroconvulsive therapy for poststroke depression. J Clin Psychiatry 47:258–260, 1986.

109. Nauta WJH: The problem of the frontal lobe: A reinterpretation. J Psychiatr Res 8:167–187, 1971.

110. Norris VK, Stephens MAP, Kinney JM: The impact of family interactions on recovery from stroke: Help or hindrance? Gerontology 30:535–542, 1990.

111. O'Rourke S, MacHale S, Signorine D, Dennis M: Detecting psychiatric morbidity after stroke. Comparison of the GHQ and the HAD Scale. Stroke 29:980–985, 1998.

112. Okada K, Kobayashi S, Yamagata S, et al: Poststroke apathy and regional cerebral blood flow. Stroke 28:2437–2441, 1997.

113. O'Sullivan RL, Fava M, Agustin C, et al: Sensitivity of the six-item depression rating scale. Acta Psychiatr Scand 95:379–384, 1997.

114. Paradiso S, Robinson RG, Arndt S: Self-reported aggressive behavior in patients with stroke. J Nerv Ment Dis 184:746–753, 1996.

115. Paradiso S, Tatsunobu O, Robinson RG: Vegetative and psychological symptoms associated with depressed mood over the first two years after stroke. Int J Psychiatry Med 27:137–157, 1997.

116. Parikh RM, Lipsey JR, Roginson RE, et al: A two year longitudinal study of poststroke mood disorders: Prognostic factors related to one and two year outcome. Int J Psychiatry Med 18:45–56, 1988.
117. Pintoff E: Bolt from the Blue. Salt Lake City, Northwest, 1992.
118. Popkin MK, Callies AL, Colon EA: A framework for the study of medical depression. Psychosomatics 28:27–33, 1987.
119. Primeau F: Post-stroke depression: A critical review of the literature. Can J Psychiatry 33:757–765, 1988.
120. Raffaele R, Rampello L, Vecchio I: Trazodone therapy of the post-stroke depression. Arch Gerontol Geriatr 5(suppl):217–220, 1996.
121. Reding MJ, Orto LA, Winter SW, et al: Antidepressant therapy after stroke. Arch Neurol 43:763–765, 1986.
122. Reding MJ, Gardner C, Hainline B, et al: Neuropsychiatric problems interfering with inpatient stroke rehabilitation. J NeuroRehabil 7:1–7, 1993.
123. Reynolds WM, Kobak KA: Reliability and validity of the Hamilton Depression Inventory: A paper-and-pencil version of the Hamilton Depression Rating Scale Clinical Interview. Psychol Assess 7:472–483, 1995.
124. Roberts L, Counsell C: Assessment of clinical outcomes in acute stroke trials. Stroke 29:986–991, 1998.
125. Robinson RG: Poststroke pathological laughing and crying: A reply to Ivan and Franco. Am J Psychiatry 151:291–292, 1994.
126. Robinson RG: Neuropsychiatric consequences of stroke. Annu Rev Med 48:217–229, 1997.
127. Robinson RG, Parikh RM, Lipsey JR, et al: Pathological laughing and crying following stroke: Validation of a measurement scale and a double-blind treatment study. Am J Psychiatry 150:286–293, 1993.
128. Robinson RG, Starr LB, Kubos KL, Price T: A two-year longitudinal study of post-stroke mood disorders: Findings during the initial evaluation. Stroke 14:736–741, 1983.
129. Robinson RG, Starr LB, Price TR: A two year longitudinal study of mood disorders following stroke: Prevalence and duration at six months follow-up. Br J Psychiatry 144:256–262, 1984.
130. Robinson RG, Szetela B: Mood change following left hemispheric brain injury. Ann Neurol 9:447–453, 1981.
131. Ross ED, Gordon WA, Hibbard M, et al: The dexamethasone suppression test, post-stroke depression and the validity of DSM-III-based diagnostic criteria. Am J Psychiatry 143:1200–1201, 1986.
132. Rosse RE, Ciolino CP: Effects of cortical lesion location on psychiatric consultation referral for depressed stroke patients. Int J Psychiatr Med 15:311–319, 1986.
133. Schneider L, Pollock VE, Lyness SA: A meta-analysis of controlled trials of neuroleptic treatment in dementia. J Am Geriatr Soc 38:555–563, 1990.
134. Schulz R, Decker S: Long-term adjustment to physical disability: The role of social support, perceived control and self-blame. Pers Soc Psychol 48:1162–1172, 1985.
135. Schultz SK, Castillo CS, Kosier JT, et al: Generalized anxiety and depression. Am J Geriatr Psychiatry 5:229–237, 1997.
136. Seligman ME: Fall into helplessness. Psychol Today 7:43–48, 1973.
137. Sharpe M, Hawton K, House A, et al: Mood disorders in long-term survivors of stroke: Associations with brain lesion location and volume. Psychol Med 20:815–828, 1990.
138. Sharpe M, Hawton K, Seagroatt V, et al: Depressive disorders in long-term survivors of stroke. Associations with demographic and social factors, functional status, and brain lesion volume. Br J Psychiatry 164:380–386, 1994.
139. Shiekh JI, Yesevage JA: Geriatric Depression Scale: Recent evidence and development of a shorter version. Clin Gerontol 5:165–173, 1986.
140. Small M, Ellis S: Denial of hemiplegia: An investigation into the theories of causation. Eur Neurol 36:353–363, 1996.
141. Sneeuw KCA, Aaronson NK, de Haan RJ, et al: Assessing quality of life after stroke: The value and limitations of proxy ratings. Stroke 28:1541–1549, 1997.
142. Stamenkovic M, Schindler S, Kasper S: Poststroke depression and fluoxetine. Am J Psychiatry 153:446–447, 1996.
143. Starkstein SE, Boston JD, Robinson RG: Mechanisms of mania after brain injury. J Nerv Ment Dis 176:87–100, 1988.
144. Starkstein SE, Cohen BS, Federoff P, et al: Relationship between anxiety disorders and depressive disorders in patients with cerebrovascular injury. Arch Gen Psychiatry 47:246–251, 1990.
145. Starkstein SE, Federoff JP, Price TR, et al: Catastrophic reaction after cerebrovascular lesions: Frequency, correlates, and validation of a scale. J Neuropsychiatry Clin Neurosci 5:189–194, 1993.

146. Starkstein SE, Federoff JP, Price TR, et al: Anosognosia in patients with cerebrovascular lesions: A study of causative factors. Stroke 23:1446–1453, 1992.
147. Starkstein SE, Mayberg HS, Preziosi TJ, et al: Reliability, validity, and clinical correlates of apathy in Parkinson's disease. J Neuropsychiatry Clin Neurosci 4:134–139, 1992.
148. Starkstein SE, Robinson RG: Aphasia and depression. Aphasiology 2:1–20, 1988.
149. Starkstein SE, Robinson RG: Neuropsychiatric aspects of stroke. In Coffey CE, Cummings JL (eds): The American Psychiatric Press Textbook of Geriatric Neuropsychiatry. Washington, DC, American Psychiatric Press, 1994.
150. Starkstein SE, Robinson RG: Mechanisms of disinhibition after brain lesions. J Nerv Ment Dis 185:108–114, 1994.
151. Starr LB, Robinson RG, Price TR, et al: Reliability, validity and clinical utility of the social functioning exam in the assessment of stroke patients. Exp Aging Res 9:101–106, 1983.
152. Stephens MAP, Kinney JM, Norris VK, et al: Social networks as assets and liabilities in recovery from stroke by geriatric patients. Psychol Aging 2:125–129, 1987.
153. Swartzman LC, Teasell RW: Psychological consequences of stroke. Phys Med Rehabil Stat Art Rev 7:179–194, 1993.
154. The EuroQol Group: EuroQol—a new facility for the measurement of health-related quality of life. Health Policy 16:199–208, 1990.
155. Thompson SC, Sobolew-Shubin A, Graham MA, et al: Psychosocial adjustment following a stroke. Soc Sci Med 28:239–247, 1989.
156. Van Straten A, de Haan RJ, Limburg M, et al: A stroke adapted version of the sickness impact profile to assess quality of life (SA-SIP30). Stroke 28:2155–2161, 1997.
157. [Reference deleted.]
158. Wade DT, Legh-Smith J, Hewer RA: Social activities after stroke: Measurement and natural history using the Frenchay Activities Index. Intl Rehabil Med 7:176–181, 1985.
159. Wade DT, Legh-Smith J, Hewer RA: Depressed mood after stroke. A community study of its frequency. Br J Psychiatry 151:200–205, 1987.
160. Ware JE, Sherbourne CD: The MOS 36-item short-form health survey (SF-36): Conceptual framework and item selection. Med Care 30:473–483, 1992.
161. Ween JE, Alexander MP, D'Esposito M, et al: Factors predictive of stroke outcome in a rehabilitation setting. Neurology 47:388–392, 1996.
162. Weinman E, Ruskin PE: Anger attacks in poststroke depression: Responses to fluoxetine. Am J Psychiatry 151:1839, 1994.
163. Williams AM: Self-report of indifference and anxiety among persons with right hemisphere stroke. Res Nurs Health 15:343–347, 1992.
164. Wyller TB, Holmes J, Laake P, et al: Correlates of subjective well-being in stroke patients. Stroke 29:363–367, 1998.
165. Yesavage JA, Brink TL, Rose TL: Development and validation of a geriatric depression scale: A preliminary report. J Psychiatr Res 17:37–49, 1983.
166. Zigmond AS, Snaith RP: The hospital anxiety and depression scale. Acta Psychiatr Scand 67:361–370, 1983.
167. Zung WW: From art to science: The diagnosis and treatment of depression. Arch Gen Psychiatry 29:328–337, 1973.

ASHOK DEVASENAPATHY, MD
VLADIMIR C. HACHINSKI, MD,
MSc, DSc (MED), FRCPC

COGNITIVE IMPAIRMENT POSTSTROKE

From the Department of Clinical
    Neurological Sciences
University of Western Ontario
London, Ontario
Canada

Reprint requests to:
Ashok Devasenapathy, MD
Department of Clinical Neurological
    Sciences
University of Western Ontario
339 Windermere Road
London, Ontario N6A 5A5
Canada

Strokes relate to cognitive impairment in different ways. They may cause, contribute to, or coexist with impaired cognition and memory problems (Fig. 1). Cognitive deficits that are causally related to strokes are commonly referred to as *vascular dementia*.[18]

The use of the generic term *vascular dementia* should be discouraged because it neither identifies an etiology that may respond to current or future treatments nor recognizes the cognitive impairment as a syndrome with a clinical spectrum of neurologic and neuropsychologic deficits.[19] An alternate approach is desirable that would identify individuals across the entire spectrum of vascular cognitive impairment, from being at high risk with no clinical symptoms (brain-at-risk stage) to having full-blown dementia.[18,19]

The concept of vascular cognitive impairment as a "dementia" implies a degenerative cause of the underlying cognitive deficits and a predominantly short-term memory deficit pattern of cognitive impairment, as seen in Alzheimer's disease. Alzheimer's disease has an unknown cause and is therefore not preventable, but strokes often have an identifiable cause that may respond to both preventive and acute therapeutic measures.[4]

Population-based studies show that cognitive deficits occur in at least 10% of persons older than 65 and in 25–50% of those older than 85.[22] Although Alzheimer's disease accounts for up to two thirds of all dementias, vascular causes form the second largest group, with a prevalence of 15–20%.[12] Epidemiologic studies show that up to

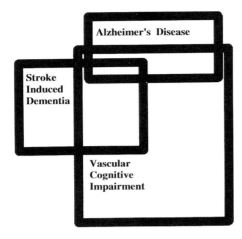

FIGURE 1. Relationship among vascular cognitive impairment and other causes of cognitive impairment.

a quarter of stroke patients may develop a vascular dementia.[39] The lack of standardized criteria for the identification of vascular cognitive impairment, and the generalized use of psychometric tests oriented to short-term memory to screen for cognition deficits in individuals with cerebrovascular disease, carries with it the risk of underestimating the true clinical magnitude of vascular cognitive impairment.[10]

The early identification and treatment of vascular dementia warrants its recognition as a clinical syndrome rather than a true dementia or a single disease.[4] Although multiple large infarcts from ischemic strokes may form one end of a clinical continuum associated with this syndrome, most patients with vascular cognitive impairment have minimal or subclinical deficits (with either vascular risk factors in isolation or clinically silent strokes from under- or untreated risk factors, i.e., the brain-at-risk stage). It is with these latter patients that preventive measures are most responsive and treatments effective.[4]

Over the last several decades, great strides have been made in the early identification and treatment of vascular risk factors that contribute to the development of heart disease and strokes. Yet, the relative risk associated with any known vascular risk factors in the development of vascular dementia remains poorly characterized and understood.[10] The clinical significance of this problem takes on a greater importance given that many elderly patients who have a nondegenerative cause for their cognitive deficits may have the early manifestation of cerebrovascular disease, which may eventually manifest as ischemic and hemorrhagic strokes.[13]

This chapter outlines the current knowledge of the epidemiology, pathophysiology, pathology, diagnosis, and treatment of vascular cognitive impairment.

EPIDEMIOLOGY

Vascular cognitive impairment accounts for 15–20% of all dementias.[22] The prevalence increases exponentially with age and varies among countries, ranging from 1.2–4.2% in persons older than 65.[5] In Western countries about 30% of patients with cognitive impairment (as shown in clinical studies of dementia that have autopsy series) have a mixed dementia, with a combination of vascular and degenerative processes rather than one isolated pathology.[10,12] However, no standard clinical or pathologic criteria exist for the identification of mixed dementia.

Patients with a history of cerebrovascular disease appear to be at considerable risk for cognitive impairment (odds ratio 5.7–31.2).[39] Up to one quarter of stroke patients develop some form of cognitive impairment after a stroke.[39] Studies show that a stroke increases the relative risk of cognitive impairment by ninefold, and the risk is highest in the age group of 70–79, with an odds ratio of 31.2, suggesting stroke is an important independent risk factor for cognitive impairment.[39]

Racial and genetic factors may be other independent risk factors for vascular cognitive impairment, with the relative risk of vascular dementia higher in certain racial groups and demographic regions, as illustrated in published case series showing a relatively higher incidence of vascular dementia in China and Japan.[25] Stroke subtypes may be another important factor. Compared to nonstroke control groups, lacunar strokes have a four- to fivefold relative risk of contributing to the development of cognitive deficits.[28] The significance of stroke subtypes in the development of vascular cognitive impairment may reflect the relative importance of vascular risk factors that are common to both the stroke subtype and the cognitive deficits. Because our current understanding of the risk factors and pathogenic mechanisms involved in the development of the different stroke subtypes is incomplete, especially in the case of lacunar strokes and subcortical white matter infarcts, the presumed benefits derived (in preventing cognitive impairment) from the early institution of primary and secondary preventive measures remain unknown.[10]

PATHOPHYSIOLOGY

Although the pathophysiology of Alzheimer's disease and vascular dementia are different, several of the neurochemical processes induced by cerebral ischemia and seen with Alzheimer's disease seem common.[3]

Patients with strokes are prone to develop Alzheimer's-type histology.[3] It is believed that vascular insults to the brain may activate or accelerate degenerative mechanisms.[36] Ischemia-induced inflammation, microglial activation, glutamate toxicity, and neuronal death are common to both of these dementias.[29] Additionally, inflammatory processes occur in both dementias and are associated with a proliferation of microglial cells as well as the production of cytokines—mainly interleukin-1-β, tumor necrosis factor-β, and neurotoxic free radicals.[11] The free radicals generated promote the aggregation of β-amyloid peptides (an important component of amyloid plaques), which is a common pathologic feature of Alzheimer's disease.[24] Additionally, mature astrocytes that normally produce nerve growth factor are affected by ischemia/degenerative processes, with the resultant production of abnormal subtypes of nerve growth factor that have a reduced capacity in maintaining extracellular homeostasis.[2] Furthermore, neuronal death from ischemia or degeneration provokes an excessive release of the amino-acid glutamate, resulting in an increase in extracellular calcium concentration.[2] Astrocytes have the important physiologic role as scavengers of excess extracellular calcium. Intracellular "calcium overload" in astrocytes results in their death, which leads to the production of neuritic (astrocytic) plaques, another hallmark of Alzheimer's disease.[2]

Cohort studies show that some patients with vascular cognitive impairment—other than from large cerebral infarcts or strategic infarcts—have a delayed onset and slow, insidious evolution of their cognitive deficit, which occurs over several months following stroke rather than as an abrupt presentation of cognitive symptoms.[39] It is likely that the degenerative pathology and processes that are common to vascular dementia and Alzheimer's disease may relate to impaired function or loss of cholinergic neurons in the basal forebrain.[31] Impaired activity of cholinergic neurons in the forebrain (basal nucleus of Meynert) has been implicated in cognitive deficits and behavioral disturbance associated with Alzheimer's disease.[31] Similar biochemical mechanisms may be important in the development of cognitive impairment associated with cerebrovascular disease.

PATHOLOGIC SUBTYPES OF VASCULAR COGNITIVE IMPAIRMENT

This chapter strives to convey a logical approach to an understanding of vascular cognitive impairment as a clinical syndrome, with neuropsychological deficits forming a continuum from the asymptomatic brain-at-risk stage to frank dementia. An overview of the cerebrovascular pathology underlying the distinctive subtypes of vascular cognitive impairment may aid in an appreciation of the complex clinical spectrum, neuropsychological deficits, and neuroradiologic features encountered in this syndrome.

Brain-at-Risk Stage

Longitudinal follow-up of asymptomatic patients with isolated vascular risk factors shows that these patient are not only at risk for strokes but also for cognitive impairment. The underlying basis for this observation remains unclear. At least some of the patients develop clinical strokes and others silent strokes that may contribute to the observed cognitive deficits.[13]

Other individuals who remain free of strokes may have chronic ongoing brain ischemia from a combination of one or more factors that may contribute to the development of ischemia-induced degenerative processes. The long-term influence of vascular risk factors or arteriosclerosis on the cerebral vessels may lead to impaired cerebral autoregulation, resulting in chronically lowered cerebral perfusion.[38] This phenomenon has been called *misery perfusion* based on positron emission tomography results that show increased cerebral oxygen extraction in patients who have normal cognition (predementia phase) but a sharp drop in the oxygen extraction value in individuals with vascular dementia.[38] Cerebral ischemia may directly or indirectly influence the normal activity of important neurochemical pathways involved in cognition.[38] Additionally, cerebral ischemia-related activation of degenerative mechanisms, as described above, may aggravate the already diminished activity of important neurotransmitters involved in cognition.[3,31]

Early and aggressive treatment of all identified vascular risk factors may be beneficial in the primary prevention of cognitive impairment from cerebrovascular disease, as suggested by studies that support the benefits (prevention of dementia) of the primary and secondary prevention of strokes and clinical trials that show the combined benefit of postmenopausal estrogen replacement therapy in women as an effective means of reducing vascular morbidity and Alzheimer's disease.[20] Current and future longitudinal population-based studies of dementia that seek to assess the benefits of treating vascular risk factors may provide more insight into the pathogenesis of vascular cognitive impairments.[5,10,37]

Strategic Infarct Dementia

Ischemic or hemorrhagic strokes that involve the dominant angular gyrus, left thalamus/basal ganglia, and temporal lobes have been associated with the abrupt onset of cognitive deficits. Small strategic infarcts in the thalamus/basal ganglia also may produce diverse neurologic and psychological manifestations, from the disruption of one or more connections to the limbic system and frontal lobes.[40] The severity of cognitive deficits associated with such strokes is often dependent on the patient's age, presence of premorbid cognitive deficits, location of the stroke, underlying cause of the stroke, and the extent of associated cerebrovascular disease. Generally, the resultant cognitive deficit remains unchanged or may improve over time.[40]

Cognitive Impairment after a Single Stroke

Some susceptible individuals develop cognitive problems after an isolated, nondebilitating clinical or silent stroke. Cerebral ischemia may activate or accelerate mechanisms that lead to the development of cerebral histopathology typically seen in Alzheimer's disease. Neurofibrillary tangles and senile plaques may cause, contribute, or have a casual association with cognitive impairment from strokes. Single large strokes involving cerebral hemispheres or the frontal lobes may produce profound cognitive impairment, behavorial changes, and complex neuropsychological deficits immediately after the stroke. In such instances, the site and volume of cerebral infarction may predict the severity of the cognitive impairment.[40]

Multi-infarct Dementia

The term *multi-infarct dementia* generally refers to the cognitive impairment that is associated with multiple large strokes or recurrent lacunar strokes.[16] The resulting pattern of cognitive deficit has been described as stepwise in its progression.[27] The Hachinski Ischemic Scale (Table 1) has been validated for use in the diagnosis of multi-infarct dementia and acts as a reliable means of differentiating multi-infarct dementia from Alzheimer's disease.[27] This scale has not been validated for use in differentiating vascular dementia from the mixed dementias, although the vascular component remains the only treatable element that is common to both types of cognitive impairment.[7]

Cerebral Leukoaraiosis and White Matter Dementia

The cerebral white matter receives perfusion from both the superficial cortical penetrating blood vessels and the deep terminal perforating vessels. By virtue of the

TABLE 1. The Ischemic Scale

Feature	Value*
Abrupt onset	2
Stepwise deterioration	1
Fluctuating course	2
Nocturnal confusion	1
Relative preservation of personality	1
Depression	1
Somatic complaints	1
Emotional incontinence	1
History or presence of hypertension	1
History of strokes	2
Evidence of associated atherosclerosis	1
Focal neurologic symptoms	2
Focal neurologic signs	2
Total score	—

* Scores of 7 or more suggest a vascular etiology for dementia; scores of 4 or less do not support a vascular etiology. (Adapted from Hachinski VC, Lliff LD, Zilkha E, et al: Cerebral blood flow in dementia. Arch Neurol 32:632–637, 1975.)

pattern of blood supply, the white matter is a watershed zone and is susceptible to ischemia from different causes.

No neuroimaging modalities are presently available that can definitely differentiate ischemic cerebral white matter disease from other nonischemic pathology. The widespread availability of cerebral magnetic resonance imaging (MRI) has resulted in a false overidentification of ischemic white matter lesions, warranting the development of the term *leukoaraiosis*.[17] Leukoaraiosis describes the nonspecific nature of the MRI signal (hyperintensity) from the cerebral white matter that is common to individuals with normal cognition (associated with or without vascular risk factors), clinically probable Alzheimer's disease, and ischemic cerebrovascular disease. This term makes no reference to the underlying pathology or neurologic/cognitive deficits.[17]

In patients with normal neurologic examinations and cognition, the most likely cause for leukoaraiosis is dilated perivascular space that surrounds the penetrating cerebral blood vessels—commonly observed in individuals with poorly controlled hypertension—or "ventricular caps" and "rims" that surround the cerebrospinal fluid cavity of the brain.[42] The latter observation is common in young individuals and is often misinterpreted as being pathologic.[42]

Patients who meet clinical criteria for probable Alzheimer's disease often have leukoaraiosis; the underlying basis for this observation includes the presence of hypertensive arteriopathy, amyloid angiopathy, and cerebral small artery disease.[42] Ischemic white matter disease may reflect the effects of long-standing vascular risk factors, including hypertension, diabetes, and impaired cerebral autoregulation.[33] An impaired cerebral autoregulatory mechanism may accompany normal aging but is more pronounced in individuals with arteriosclerosis of the cerebral vessels.[37] Patients with dementia and other neurodegenerative disorders that are associated with cell loss in the midbrain/brain stem autonomic nuclei often have more pronounced postural hypotension with a predisposition for recurrent acute drops in cerebral perfusion.[37] Postural drops in blood pressure from ischemic heart disease and low cardiac output states, such as angina, and atrial fibrillation, often accompany normal aging and may worsen preexisting white matter ischemia.[33]

Patients with clinical evidence of diffuse or focal neurologic deficits may also have leukoaraiosis.[37] Some of these patients have cognitive deficits that may reflect different stages of ischemic injury to the white matter tracts, with resultant disconnection of the association pathways, to the overlying cerebral cortex, between hemispheres and subcortical gray nuclei.[9] Additionally, such patients often have radiologic evidence of strokes in the thalamus/basal ganglia that may compound the observed cognitive deficits.[38] Gait problems and bowel/bladder incontinence may accompany later stages of this process.[21] Emotional incontinence, such as with pseudobulbar phenomena, usually suggests bilateral involvement of the connections between the brain stem, frontal association cortex, and thalamus.[21] Although hypertension-induced microvascular infarcts (lacunar strokes) with recurrent subcortical ischemic strokes ("etat lacunare" or lacunar state) may be a rare cause for such symptoms, other recently identified stroke syndromes that are often associated with these symptoms include CADASIL (cerebral autosomal dominant arteriopathy with subcortical strokes and ischemic leukoencephalopathy),[41] lupus anticoagulant/antiphospholipid antibody syndrome, and the systemic autoimmune diseases.[6]

There is little evidence to suggest that Binswanger's disease is a distinct pathologic entity. Its clinical features, including cognitive problems, gait disorder, emotional incontinence, and bowel/bladder incontinence, are common to all subcortical vascular dementias.[32]

Subcortical vascular dementias have a common pattern of cognitive deficits that includes slowing of information-processing and impaired memory with poor sustained attention. Expressive language deficits are common and include poor generation of word lists, impaired verbal fluency, and impaired motor programming with impersistence and preservation. Additionally, poor concentration and impaired immediate memory result in difficulties with set shifting that may be characterized by the poor retrieval of information but intact recognition.[21]

The pathologic lesions in the subcortical vascular dementias are felt to affect the circuitry interconnecting the caudate nuclei, globus pallidus, thalamus, and frontal lobes. Gait problems often accompany the cognitive impairment and are the result of the involvement of frontal subcortical and periventricular white matter with the disruption of the thalamocorticomediocapsular pathways.[21]

RISK FACTORS

Although it is widely believed that the risk factors for vascular cognitive impairment are the same as those for cerebrovascular disease, the relative risk associated with any individual risk factor involved in the development of vascular dementia remains unclear.[37] Strokes and age are the most important independent predictors of vascular cognitive impairment.[37] A racial predilection for vascular cognitive impairment remains unproven.[4,10] Although asians may have a higher prevalence of this form of cognitive impairment than caucasians, the lack of uniformly accepted criteria for the diagnosis of vascular dementia may result in the underestimation of the prevalence of vascular dementia and mixed dementia in western countries.[10]

The relative risk associated with the other major vascular risk factors is even less clear. Systolic hypertension may be an important risk factor, but a meta-analysis of different population-based prevalence studies in vascular dementia shows inconclusive results.[30] An unclear understanding of the relative importance of risk factors involved in the development of vascular cognitive impairment may be a direct reflection of the lack of a uniformly accepted research criterion for vascular dementia and the heterogeneous nature of vascular cognitive impairment.[4,10]

CLINICAL CRITERIA FOR THE DIAGNOSIS OF VASCULAR DEMENTIA

The last three decades have witnessed an increased interest in the prevention and early treatment of cerebrovascular disease. Researchers have tried to develop clinical criteria for the diagnosis of vascular dementia that can be applied to research and clinical practice. Yet, the "dementia" concept of vascular cognitive impairment still prevails and hinders the development of clinical criteria that may be accepted uniformly.[10]

In the 1970s, the widespread understanding that cerebrovascular disease was preventable prompted the development of the Ischemic Scale (see Table 1) to help differentiate multi-infarct dementia from the degenerative dementias.[7,27] Since then this scale, either in its original or modified forms, has been applied to operationalize the many available clinical criteria for vascular dementia. This scoring system has been validated for use in the differentiation of pure Alzheimer's disease from definitive vascular dementia, but it lacks sensitivity in the diagnosis of mixed dementia.[7]

The five clinical criteria that are commonly used in clinical research for the diagnosis of vascular dementia can be categorized into two groups: The first set of criteria includes the *Diagnostic and Statistical Manual of Mental Disorders* (DSM-IV) and the International Classification of Disease (ICD-10) criteria for multi-infarct dementia

TABLE 2. Diagnostic Criteria for Vascular Dementia According to the DSM-IV

A. The development of multiple cognitive deficits manifested by both of the following:

  1. Memory impairment (impaired ability to learn new information or recall previously learned information)

  2. One or more of the following cognitive disturbances:
- Aphasia
- Apraxia
- Agnosia
- Disturbances in executive functioning

B. Memory and other cognitive deficits cause significant impairment in social or occupational functioning and demonstrate a significant decline from a previous level of functioning.

C. Focal neurologic signs and symptoms (e.g., exaggeration of deep tendon reflexes, extensor plantar response, pseudobulbar palsy, gait abnormalities, weakness of an extremity) or laboratory evidence indicative of cerebrovascular disease (e.g., multiple infarcts involving cortex and underlying white matter) that are judged to be etiologically related to the disturbance.

D. The deficits do not occur exclusively during the course of delirium.

Adapted from American Psychiatric Association: Diagnostic and Statistical Manual of Mental Disorders. 4th ed. Washington, DC, APA, 1994.

and Alzheimer's disease.[1,44] They are similar and place great emphasis on "long tract signs" and focal neurologic deficits as key elements in the diagnosis of vascular dementia (Tables 2 and 3).[1,44] The second group includes those developed by the California Alzheimer's Disease Diagnosis and Treatment Centers (CADDTC) (Table 4), the National Institute of Neurological Disease and Stroke (NINDS), and the Association Internationale pour la Research et L'Enseignement en Neuroscience (AIREN).[8,34] The NINDS and AIREN criteria have risen from the DSM-IV and ICD-10 criteria in an attempt to better facilitate operationality of the clinical criteria. Both the NINDS and AIREN are based on clinical and neuroimaging features of cerebral infarct but fail to acknowledge cerebral hemorrhage and anoxic injuries. All clinical criteria make no attempt to identify patients at the brain-at-risk stage, where intervention would be most desirable.[4,8,34]

TABLE 3. Diagnostic Criteria for Alzheimer's Disease, According to the DSM-IV

A. The development of multiple cognitive deficits manifested by both of the following:

  1. Memory impairment
  2. One or more of the following cognitive disturbances:
- Aphasia
- Apraxia
- Agnosia
- Disturbance in executive functioning

B. The cognitive deficits in criteria A1 and A2 cause significant impairment in social or occupational functioning and demonstrate a significant decline from a previous level of functioning.

C. The course is characterized by gradual onset and continuing cognitive decline.

D. The memory and other cognitive deficits are not caused by any of the following:
  1. Other central nervous conditions that cause progressive deficits in memory and cognition
  2. Systemic conditions that are known to cause dementia
  3. Substance-induced conditions

E. The deficits do not occur exclusively during the course of delirium.

F. The disturbance is not better accounted for by another disorder.

Adapted from American Psychiatric Association: Diagnostic and Statistical Manual of Mental Disorders. 4th ed. Washington, DC, APA, 1994.

TABLE 4. Criteria for Ischemic Vascular Dementia (IVD) from the State of California Alzheimer's Disease Diagnostic and Treatment Centers

I. **Dementia**

Dementia is a deterioration from a prior known or estimated level of function sufficient to interfere broadly with the conduct of the patient's customary affairs of life, which is not isolated to a single narrow category of intellectual performance and which is independent of level of consciousness.

This deterioration should be supported by historical evidence and documented by either bedside mental status testing or, ideally, by more detailed neuropsychological exam, using tests that are quantifiable, reproducible, and for which normative data are available.

II. **Probable IVD**

A. The criteria for the clinical diagnosis of probable IVD includes *all* of the following:
 1. Dementia
 2. Evidence of two or more ischemic strokes by history, neurologic signs, and/or neuroimaging studies (CT or T1-weighted MRI) or occurrence of a single stroke with a clearly documented temporal relationship to the onset of dementia
 3. Evidence of at least one infarct outside the cerebellum by CT or T1-weighted MRI
B. The diagnosis of probable IVD is supported by
 1. Evidence of multiple infarcts in brain regions known to affect cognition
 2. A history of multiple transient ischemic attacks
 3. History of vascular risk factors (e.g., hypertension, heart disease, diabetes mellitus)
 4. Elevated Hachinski Ischemic Scale (original or modified version)
C. Clinical features that are thought to be associated with IVD, but await further research, include
 1. Relatively early appearance of gait disturbances and urinary incontinence
 2. Periventricular and deep white matter changes on T2-weighted MRI that are excessive for age
 3. Focal changes in electrophysiologic studies (e.g., EEG, evoked potentials) or physiologic neuroimaging studies (e.g., SPECT, PET, NMR, spectroscopy)
D. Other clinical features that do not constitute strong evidence either for or against a diagnosis of probable IVD include
 1. Periods of slowly progressive symptoms
 2. Illusions, psychosis, hallucinations, delusions
 3. Seizures

E. Clinical features that cast doubt on a diagnosis of probable IVD include
 1. Transcortical sensory aphasia in the absence of corresponding focal lesions on neuroimaging studies
 2. Absence central neurologic symptoms/signs, other than cognitive disturbances
 3. Possible IVD

III. **Possible IVD**

A clinical diagnosis of possible IVD may be made when there is dementia and at least one of the following:

A. A history or evidence of a single stroke (but not multiple strokes) without a clearly documented temporal relationship to the onset of dementia
B. Binswanger's syndrome (without multiple strokes) that includes all of the following:
 1. Early onset urinary incontinence not explained by urologic disease, gait disturbance (e.g., parkinsonian, magnetic, apraxia, or "senile" gait) not explained by peripheral cause
 2. Vascular risk factors
 3. Extensive white matter changes on neuroimaging

IV. **Definite IVD**

A diagnosis of definite IVD requires histopathologic examination of the brain plus

A. Clinical evidence of dementia
B. Pathologic confirmation of multiple infarcts, some outside the cerebellum

Note: If there is evidence of Alzheimer's disease or some other pathologic disorder that is thought to have contributed to the dementia, a diagnosis of mixed dementia should be made.

V. **Mixed dementia**

A diagnosis of mixed dementia should be made in the presence of one or more other systemic or brain disorders that are thought to be causally related to dementia.

The degree of confidence in the diagnosis of IVD should be specified as *possible, probable,* or *definite,* and other disorder(s) contributing to the dementia should be listed. For example: "mixed dementia due to probable IVD and possible Alzheimer's disease or mixed dementia due to definite IVD and hypothyroidism." Also indicate:
Location: Cortical white matter, periventricular, basal ganglia, thalamus
Size: Volume
Distribution: Large, small, or microvessel
Severity: Chronic ischemia versus infarction
Etiology: Embolism, atherosclerosis, arteriosclerosis, cerebral amyloid angiopathy, hypoperfusion

Adapted from Chui HC, Victoroff JI, Margolin D, et al: Criteria for the diagnosis of ischemic vascular dementia proposed by the State of California Alzheimer's Disease Diagnostic and Treatment Centers. Neurology 42:473–480, 1992.

The NINDS, AIREN and the CADDTC clinical criteria categorize the certainty of diagnosis of vascular dementia as probable, possible, and definite. A definite diagnosis requires tissue diagnosis either from autopsy or brain biopsy. All of the clinical criteria require a causal role for strokes in cognitive impairment.[8,34] None of the criteria recognizes the mixed dementias, which become increasingly common with advancing age and occur in up to a third of patients with cognitive impairment.[10]

Neurology and Neuropsychology of Vascular Cognitive Impairment

Because the vascular dementias form a syndrome, patients with a diagnosis of vascular cognitive impairment need not have multifocal neurologic deficits or bilateral corticospinal tract signs. The reverse of the above statement can also apply, because patients with bilateral neurologic signs from brain stem strokes or cervical disc disease may have normal cognition.[4,10] Therefore, clinicians should use caution in relating the presence or absence of neurologic signs found on examination to a diagnosis of vascular cognitive impairment.

Although patients with strategic cerebral infarcts and multi-infarct dementia may have diverse neurologic signs and neuropsychological deficits, most patients with vascular cognitive impairment have neurologic examinations and cognitive deficits that suggest a subcortical dementia.[34] Some patients may develop short-term memory problems or experience worsening of ongoing memory problems from their cerebrovascular disease.[26]

Neuropsychological tests, such as the Mini-Mental State Exam (MMSE), are poor in screening for the cognitive impairment that is associated with cerebrovascular disease.[26,34] The MMSE emphasizes memory and language and lacks the visual recognition portion of the clinical test.[26,34] Studies show patients with vascular dementia typically do poorly on test items that are influenced by frontal and subcortical mechanisms that are involved in executive functions, verbal fluency, attention, and motor performance.[26]

Psychometric tests sensitive to identifying the spectrum of cognitive deficits associated with vascular dementia include the Mattis Dementia Rating Scale, motor performance subsets; Wechsler Adult Intelligence Scale-Revised (WAIS-R), picture arrangement subsets; Wechsler Aphasia Battery (WAB), writing subsets; the WAIS-R object assembly subsets; and the WAB block design subsets. Patients with early Alzheimer's dementia do poorly on tests such as the WAB repetition subsets, while patients with more severe Alzheimer's disease do poorly on story recall tests.[26]

The cognitive deficits associated with the mixed dementias remain poorly characterized, primarily due to an underestimation of the clinical magnitude of this disorder.[34]

Diagnosis and Treatment of Vascular Dementia: A New Approach

Patients with silent or symptomatic cerebrovascular disease and vascular risk factors warrant treatment of all modifiable risk factors regardless of whether the risk factors are symptomatic, because such patients appear to be at considerable risk not only for strokes but also for vascular cognitive impairment.[4,10,19]

Regardless of whether vascular risk factors are causal or "casual" in the development of vascular dementia, the treatment of these risk factors remains the only way to prevent "premature senility" from cerebrovascular disease.[10,19] Although epidemiologic studies show conflicting results for the relative importance of any individual vascular risk factor that may contribute to the development of vascular dementia, all studies show that the prevention of stroke may be the only means of preventing vascular cognitive impairment. Other than hemorrhagic strokes from vascular malformations and amyloid angiopathy that have little or no primary prevention, most ischemic strokes are the result of long-standing poorly controlled or poorly treated risk factors.[40] Therefore, the aggressive and early treatment of all major risk factors, especially in all individuals older than 50, may be the only means of preventing or reducing the incidence and severity of vascular and cognitive impairment (see chapter entitled "Recent Advances in Stroke Prevention and Treatment").

Cognitive Impairment and Stroke Rehabilitation

A rational approach toward the optimal treatment of all patients with nondebilitating strokes should include periodic neuropsychological assessments to determine the individual stroke patient's rehabilitation requirements. Functional MRI may be an important research tool in this regard and may serve as a "physiologic" instrument that can assess neuronal plasticity and functional recovery in the brain regions of interest.[14,35] Functional MRI techniques may also aid in assessing the beneficial effects of novel pharmacologic agents and rehabilitation techniques that may potentially enhance functional recovery from strokes.[35]

Pharmacologic agents may serve as a future adjuvant to standard rehabilitation protocols. Amphetamines have been shown to accentuate learning and improve functional recovery in stroke patients. Synthetic compounds with pharmacologic effects on dopamine receptors similar to the parent drug, with less potential for abuse and tolerance, are currently in development for use in stroke rehabilitation.[23]

Phase II and III trials have been completed for the use of propentofylline in vascular dementia and Alzheimer's disease. Its presumed neurologic effects are on the excitotoxic/inflammatory mechanisms involved in the development of vascular dementia and Alzheimer's disease. This drug holds similar promise for serving as an agent that may prevent or reduce the symptoms of cognitive impairment associated with cerebrovascular disease.[15]

CONCLUSION

Vascular dementia is the only form of dementia that is preventable, but there is little agreement concerning the way it should be defined. The "dementia" concept of vascular cognitive impairment still widely prevails and hinders the acceptance of this disorder as a vascular syndrome that is associated with a diverse spectrum of clinical manifestations rather than a single disease or a true dementia. Although dementia may be a finite manifestation at one end of the spectrum, premature senility can be prevented by instituting appropriate interventions at the asymptomatic brain-at-risk stage. Hence, there is the need for a redefinition of the limited term *vascular dementia* to the more general term *vascular cognitive impairment*. Using this approach will facilitate the development of clinical and research criteria that can identify all patients at risk for vascular cognitive impairment.

Knowledge of the primary and secondary prevention of cerebrovascular disease has tremendously expanded over the last three decades; however, the risk factors for vascular cognitive impairment remain unclear. This may reflect the fact that currently used research methodology in vascular dementia fails to consider the heterogeneous nature of vascular cognitive impairment as a syndrome rather than a single disease. Although much overlap exists in the pathophysiology and clinical symptoms associated with vascular cognitive impairment and Alzheimer's disease, the factors that initiate the development of Alzheimer's disease remain ill defined. Cognitive impairment from strokes is clearly the result of vascular risk factors and strokes. Clinical studies show strokes can be prevented with the early institution of primary and secondary prevention. Hence, the only current way to prevent premature senility from vascular cognitive impairment lies in the judicious and aggressive treatment of all vascular risk factors.

Research in the basic medical sciences has led to the development of pharmacologic agents that act on ischemia-induced excitotoxic mechanisms that may have a critical role in the development of some forms of vascular cognitive impairment. The widespread clinical application of such agents warrants the development of clinical criteria that will aid in the early identification of vascular cognitive impairment.

REFERENCES

1. American Psychiatric Association: Diagnostic and Statistical Manual of Mental Disorders. 4th ed. Washington, DC, APA, 1994.
2. Beal M, Flint M: Mechanisms of excitotoxicity in neurological disease. FASEB J 6:3334–3338, 1991.
3. Bowen DM, Davison AN: Can the pathophysiology of dementia lead to rational therapy? In Crook T, Bartus R, Ferris S, Gershon S (eds): Treatment Development Strategies for Alzheimer's Disease. Madison, CT, Mark Powley Associates, 1986, pp 36–66.
4. Bowler JV, Hachinski V: Vascular cognitive impairment: A new approach to vascular dementia. Baillieres Clin Neurol 4:357–376, 1995.
5. Brayne HR: Epidemiology of vascular dementia. Neuroepidemiology 14:240–257, 1995.
6. Chakravarthy K, Fountain G, Marry P, et al: A longitudinal study of anticardiolipin antibodies in polymyalgia rheumatica and giant cell arteritis. J Rheumatol 22:1694–1697, 1995.
7. Chui HC: Dementia: A review emphasizing clinico-pathological correlations and brain-behavior relationships. Arch Neurol 46:806–814, 1989.
8. Chui HC, Victoroff JI, Margolin D, et al: Criteria for the diagnosis of ischemic vascular dementia proposed by the State of California Alzheimer's Disease Diagnostic and Treatment Centers. Neurology 42:473–480, 1992.
9. Cummings JL: Vascular subcortical dementias: Clinical aspects. Dementia 5:3–4, 177–180, 1994.
10. Devasenapathy A, Hachinski VC: Vascular Cognitive Impairment: A New Approach. Petersfield, UK, Wrightson Biomedical Publishing, 1997.
11. Djuricic BM, Kostic VS, Mrusulja BB, et al: Prostanoids and ischemic brain edema: Human and animal study. Ann N Y Acad Sci 559:435–437, 1989.
12. Ebly EM, Parhad IM, Hogan DB, Fung TS: Prevalence and types of dementia in the very old: Results from the Canadian Study of Health and Aging. Neurology 44:1563–1600, 1994.
13. Ferruci L, Gurainik JM, Salive ME, et al: Cognitive impairment and the risk of stroke in the older population. J Am Geriatr Soc 44:237–241, 1996.
14. Goldman-Rakie PS: Cellular basis of working memory. Neuron 14:477–485, 1995.
15. Grome JJ, Rudolphi K, Harper AM: Cerebrovascular effects of a xantine derivative propentofylline (HWA 285). Drug Rev Res 5:111–121, 1985.
16. Hachinski VC, Lassen NA, Marshall J: Multi-infarct dementia: A cause for mental detonation in the elderly. Lancet 11:207–210, 1974.
17. Hachinski VC, Potter P, Merskey H: Leukoaraiosis: An ancient term for a new problem. Can J Neurol Sci 13(suppl 4):533–534, 1986.
18. Hachinski VC: Preventable senility: A call for action against the vascular dementias. Lancet 340:645–648, 1992.
19. Hachinski VC: Vascular dementia: A radical redefinition. Dementia 5:130–132, 1994.
20. Henderson VW: Estrogen, cognition, and a woman's risk of Alzheimer's disease. Am J Med 103:11S–18S, 1997.
21. Hennerici MG, Oster M, Cohen S, et al: Are gait disturbances and white matter degeneration early indicators of vascular dementia? Dementia 5:197–202, 1994.
22. Heyman A, Wilkinson WE, Stafford JA, et al: Alzheimer's disease: A study of epidemiological aspects. Ann Neurol 15:335–341, 1984.
23. Hornstein A, Lennihan L, Seliger G, et al: Amphetamines in recovery from brain injury. Brain Inj 10:145–148, 1996.
24. Jarrett JT, Landsbury PT Jr: Seeding "one dimensional crystallization" of amyloid: A pathogenic mechanism in Alzheimer's disease and scrapie? Cell 73:1055–1058, 1993.
25. Kasahara H, Sasahara R: Diagnostic criteria of cerebral vascular dementia: DSM-III-R, ICD-10-JCM, ischemic score and vascular score for differential diagnosis from SDAT. Nippon Rinsho 51(suppl):443–451, 1993.

26. Kertesz A, Clydesdale S: Neuropsychological deficits in vascular dementia vs. Alzheimer's disease. Frontal lobe deficits prominent in vascular dementia. Arch Neurol 51:1226–1231, 1994.

27. Loeb C, Gandolfo C, Bino G: Intellectual impairment and cerebral lesions in multiple cerebral infarcts: A clinical-computed tomography study. Stroke 19:560–565, 1988.

28. Loeb C: Dementia due to lacunar infarctions: A misnomer or a clinical entity? Eur Neurol 35:187–192, 1995.

29. McGeer PL, Rogers J: Anti-inflammatory agents as a therapeutic approach for Alzheimer's disease. Neurology 42:447–449, 1992.

30. Munson RJ, Bowler J, Pablo M, et al: The importance of quantification of risk factors for stroke and dementia. Stroke 29:321, 1998.

31. Palmer AM, Gershon S: Is the neuronal basis of Alzheimer's disease cholinergic or glutamatergic? FASEB J 4:2745–2752, 1990.

32. Pantoni L, Garcia JH: The significance of cerebral white matter abnormalities 100 years after Binswanger's report. A review. Stroke 26:1293–1301, 1995.

33. Raiha I, Tarvonen S, Kurki T, et al: Relationship between vascular factors and white matter low attenuation of the brain. Acta Neurol Scand 87:286–289, 1993.

34. Roman GC, Tatemichi TK, Erkinjuntii T, et al: Vascular dementia diagnostic criteria for research studies. Report of the NINDS-AIREN international workshop. Neurology 43:250–260, 1993.

35. Rueckert L, Appollonio I, Grafman J, et al: Magnetic resonance imaging functional activation of left frontal cortex during covert word production. J Neuroimaging 4:67–70, 1994.

36. Siesjo BK, Agardh CD, Bengtsson F: Free radicals and brain damage. Cerebrovasc Brain Metab Rev 1:165–211, 1989.

37. Skoog I: Risk factors for vascular dementia: A review. Dementia 5:137–144, 1994.

38. Sultzer DL, Mahler ME, Cummings JL, et al: Cortical abnormalities associated with subcortical lesions in vascular dementia. Clinical and positron emission tomographic findings. Arch Neurol 52:773–780, 1995.

39. Tatemichi TK, Desmond DW, Mayeux R, et al: Dementia after stroke: Baseline frequency, risks and clinical features in a hospitalized cohort. Neurology 42:1185–1193, 1992.

40. Tatemichi TK, Desmond DW, Prohovnik I: Strategic infarcts in vascular dementia. A clinical and brain imaging experience. Arzneimittelforschung 45:371–385, 1995.

41. Tournier-Lasserve E, Joutel A, Melki J, et al: Cerebral autosomal dominant arteriopathy with subcortical infarcts and leukoencepholopathy maps to chromosome 19q12. Nature Genet 3:256–259, 1993.

42. Willin A, Blenow K: Pathogenetic basis of vascular dementia. Alzheimer Dis Assoc Disord 15:91–102, 1991.

43. Verney M, Duyckaerts C, Pierot L, et al: Leuko-araiosis. Dev Neurosci 13:245–250, 1991.

44. World Health Organization: The Neurological Adaptation of the International Classification of Disease (ICD-10NA). Geneva, World Health Organization, 1991.

COLLEEN CHURCHILL, BSW, MSW

SOCIAL PROBLEMS POSTSTROKE

From the Rehabilitation Unit
London Health Sciences Center
London, Ontario
Canada

Reprint requests to:
Colleen Churchill, BSW, MSW
Rehabilitation Unit
London Health Sciences Center
University Campus
339 Windermere Road
London, Ontario N6A 5A5
Canada

A stroke is characterized by rapidly developing signs of focal cerebral dysfunction of vascular origin lasting more than 24 hours. Stroke includes infarcts due to atherothrombosis or emboli as well as intracerebral and subarachnoid hemorrhages. Stroke is the third leading cause of death in western society, after heart disease and cancer, and the most important cause of permanent handicaps.[6,21] The annual incidence of stroke is about 1–2 per 1000 persons, which amounts to half a million new cases in the United States annually.[40,69] The annual cost of caring for stroke patients is $14 billion.[63] Stroke survivors live an average of 7 years after stroke.[2,38]

Stroke survivors experience stress from three sources. First, they are subject to the same stressful life events as anyone in the general population. Secondly, they are subject to the serious illness event of the stroke itself. Thirdly, and perhaps most importantly, their life is often irrevocably changed. Upon returning home, stroke survivors are frequently confronted with change in functional performance, family roles, social life, and employment status. The events tend to be negative and beyond the individual's control, which, combined with the frequent suddenness of the event, add to the resultant stress.[47]

Despite the seriousness of stroke disorders, many stroke survivors and their family members are poorly informed about the nature of the disease, recovery, treatment,[3,45] and the availability of social services.[48] Of the estimated 1.7 million stroke survivors in the United States,[69] 15% require long-term institutional care[31] and 70% experience significant functional disability in the realms of mobility, activities of daily living (ADL), social integration, and gainful employment.[32]

TABLE 1. Psychosocial Problems Following Discharge after Stroke

Problem	Percentage of Patients
Social isolation	56%
Decreased community involvement	43%
Economic strain causing a lifestyle alteration	46%
Disruption of family functioning	52%
Major depression	37%
Anxiety/anger	32%

Adapted from Feibel JH, Berk S, Joynt RJ: The unmet needs of stroke survivors [abstract]. Neurology 29:592, 1979.

Hence, the burden of disability is frequently high, emphasizing the need for social supports.

What is often not appreciated about a stroke is its significant effect on the immediate family. The management of stroke patients often focuses on the acute care phase, when patients receive full and comprehensive treatment. Later sequelae, particularly psychosocial problems, are frequently downplayed by health care professionals, who often lack the resources to adequately deal with them. As a result, the psychological and social consequences of stroke often do not receive appropriate attention.

Feibel et al. reviewed 85 patients with an acute stroke within 6 months after discharge.[25] Among the patients there was a significant incidence of psychosocial problems, including social isolation, decreased community involvement, new economic strain, disruption of family functioning, major depression, anxiety, and anger (Table 1). Major depression was present in more than a third of patients but was rarely treated. None of the patients used the existing stroke support groups or psychological or family services. Feibel's study demonstrated the need for careful follow-up of stroke patients after discharge and the need for ongoing psychosocial support on entering the community. This chapter focuses on family and social issues that further complicate the lives of stroke patients over the long term.

CAREGIVER INVOLVEMENT POSTSTROKE

Family Problems

The effects of a stroke on the patient's family are not often fully appreciated. A stroke in one family member inevitably affects the well-being of the entire family. However, contrary to popular belief, most families are supportive. Reasons for refusal to take the stroke patient home include the fact that the family relationship was poor prior to the stroke, major barriers to home care exist (e.g., spouse with poor health), or the family was disenchanted with previous home support or lack of community resources.

Caregiver's Stress

The brunt of the long-term care of the stroke survivor falls onto family caregivers and, in particular, one primary caregiver. In a review on caregiving provided to frail elderly individuals, Silverstone and Horowitz pointed out that no family caregiving system exists; rather, one family member is the primary caregiver and the primary provider of direct care.[54] The primary caregiver will usually be the spouse and, otherwise, an adult child. Only in the absence of a spouse or child do other relatives, friends and neighbors become primary caregivers. However, apart from the primary caregiver, other family members generally play only minor roles.[40,60] Brocklehurst et al. noted that although friends and relatives provide the primary caregiver with significant support shortly after discharge home, they offered little help 1 year after the stroke.[13] If new care demands develop, the family and, in particular, the primary caregiver must meet those demands.[50]

When the care demands of the stroke survivor become overwhelming or adequate support is not available, institutionalization may follow. Elderly individuals enter chronic care facilities more often because of deterioration of the caregiver's health or decompensation in the face of continuous stress than because they need increased levels of care.[11,17,34]

Adjustment Problems for Caregivers

Family members providing care for stroke victims face their own adjustment problems, because their own personal needs are often sacrificed to meet the needs of the stroke survivor. In the case of stroke, Silverstone and Horowitz noted that families often need to provide skilled nursing assistance for which they are not experienced and for which they have received no training.[54] They often have no choice but to learn by trial and error.[50] Kulkarni et al. observed that patients' physical dependency is two to six times greater at home than in hospital.[41] The help provided by home services is often not adequate. Pound et al. noted that 61% of caregivers are dissatisfied with home services in the United Kingdom.[50] Mobility may be limited, and traveling becomes a difficult chore. Brocklehurst et al. and Sanford both noted that lifting problems were not tolerated well by caregivers.[13,52] There are generally limited opportunities for rest, putting the primary caregiver under great stress.

Spouses provide the most extensive and comprehensive care and tolerate greater levels of disability than other caregivers; however, they also report the highest level of stress compared to other caregivers.[54,61] One study conducted 2–3 years after the stroke found that 36% of stroke victims and 32% of primary caregivers had not adjusted to the stroke;[33] it did not always follow that if the stroke survivor had adjusted the primary caregiver had also done so. Family roles often become reversed, as other family members struggle to fill the void left by the stroke survivor. For instance, the wife of a stroke victim may have to perform tasks previously performed by her husband. A child may need to become a parent to his or her parents.

In a study of stroke survivors and spouses 3–8 years after the stroke, Coughlan and Humphrey noted that 41% of patients and 32% of spouses reported much less enjoyment of life.[18] Patients' loss of enjoyment was attributed primarily to residual disabilities, loss of independence, and lack of occupation. For spouses, the chief causes of loss of enjoyment were loss of companionship, increased domestic responsibility, and interference with leisure and social activities. Webster and Newhoff noted that stroke patients experienced a variety of common problems, including needing to assume duties formerly assigned to the spouse, lack of people to confide in or talk to, and lack of personal time alone.[67]

Caregivers of stroke survivors have higher rates of depression and greater rates of deterioration of their own health.[39] Caregivers at greatest risk of ongoing depression are the spouses of younger, more severely impaired patients with lower household incomes, smaller social networks, and lower levels of future optimism and expectation.[61] Adjustment by the caregiver, generally the spouse, is not related to the severity of the patient's disability in terms of paralysis, level of activities of daily living functioning, or severity of aphasia, although caregivers of aphasics in general have more difficulty adjusting.[39] Kinsella and Duffy suggest that adjustment by the caregiver is most often influenced by the presence or absence of behavioral problems in the stroke survivor.[39] In contrast, Evans and Northwood reported that the burden of caregivers is associated more with changes in stability and family support than with patient behavior problems.[20] Mykyta identified communication difficulties, altered role relations, overprotection, and guilt as common problems for the primary caregivers of stroke patients.[49] In the case of younger stroke patients, the primary caregiver often has the added responsibility of caring for children.

Stroker[59] studied the impact of a disabled family member on his or her significant other. Although this study was of a descriptive nature and consisted of a small sample size, the subjects were coping relatively well but had some difficulty with feeling overprotective and overcommitted to the disabled family member.

To determine the effects of stress on the mood of the primary caregiver, Wade et al.[66] conducted a 2-year longitudinal study of a community sample of patients. Increased anxiety was the most commonly reported change 6 months after the stroke. Significant depression was also seen in 11–13% of caregivers over the first 2 years after the stroke. Therefore, treatment should aim at reducing the caregiver's depression, minimizing family dysfunction, and increasing the family's knowledge about stroke.[23]

Recent research has been optimistic regarding the impact of stroke and disability on family support or caregivers. Bishop et al. indicated that couples in a stroke sample did not differ from couples in a matched community sample on level of morale, family functioning, or subjective health rating.[8] Unks found that elderly wives of stroke patients had morale scores that were comparable with those of the general public.[62] Silliman et al. reported that relatives felt better about themselves because they had learned to manage the illness.[53] Mackay and Nias reported that most families reported a closer relationship with the patient and that most patients were moderately happy and confident.[46]

Although good family functioning is possible following a stroke in one of the family members, stroke survivors and families will continue to have problems with practical concerns such as transportation and socialization. As time progresses following the stroke, caregivers may become less well adjusted.[39]

Family Adjustment Stages

Stages of family adjustment following a severe disability have been identified (Table 2).[10,12,33] Silverstone and Horowitz noted that when a healthy, elderly individual suddenly becomes disabled, a severe family crisis ensues.[54] Denial among family members that the neurologic deficits may be permanent is common in the first few months following a stroke. Initial relief over survival and hope for a complete recovery eventually turn to feelings of despair when the desired recovery fails to take place. At this point, a spouse or other caregiver may be able to express anger or resentment toward the stroke victim. As time progresses, family members accept or learn to cope with the permanence of the disability.

Behavioral Issues

Numerous emotional and behavioral disorders occur following a stroke. Depression is the most common, affecting up to 40% of patients. Other poststroke emotional/behavioral disorders include mania, bipolar disorder, anxiety disorder, apathy, and pathologic crying.[51]

TABLE 2. Stages of Family Adjustment to Severe Disability

Acute reaction
  Shock and confusion
  Relief that the patient did not die
  High anxiety

Rehabilitation and treatment
  Denial of permanence of disability
  High expectations of recovery
  Family members often express helplessness and anxiety by questioning the competence of care, but
    they are reluctant to openly criticize
  Fears about future
  Grieving

Acceptance of disability
  Full acceptance of permanence of the disability
  Family attitude changes to actively seeking means to better accommodate to changes in the patient-
    family system
  Information previously denied or rejected is now readily accepted
  Feelings of frustration, despair, and depression
  Hidden and guilt-ridden feelings of anger and hostility can now be expressed toward the patient

Brocklehurst et al. noted that the major problems for primary caregivers were related to the stroke survivor's behavior: the need for constant supervision and loss of sleep due to nocturnal restlessness.[13] Coughlan and Humphrey found that personality changes were noted by the caregiver in two of three stroke survivors 3–8 years after the stroke.[18] The change was for the better in 5%, for the worse in 82%, and not clear in 13%. The main changes were irritability and loss of self-control, lower frustration tolerance, emotional lability, self-centeredness, and reduced initiative. Marked personality changes were reported in a quarter of the patients.[18]

Education and Counseling for Caregivers

Because stroke is a recurrent disease—with the risk increasing fivefold after the initial stroke—education and participation of the family is of utmost importance.[29] Limited family education and counseling in the early stages following a stroke results in significantly better stroke-related knowledge, problem-solving, communication, and global family functioning compared to controls.[22] With time, a new equilibrium develops as the family adjusts roles to accommodate the changed capabilities of the disabled family member. However, this new equilibrium may take years to establish, and the family can decompensate under the burden of care required by stroke survivors. Family coping and reintegration often depend on how well family members communicate and solve problems.[22]

van Veenendaal et al. provided a questionnaire to stroke patients, their families, and health professionals.[64] Questionnaires returned by 44 stroke survivors and 44 family members showed that both stroke survivors and family members want to receive information from talking with professionals more frequently rather than from pamphlets and books. The study showed that stroke survivors were moderately informed (Table 3), but family members were less informed than stroke survivors (Table 4). Generally, family members reported wanting more information than stroke survivors. Family members reported a relatively low need for information about sexual activity and bladder problems. Their greatest need was for information concerning where to apply for help coping with stress, strategies to manage activities of daily life, and strategies to reduce the chance of a new stroke.[64]

TABLE 3. The Highest Rated Items (and Percentages) in Received and Desired Information of Stroke Survivors

Received No Information About	Received a Lot of Information About	Desire No Information About	Desire a Lot of Information About
How a stroke may affect sexual activity (65.0%)	Diagnosis (50.0%)	What is going to happen when I leave the hospital (35.5%)	Reducing the chance of a new stroke (84.4%)
Bladder problems (60.5%)	What is being done for the stroke survivor (37.5%)	Changes in touch (34.4%)	Risk factors for stroke (75.0%)
Changes in touch (52.8%)	Risk factors (37.5%)	How a stroke may affect sexual activity (32.3%)	Causes of stroke (71.9%)
Problems with vision (51.2%)	Causes of stroke (35.9%)	Problems with vision (32.2%)	Diagnosis (67.6%)
Coping with stress (42.1%)	Talking and walking difficulties (32.5%)	Problems with concentration (31.3%)	What is done for the stroke survivor, walking difficulties, and rehabilitation process (61.3%)

Adapted from van Veenendaal H, Grinspun RD, Adriaanse H: Educational needs of stroke survivors and their family members, as perceived by themselves and by health professionals. Patient Educ Counsel 28:265–276, 1996.

Families of stroke patients may need considerable support for many years after the stroke.[33] Holbrook points out that stroke survivors and their families need continuity of care so that they will know to whom to turn for help when new problems develop.[33]

TABLE 4. The Highest Rated Items (and Percentages) in Received and Desired Information of Family Members

Received No Information About	Received a Lot of Information About	Desire No Information About	Desire a Lot of Information About
How a stroke may affect sexual activity (69.2%)	Walking difficulties (62.3%)	How a stroke may affect sexual activity (38.9%)	Reducing the chance of a new stroke (83.3%)
Changes in touch (69.2%)	Diagnosis (47.4%)	Bladder problems (27.8%)	Risk factors for stroke (77.8%)
Spending leisure time (60.5%)	What is being done for the stroke survivor (46.2%)	Activities of daily living (22.2%)	Causes of stroke (77.8%)
Bladder problems (60.5%)	Risk factors for stroke (43.6%)	Problems with vision (20.0%)	What is done for the stroke survivor (77.8%)
Activities of daily living (56.4%)	Medication (41.0%)	What is going to happen when the stroke survivor leaves the hospital (20.0%)	Diagnosis (75.0%)

From van Veenendaal H, Grinspun RD, Adriaanse H: Educational needs of stroke survivors and their family members, as perceived by themselves and by health professionals. Patient Educ Counsel 28:265–276, 1996; with permission.

QUALITY OF LIFE AFTER STROKE

Stroke is an unexpected event with an unpredictable recovery. Stroke survivors returning home frequently find it difficult to perform tasks they could simply or automatically perform prior to the stroke, which produces fear and anxiety regarding the future. There is a growing consensus that quality of life is an important health care outcome.[26,28]

Goodstein noted that the psychological and social impact of stroke on the individual is devastating.[30] In a study of disablement and quality of life following stroke, Ahlsio et al. found that stroke survivors still experienced tiredness, memory difficulties, impairment of motor function, vertigo, and had limited opportunities for leisure and social functions.[1] They also found that subjective measurement of quality of life failed to improve with time, even if independence and the ability to perform activities of daily living improved dramatically. Quality of life was influenced by physical and psychological factors, including concentration and memory. Sjogren suggested that life quality is closely related to leisure activities.[56] He found that the stroke survivors participated in leisure activities less frequently following their stroke, and these individuals became discontented.

Kwa and Limburg studied 129 patients to investigate the role of cognitive impairment in the quality of life of patients after stroke; 75% of the sample completed all the tests.[42] The authors noted that "ischaemic stroke patients with substantial infarct volumes, aphasia, impaired motor function, ADL disability, disturbed global functional health and impaired cognitive function had poorer quality of life after 3 months or more compared with patients without these characteristics."[42]

Lawrence and Christie studied 45 people who had had a stroke 3 years previously.[44] The patients were interviewed along with their families and close friends. The stroke had devastated many people's lives: patients and caregivers ceased work prematurely, their interpersonal relationships deteriorated, and more than 70% viewed their future with uncertainty or gloom. Physical disability itself was less important than individual's responses to their disability; inappropriate and dysfunctional responses were present in more than half the sample. Astrom et al. concluded that major depression early after stroke, functional disability, and an impaired social network interacted to reduce life satisfaction for long-term survivors of stroke.[5]

It is apparent that quality of life and leisure activities diminish to a considerable degree following a stroke. There is a need for a greater awareness about how a stroke affects a person's perceived quality of life.

Socialization

Lack of socialization is a common complaint of many stroke victims and their caregivers. Feibel and Springer measured socialization by compiling five categories of social activities: work, hobbies/sports, pastimes, community activities, and socializing.[24] A total of 27% of stroke patients reported at least a two thirds reduction in socialization, and another 36% reported a reduction of one third to two thirds. Isaacs et al. found that socialization was a key factor in adjustment.[37] They reported that no stroke patient went out by public transportation during the first 6 months. Of the 21 patients who were surveyed after 1 year, only one stroke survivor went out of the house on more than 100 occasions, 11 went out 10–100 times, and nine went out fewer than 10 times or not at all. Holbrook found that 72% of primary caregivers reported that the stroke had an adverse effect on their social life.[33]

Physical disability itself appears to be the major factor leading to loss of socialization.[15,65] Although physical disabilities such as hemiplegia and urinary incontinence frequently limit social contacts, factors such as self-consciousness about impaired mobility, communication problems, depression, or other sequelae of stroke frequently also prevent stroke patients from resuming their previous social activities.

Hyman reported that social reintegration was more problematic for women and for those with more education, possibly because women and men have different body images. Research has indicated a relationship between body image and feelings of stigma and outcome of physical rehabilitation.[35]

Labi et al. found that many stroke survivors do not return to a normal social life, even after physical disability has ceased to be a serious obstacle.[43] Stroke survivors who lived alone were less likely than those who live with a family to experience decreased outside socialization. It is felt that family support is important initially, but family members may later become overprotective to the detriment of the stroke survivor's long-term adjustment. A study by Astrom et al. provided prospective data regarding the global situation in a population-based sample of long-term survivors of stroke as well as information on the development of changes over time.[5] Compared with the general elderly population, patients 3 years after a stroke had more psychiatric symptoms, lower functional ability, and a pronounced reduction of life satisfaction. Contacts with close family members were maintained over the 3-year follow-up period. However, contact with other relatives, friends, and neighbors declined early after the stroke and remained lower than in the general elderly population.

These studies reveal the importance of psychosocial intervention prior to a stroke survivor's discharge from the hospital and the need for ongoing psychosocial intervention while in the community. Patient and family counseling may lessen some of these difficulties. Fortunately, greater emphasis has been placed on community resources for stroke victims and their spouses with the availability of senior centers, public transportation for the disabled, easier access to public places, and support groups, all of which aid in socialization.

Social support has been shown to act as a buffer against stress in a variety of circumstances.[16] Although the relationship between social support and positive health outcome seems to be well-established, social support intervention may be difficult to implement.[19]

Functional Consequences

While stroke rehabilitation programs do not appear to influence neurologic or intrinsic recovery, they do increase stroke survivors' level of independence. About 90% of patients undergoing intensive rehabilitation eventually return home.[55,57,58] Following a stroke, an individual may be unable to perform ADLs, may lack mobility skills, and may be unable to communicate. These ADL skills are often reacquired through exposure to an intensive rehabilitation environment designed to maximize the stroke patient's independence. Being able to transfer independently or pull up one's pants after toileting may seem like mundane issues, but the ability to perform these types of tasks often determines whether stroke survivors will be able to remain in their own homes or require institutionalization. The difference in quality of life to the individual stroke victim and eventual monetary savings to society are obvious.

Rehabilitation nurses and therapists encourage patients to dress, groom, and transfer themselves even though it may take longer than if the attendant assisted them. Patients are frequently capable of performing activities in the hospital that they seem unable to perform at home.[4] This may occur because the patient is depressed and lacks motivation or because the relatives find it easier to perform the tasks themselves.[33] In their attempts to be supportive, family members may make patients dependent again by not allowing them to perform these activities.[27] Families must be warned that their good intentions may lead to deterioration in the stroke survivor's level of independence. Often because of lack of resources and inadequate follow-up, these issues remain unresolved and many of the gains acquired through intensive rehabilitation efforts may be lost.

Driving

Resumption of driving often represents the final step toward independence and reintegration into the community. However, driving a car is one of the most complicated of learned skills, requiring good vision and intact reflex responses, rapid decision making, and careful attentiveness. If one or more of these factors is impaired, the individual's driving skills need to be retested or a decision made that the patient not drive. In the case of significant hemineglect or homonymous hemianopsia, patients should not be allowed to drive. A recent seizure is also a contraindication to driving. Ensuring that the car has an automatic transmission, power steering, and power brakes makes driving easier and safer.

In their review of acquired brain damage in driving, Zomeren et al. reached the following conclusions:[70]

1. About half of the subjects they studied still held a valid driver's license;

2. Brain-damaged drivers could not, in general, be seen as risky drivers, although some individuals showed decreased driving skill and risky behavior in traffic; and

3. Statistics showed no increase in traffic violations or accidents in groups of patients with acquired brain lesions or disease.

Problems noted in brain-damaged drivers include visual-spatial impairment, impassivity, and poor judgment of traffic situations. If health professionals find it difficult to judge the patient's ability to resume driving or have concerns about their competence to drive, the patient must undergo a formal driving assessment. The most common reason for not driving is a homonymous hemianopsia. When there are concerns about vision, a careful visual field assessment by an ophthalmologist should be a prerequisite to driving. In the case of stroke patients, the driving assessment is best conducted with a specialized program that can accurately assess operational skills and cognitive ability to operate a motor vehicle.

Vocational Issues

In the United States, 29.6% of all strokes occur in persons younger than 65 and 25.9% in persons 45–65 years old.[69] Studies have found that the number of patients returning to work after stroke ranges from 3–84% (Table 5).

Vocational counseling should be considered for all patients employed at the time of their stroke. For those with significant deficits, the decisions to return to employment may need to be delayed for several months to allow maximum neurologic and functional recovery to occur. The remaining skills of the stroke survivor must be carefully measured against the demands of the job. However, many stroke survivors are not successful in returning to work.

In the study by Coughlan and Humphrey of 170 surviving stroke patients 3–8 years after a stroke, all patients were younger than 65 at the time of their stroke. Of those still younger than 65 at follow-up, only 30% of the men were in paid employment, most of whom had reduced the number of hours they worked or had changed the nature of their work. Of the women younger than 60 at the time of follow-up,

TABLE 5.   Return to Work after Stroke: Review of 16 Studies

Investigators	Number of Patients	Return to Work (%)	Ages (Years)	Definition of Work*
Adunsky et al., 1992	30	81	20–45	FE, other
Black-Schaffer & Osberg, 1990	79	49	21–65	FT, PT, HM, US
Bogousslavsky & Regli, 1987	41	81	< 30	FT
Coughlan & Humphrey, 1982	170	33	< 65	FT, PT
David & Heyman, 1960	67	24	26–70 or older	FE
Feldman et al., 1962	38	3	36–82	CE
Fugl-Meyer, Jaasko & Norlin, 1975	83	41	< 65	FT, HM, PT
Heinemann et al., 1987	364	11	> 20	Unspecified
Hindfelt & Nilsson, 1977	52	84	16–40	FT, PT
Howard et al., 1985	379	19	< 55–older than 66	FE
Kotila et al., 1984	58	55	< 65	CE, HM, US
Mackay & Nias, 1979	45	38	< 65	Unspecified
Marquardsen, 1969	269	41	< 70	FT, HM, PT
Smolkin & Cohen, 1974	74	32	Mean 47	CE
Waltimo et al., 1980	71	21	< 65	Unspecified
Weisbroth, Esibill & Zuger, 1971	62	37	< 65	CE

* FE = former employment, FT = full-time competitive employment, PT = part-time competitive employment, HM = homemaking, US = full-time university level study, CE = competitive employment
Adapted from Black-Schaffer RM, Lemieux L: Vocational outcome after stroke. Top Stroke Rehabil Spring 1994.

only 17% were in paid employment. Patients without hemiplegia were employed significantly more often (11 of 18, or 61%) than those with left hemiplegia (9 of 32, or 28%) or right hemiplegia (2 of 37, or 5%).[1,7]

In a study of 379 patients who were employed before cerebral infarction and living 1 year afterward, Howard et al. attempted to determine what factors influenced return to work.[35] Age, occupation, degree of disability, race, and the hemisphere infarcted were found to be significant. Younger patients with less disability were more likely to return to work. Patients employed in professional managerial positions were more likely to return to work than patients in blue-collar or farming positions.

Brooks et al. found that only 29% of stroke survivors returned to work after a 7-year period.[14] Isaacs et al. followed 29 stroke survivors for 3 years or until they died.[37] Before admission, 11 stroke patients had been in full-time employment and eight had full household duties. After discharge, none returned to any form of employment, one returned to full household duties, and two to partial duties.

Black-Schaffer and Lemieux found that whether a patient returns to work after stroke depends on many factors, including three factors related to severity of functional impairment and one related to lifestyle prior to alcohol use.[9]

These studies demonstrate that stroke survivors tend to not return to their previous employment. The inability to return to work frequently leads to financial and emotional concerns for stroke survivors and their family members.

Little research has been conducted as to which programs and techniques increase the likelihood of a stroke survivor's returning to the workforce. In the past, efforts have been made through neuropsychological evaluation, cognitive rehabilitation, physiotherapy, and psychological counseling to enhance the patient's ability to return to work. A relatively new approach to job retraining has been explored by Wehman et al.[68] Their study found that the program, supportive employment, allowed more stroke survivors to return to work. The concept of supported employment consists of intensive time-limited training and compensatory strategies that are provided at the job site, followed by extended assessment and support services to assist with job retention.[68] Supportive employment requires further research to demonstrate its overall effectiveness in helping stroke survivors return to employment. Further discussion on return to work poststroke is found in the chapter entitled "Rehabilitation of Younger Stroke Patients."

SOLUTIONS

There are no easy solutions to the social problems that develop following a stroke. Greater attention to these problems on the part of health professionals would help both patients and families adjust to these difficulties. It is apparent that an improvement in outpatient services, day hospitals, maintenance therapy programs, long-term patient and family counseling, intermittent relief admissions or respite care, and a long-term multidisciplinary follow-up clinic would help to ease or alleviate many of the social problems that stroke patients experience.

Continuity of care following discharge is essential. Patients need to have professionals available, if only for information, to help them deal with crises. This is best done by the original rehabilitation team. Community support groups also are of great benefit in providing socialization. More research into the long-term impact of stroke on social functioning is needed.

ACKNOWLEDGMENT

Special acknowledgment is extended to Miss Sue Merritt for her secretarial support during the preparation of this manuscript.

REFERENCES

1. Ahlsio B, Britton M, Murray V, Theorell T: Disablement and quality of life after stroke. Stroke 15:886–890, 1984.
2. Anderson TP, McClure WJ, Athelson G, et al: Stroke rehabilitation: Evaluation of its quality by assessing patient outcomes. Arch Phys Med Rehabil 59:170–175, 1978.
3. Anderson R: The unremitting burden on carers. BMJ 294:730–747, 1987.
4. Andrews K, Stewart J: Stroke recovery: He can but does he. Rheum Rehabil 18:43–48, 1979.
5. Astrom M, Asplund K, Astrom T: Psychosocial function and life satisfaction after stroke. Stroke 23:527–531, 1992.
6. Barnett HJM, Mohr JP, Stein BM, Yatsu FM: Stroke: Pathophysiology, Diagnosis and Management. 2nd ed. New York, Churchill Livingstone, 1992.
7. Binder LM: Emotional problems after stroke. Stroke 15:174–177, 1984.
8. Bishop D, Epstein NB, Keitner G, et al: Stroke: Morale, family functioning, health status and functional capacity. Arch Phys Med Rehabil 67:84–87, 1986.
9. Black-Schaffer RM, Lemieux L: Vocational outcome after stroke. Top Stroke Rehabil Spring:74–86, 1994.
10. Bleiberg J: Psychological and neuropsychological factors in stroke management. In Kaplan PE, Cerullo LJ (eds): Stroke Rehabilitation. Stoneman, MA, Butterworth, 1986, pp 210–212.
11. Boxell J, McKercher G: Needs of caregivers of elderly attending day hospital. Can Fam Physician 36:45–49, 1990.
12. Bray GD: Reactive patterns in families of the severely disabled. Rehabil Counsel Bull Mar:236–239, 1977.
13. Brocklehurst JC, Morris P, Andrews K, et al: Social effects of stroke. Soc Sci Med 15:35–39, 1981.
14. Brooks N, McKinlay W, Symington C, et al: Return to work within the first seven years after head injury. Brain Injury 1:5–19, 1987.
15. Christie D: Aftermath of stroke: An epidemiological study in Melbourne, Australia. J Epidemiol Community Health 36:123–126, 1982.

16. Cobb S: Social support as a moderator of life stress. Psychosom Med 38:300–314, 1976.
17. Colerick EJ, George LK: Predictors of institutionalization among caregivers of patients with Alzheimer's disease. J Am Geriatr Soc 34:493–498, 1986.
18. Coughlan AK, Humphrey M: Presenile stroke: Long-term outcome for patients and their families. Rheumatol Rehabil 21:115–122, 1982.
19. Cwikel J, Israel B: Examining mechanisms of social support and social networks: A review of health-related intervention studies. Public Health Rev 15:159–193, 1987.
20. Evans RL, Northwood L: Social support needs in adjustment in stroke. Arch Phys Med Rehabil 64:61–64, 1987.
21. Evans RL, Miller RM: Psychosocial implications and treatment of stroke. Social Casework 40:242–247, 1984.
22. Evans RL, Matlock AL, Bishop DS, et al: Family intervention after stroke: Does counseling or education help? Stroke 19:1243–1249, 1988.
23. Evans RL, Bishop DS, Haselkorm JK: Factors predicting satisfactory home care after stroke. Arch Phys Med Rehabil 72:144–147, 1991.
24. Feibel JH, Springer CJ: Depression and failure to resume social activities after stroke. Arch Phys Med Rehabil 63:276–278, 1982.
25. Feibel JH, Berk S, Joynt RJ: The unmet needs of stroke survivors [abstract]. Neurology 29:592, 1979.
26. Fuhrer M: Subjective well-being: Implications for medical rehabilitation outcomes and models of disablement. Am J Phys Med Rehabil 73:358–364, 1994.
27. Garraway WM, Akhtar AJ, Hockey L, Prescott RJ: Management of acute stroke in the elderly: Follow-up of a controlled trial. BMJ 28:827–829, 1980.
28. Gill TM, Feinstein AR: A critical appraisal of the quality of quality of life measurements. Aging 5:188–192, 1976.
29. Goldberg G, Berger G: Secondary prevention in stroke: A primary rehabilitation concern. Arch Phys Med Rehabil 69:32–40, 1988.
30. Goodstein RK: Overview: Cerebrovascular accident and the hospitalized elderly—a multidimensional clinical problem. Am J Psychiatry 140:141–147, 1983.
31. Gresham GE, Phillips TF, Wolf PA, et al: Epidemiologic profile of long-term stroke disability: The Framingham study. Arch Phys Med Rehabil 60:487–491, 1979.
32. Gresham GE, Fitzpatrick TE, Wolf PA, et al: Residual disability in survivors of stroke: The Framingham study. N Engl J Med 293:954–956, 1985.
33. Holbrook M: Stroke and emotional outcome. J R Coll Physicians Lond 16:100–104, 1982.
34. Horowitz A: Family caregiving to the frail elderly. Annu Rev Gerontol Geriatr 5:194–246, 249–282, 1985.
35. Howard G, Till JS, Toole JF, et al: Factors influencing return to work following cerebral infarction. JAMA 253:226–232, 1985.
36. Hyman MD: Stigma of stroke: Its effects on performance during and after rehabilitation. Geriatrics 26:132–141, 1971.
37. Isaacs B, Neville Y, Rushford I: The stricken: The social consequences of stroke. Age Ageing 5:188–192, 1976.
38. Kannel WE, Wolf PA, Verter J: Risk factors for stroke. In Smith RR (ed): Stroke and the Extracranial Vessel. New York, Raven Press, 1984, pp 47–57.
39. Kinsella GJ, Duffy FP: Psychosocial readjustment in the spouses of aphasic patients. Scand J Rehabil Med 11:129–132, 1979.
40. Kistler JP, Ropper AH, Heros RC: Therapy of ischemic cerebral vascular disease due to atherothrombosis. N Engl J Med 311:100–105, 1984.
41. Kulkarni JR, Chamberlain MA, Porritt R: Dependency in rehabilitation: A comparative study of dependency in hospital and at home. Int J Rehabil Res 15:63–68, 1992.
42. Kwa VIH, Limburg M, deHaan RJ: The role of cognitive impairment in the quality of life after ischaemic stroke. J Neurol 243:599–604, 1996.
43. Labi M, Phillips P, Gresham G: Psychosocial disability in physically restored long-term stroke survivors. Arch Phys Med Rehabil 61:561–565, 1980.
44. Lawrence L, Christie D: Quality of life after stroke: A three year follow up. Age Ageing 8:167–172, 1979.
45. Lomer M, McLennan DL: Informing hospital patients and their relatives about stroke. Clin Rehabil 1:33–37, 1987.
46. Mackay A, Nias BC: Strokes in the young and middle-aged: Consequences to the family and to society. J R Coll Physicians Lond 13:106–112, 1979.
47. McFarlane AH, Norman GR, Streiner DL, et al: Longitudinal study of influence of psychosocial environment on health status: Preliminary report. J Health Soc Behav 21:124–133, 1980.

48. McLean J, Roper-Hall A, Mayer P, Main A: Service needs of stroke survivors and their informal carers: A pilot study. J Adv Nurs 16:559–564, 1991.
49. Mykyta LJ: Caring for relatives of stroke patients. Age Ageing 5:87–90, 1976.
50. Pound P, Compertz P, Ebrahim S: Development and results of a questionnaire to measure carer satisfaction after stroke. J Epidemiol Community Health 47:500–505, 1993.
51. Robinson R: Neuropsychiatric consequences of stroke. Annu Rev Med 48:217–229, 1997.
52. Sanford J: Tolerance of debility in elder dependents by supports at home: Its significance for hospital practice. BMJ 3:471–473, 1975.
53. Silliman RA, Fletcher RH, Earp JL, Wagner EH: Families of elderly stroke patients: Effects of home care. J Am Geriatr Soc 34:643–648, 1986.
54. Silverstone B, Horowitz A: Issues of social support: The family and home care. In Dunkel RE, Schmidley JW (eds): Stroke in the Elderly. New York, Springer, 1987, pp 169–185.
55. Sivenins J, Pyorala K, Heinonen OP, et al: The significance of intensity of rehabilitation of stroke—a controlled trial. Stroke 16:928–931, 1985.
56. Sjogren K: Leisure after stroke. Int Rehabil Med 4:80–87, 1982.
57. Smith ME, Garraway WM, Smith DL, Akhtar AJ: Therapy impact on functional outcome in a controlled trial of stroke rehabilitation. Arch Phys Med Rehabil 63:21–24, 1982.
58. Strand T, Asplund K, Erikksson S, et al: A non-intensive stroke unit reduces functional disability and the need for long-term hospitalization. Stroke 15:29–34, 1985.
59. Stroker R: Impact of disability on families of stroke clients. Neurosurg Nurs 15:360–365, 1983.
60. Tobin SS, Kalys R: The family in the institutionalization of the elderly. J Soc Iss 37:145–157, 1981.
61. Tompkins CA, Schulz R, Ran MT: Post-stroke depression in primary support persons: Predicting those at risk. Consult Clin Psychol 56:502–508, 1988.
62. Unks RP: The relative influence of social, physical, and psychological factors on the morale and life satisfaction of elderly wives of stroke patients. Dissert Abstr Int 44:2585, 1985.
63. U.S. Department of Health and Human Services: Stroke Hope through Research. Bethesda, MD, National Institutes of Health, 1983, NIH publication 83-2222.
64. van Veenendaal H, Grinspun RD, Adriaanse H: Educational needs of stroke survivors and their family members, as perceived by themselves and by health professionals. Patient Educ Counsel 28:265–276, 1996.
65. Wade D, Langton-Hewer R, Skilbeck C, David R (eds): Stroke: A Critical Approach to Diagnosis, Treatment, and Management. Chicago, Year Book, 1985.
66. Wade D, Legh-Smith J, Hewer R: Effects of living with and looking after survivors of a stroke. BMJ 293:418–420, 1986.
67. Webster EJ, Newhoff M: Intervention with families of communicatively impaired adults. In Beasley DS, Davis GA (eds): Aging: Communication Processes and Disorders. New York, Grune & Stratton, 1981, pp 229–240.
68. Wehman P, Inlow D, Altman A, et al: Return to work for individuals recovering from stroke or traumatic brain injury: Three case studies. Can J Rehabil 5:45–50, 1991.
69. Weinfeld FD, et al: National survey of stroke. Stroke 12(suppl 1):I1–I90, 1981.
70. Zomeren AH, Brouwer WH, Minderhound JM: Acquired brain damage and driving: A review. Arch Phys Med Rehabil 68:697–705, 1987.

ROBERT W. TEASELL, MD, FRCPC
MARC McRAE, MSc

THE REHABILITATION OF YOUNGER STROKE PATIENTS

From the Department of Physical
  Medicine and Rehabilitation
University of Western Ontario
London, Ontario
Canada

Reprint requests to:
Robert W. Teasell, MD
London Health Sciences Center
University Campus
339 Windermere Road
London, Ontario N6A 5A5
Canada

Stroke is generally regarded as a condition of the elderly. In persons younger than 50, stroke is relatively uncommon.[36] For individuals 50–64 years old, stroke occurs at a rate of approximately 3 per 1,000 persons; from 65–74 years, approximately 12 per 1,000 persons; and for persons older than 79, approximately 25 per 1,000.[1,9,10,35,43,48] Of all strokes, 25.9% occur in patients 45–65 years old, and only 3.7% reportedly occur before the age of 45.[56] Similarly, it has been reported that 3–4% of strokes occur in patients 40 years or younger.[2,19,40] This chapter explores some unique challenges associated with the rehabilitation of young stroke patients.

ETIOLOGY OF STROKE

Strokes are markedly uncommon in patients younger than 30 and are generally related to unusual causes of strokes, such as migraines, hematologic disorders, developmental cardiac difficulties, and arterial dissection. The role of low-dose contraceptives in causing stroke has been controversial, but recent evidence has suggested it does not play a significant role in increasing stroke risk.[41] The same can be said of mitral valve prolapse. After 30 years of age, atherosclerosis begins to play an increasingly important role in the causation of a stroke, and once patients older than 40 are included, the number of strokes attributable to atherosclerosis rises almost exponentially.

In 1987 Bogousslavsky and Regli studied the cause and prognosis of ischemic stroke in 41 patients younger than 30.[8] Mitral valve prolapse and arterial dissection were responsible for 51% of the infarctions. Twelve patients were diagnosed as having mitral valve prolapse, which was presumed to be the cause of their stroke, and nine suffered an arterial dissection. Migrainous infarction was felt to be the likely cause of stroke in 15%. Uncommon etiologies accounted for 34% of the infarctions. Atherosclerosis played a role in only two of the patients. Three patients (7.3%) died of acute causes. The diagnosis of mitral valve prolapse would likely be made differently if the study were performed now.

Barinagarrementeria et al. extensively studied 300 consecutive patients younger than 40 with cerebral infarction.[3] Etiologies included unknown causes in 32%, nonatherosclerotic vasculopathy in 27%, cardioembolism in 24%, hematologic disturbance in 10% (including 11 patients with a deficiency of natural anticoagulant proteins), premature atherosclerosis in 3%, and migraine in 3%. The authors stated that atherosclerosis was an uncommon cause of cerebral infarction in patients younger than 40.

A prospective registry of cerebral infarction in young adults at the University of Iowa studied 286 patients 15–45 years old. An atherosclerotic etiology is implicated in 26.9%, a nonatherosclerotic vasculopathy in 23.1%, cardioembolism in 21.7%, a hematologic etiology in 12.2%, and undetermined causes in 16.1%.[33] This study did not include hemorrhagic strokes. Atherosclerosis was a more common etiology. The difference may, at least in part, be attributable to the greater predominance of atherosclerosis in patients between ages 40–45 as well as the fact that atherosclerotic stroke increases almost exponentially with increasing age.

Meyer et al. have noted that, despite significant overlap in stroke etiology in young adults and middle-aged and elderly adults, there are differences between the groups.[38] While ischemic strokes still account for about half of strokes in young adults, there is an increased incidence of hemorrhagic strokes relative to middle-aged and elderly adults. Spontaneous intracerebral hemorrhage and subarachnoid hemorrhage account for about half of strokes in young adults. In comparison 80–85% of strokes in older populations are ischemic and 15–20% hemorrhagic.[38]

Bevan et al. conducted a retrospective study of 113 young stroke patients ages 15–45 who were admitted to a Vermont hospital over a 6-year period.[5] Intracerebral hemorrhage accounted for 46 (41%) of the young strokes, and they were the result of a wide variety of etiologies. Subarachnoid hemorrhage was a cause of stroke in 14 (17%) while cerebral infarctions accounted for 48 (42%) cases, the majority due to cardiac emboli and premature atherosclerosis. Mitral valve prolapse, use of oral contraceptives, alcohol consumption, and migraines were infrequent sole causes of cerebral infarction in the absence of other risk factors.[5] Ferro and Crespo retrospectively studied 254 young stroke patients age 50 and younger.[18] Eight etiologic categories were identified: in 89 (35.0%) stroke was attributed to cerebral atherosclerosis; 78 (30.7%), including 54 with valvular heart disease, were cardiac emboli; 21 (8.3%) were a consequence of intracerebral hemorrhage; 14 (5.5%) vasospasm; 9 (3.5%) occurred during puerperium or pregnancy or were attributed to oral contraceptives; 5 (2.0%) were attributed to hematologic diseases; 8 (3.1%) to nonatherosclerotic cerebral vasculopathy; and 39 (15.4%) were of unknown etiology. Cardiac embolism was the most common cause of stroke in patients younger than 40, and atherosclerosis was the most frequent etiology among patients 41–50 years old.[18]

Race may be an important factor in the etiology of stroke in young patients. Qureshi et al. studied all stroke patients admitted to an Atlanta hospital over 4½ years. Of 248 eligible young stroke patients, 219 were black. Hypertension was associated with stroke more commonly in blacks than in nonblack patients (55% vs. 24%, p = 0.003). Hypertensive intracerebral hemorrhage (64%) was the most common subtype of intracerebral hemorrhage, and lacunar infarction among young black stroke patients suggested accelerated hypertensive arteriolar (small vessel) disease, likely due to poorly controlled hypertension.[42] In a study of 296 cases of ischemic stroke among black and white adults age 18–44 compared to 1220 controls, Rohr et al. found that diabetes mellitus, hypertension, and current cigarette smoking were important risk factors for stroke, with the latter two factors particularly important risk factors in young blacks.[44]

In summary, stroke among younger patients is uncommon. Hemorrhagic strokes and strokes of unknown etiology or due to unusual causes are more common in younger than older patients. In contrast, ischemic strokes, particularly atherosclerosis, predictably account for a lower percentage of strokes in young people. Oral contraceptives and mitral valve prolapse are no longer regarded as important causes of strokes in young people. Racial factors may increase the risk of stroke in younger individuals.

RECOVERY AND PROGNOSIS IN THE YOUNG STROKE PATIENT

Young stroke patients demonstrate greater neurologic and functional recovery and hence have a better prognosis. Falconer et al have noted that older age is generally associated with poorer rehabilitation outcomes, particularly for the oldest patients.[16] Older patients' limitations include less physiologic reserve for recovery and a higher prevalence of comorbid conditions, particularly cognitive impairment. These factors have been associated with poorer rehabilitation outcomes,[17,30,47] which may explain why younger patients fare so much better.

Ferro and Crespo found that about a third of the young aphasic patients they studied recovered completely, a third improved, and a third continued to have a significant unresolved language deficit.[18] Recovery was better than had been reported for non–age-selected aphasia populations. Complete recovery and significant improvement have been observed in young patients more than 6 months after a stroke, but complete recovery is rare in older stroke patients.

In a study of 300 stroke patients younger than 40, Barinagarrementeria et al. found that 25% made a full recovery, 47% made a partial but nondisabling recovery, 26% had a disabling stroke after a partial recovery, and 1% died.[3] A total of 85% of the patients were followed for at least 3 months. Thirteen patients (4%) had suffered recurrent cerebral infarctions (4%).

The youngest patients have an even better prognosis. For a mean of 46 months, Bogousslavsky and Regli followed their stroke patients who were younger than 30.[8] Three had died acutely. The annual incidence of death was 0.7% and that of recurrent stroke also 0.7%. Only one patient who survived the acute phase died during follow-up. This patient died of renal failure due to systemic lupus erythematosus 48 months after the stroke. One patient, who likely had intracerebral arteritis, had another stroke 10 months after the initial event. The authors noted that although mortality early after stroke was not negligible, the prognosis was good following the acute stage.

Kapelle et al. performed a follow-up assessment of 296 15- to 45-year-old patients with ischemic stroke who had been referred to a tertiary medical center.[27] The calculated annual mortality from vascular death was 1.7%. Young patients, especially those with small-vessel stroke or stroke of unknown etiology, fared significantly better than those who were older or who had large-vessel strokes of unknown etiology.

Adunsky et al. studied 35 young stroke patients who were admitted to an Israeli rehabilitation unit over 6 years.[2] The mean time to admission was almost 1 month, and patients remained on rehabilitation an average of almost 3 months. Nevertheless, a significant difference between activity of daily living (ADL) scores at admission and discharge were noted (p < 0.01) but not between discharge and follow-up. At discharge the patients had demonstrated significant improvements, with relatively high scores for functional ability as measured by ADLs and independent ambulation. The authors explained this "relatively lower degree of functional impairment" by the fact that the younger patients did not have the same degree of comorbidity or cognitive problems as elderly stroke patients.

Snyder and Ramirez-Lassepas studied 38 men and 23 women age 16–49 who had a cerebral infarction.[52] They identified five groups:

1. Premature atherosclerosis was identified as the cause of stroke in 29 patients. Cases were characterized by marked male predominance, a high frequency of risk factors, a mortality rate of 23.9%, and a recurrence rate of cerebrovascular disease of 41.6% within a mean follow-up of 2.4 years.

2. Seven women on hormonal replacement when they had their cerebral infarction suffered only one transient ischemic attack (TIA) during a 2.9-year mean follow-up period.

3. Cardiac emboli were causative in seven patients who nevertheless remained asymptomatic while on anticoagulants; one patient subsequently had a stroke after anticoagulants were discontinued.

4. Five patients had miscellaneous causes of stroke, and prognosis varied with the underlying etiology.

5. Thirteen patients had no identifiable etiology; over a mean follow-up of 3 years there was one TIA and one further cerebral infarction.

For 13–26 years, Hindfelt and Nilsson followed 74 young adults who suffered an ischemic stroke and survived the first month following stroke onset.[23] Patients ranged in age from 16–40, and the mean age at the onset of stroke was 29.5. At follow-up, 12 of the patients were dead, mostly from severe underlying disease complicated by the ischemic stroke. Death was unrelated to cerebrovascular disease in three cases. Only 10 of the remaining 62 patients experienced moderate or severe deficits, and the rest had no or minor persistent handicaps. Eight of the patients had experienced internal carotid or proximal cerebral artery occlusions. Among the surviving 62 patients, seven had experienced recurrent ischemic events (three reinfarctions, four TIAs). These seven patients already had risk factors for cerebrovascular disease at the time of their primary stroke. The authors concluded that the long-term prognosis for ischemic stroke in the young adult is favorable. The recovery from neurologic deficits was determined to be good, with a low recurrence risk of 1.1–1.2% annually; exceptions are occlusions within the internal carotid and middle cerebral arteries.[23]

Rozenthul-Sorekin et al. determined that 253 people age 17–49 with first strokes were admitted to all Israeli hospitals during a single year.[45] The age- and sex-adjusted stroke incidence rate was 10.36/1,000,000 per year, and the incidence in males was almost double that of females. The fatality rate for all stroke types within the first 4 weeks poststroke was 9.9%, with the rate for hemorrhagic strokes being much greater than for ischemic strokes. Of the young stroke survivors, 20.6% were moderately disabled and 19% were severely disabled.[45]

In summary, young stroke patients make better neurologic recoveries, develop less disability, and are less likely to have further strokes than older stroke patients.

REHABILITATION OF YOUNG STROKE PATIENTS

Rehabilitation is generally the same for young and older stroke patients. The major difference in rehabilitation lies in the differing nature of neurologic recovery and associated social issues, such as the nature of family supports, the presence or absence of young children, marital stress, and return to work.

In their study of patients 15–45 years old with ischemic strokes, Kapelle et al. found that almost half of 212 patients in whom quality of life scores were obtained after a mean follow-up of 6 years reported residual problems with physical or social functioning. [27] More than a quarter of the patients rated quality of life poor in these spheres. Almost half were diagnosed as depressed.[27] Hindfelt and Nilsson found seven of their surviving 62 young patients to be depressed; three of them had suffered a depression prior to the onset of their stroke, and four manifested overt depressive illnesses without a preceding history of similar symptomatology prior to their strokes.[23] In one patient the depression had been associated with psychotic traits. Three patients were alcoholics.

Family Stress

Younger stroke patients generally need caregivers less than elderly stroke patients because they have a tendency to make a more complete neurologic and functional recovery.[23] However, caregivers may be more readily available for younger stroke patients because their spouses and parents are more likely to be alive and able to assist. For all stroke patients, apart from the primary caregiver, other family members generally play only minor roles[24,54] (see chapter entitled "Social Problems Poststroke").

In their study of stroke patients 16–40 years old, Hindfelt and Nilsson reported that at follow-up an average of 17.7 years after stroke onset, family relations were "socially uncomplicated," and divorce as a consequence of the stroke occurred in only one case.

Mackay and Nias studied 90 stroke patients younger than 65.[34] Half of the 90 patients were working at the time of their stroke. However, only 17 had returned to work within 6 months of their stroke, and there was a mean loss of 111 working days per working patient. At 6 months, 27 of the patients had died. Of the 63 survivors, only two had to be institutionalized. Another 28 returned home to be cared for by their relatives. Their 28 primary caregivers included 19 wives, three husbands, four daughters, one sister, and one brother. Eight had to abandon their jobs to care for the patient, two had to work reduced hours, and two others were unable to work normal hours, and the remaining 16 relatives had not been working previously. Of the 28 relatives, 25 had to spend most or all of their time at home, two had to move into alternative housing to accommodate the patient, 12 abandoned their usual summer vacation, and eight were reported to be feeling emotionally depressed.[34]

Institutionalization

For stroke patients with significant disabilities and insufficient social supports, institutionalization becomes an important consideration. Placement of individuals in chronic care facilities most often occurs because of lack of a supportive caregiver, but institutionalization is required infrequently in young stroke patients. In our review of young stroke rehabilitation patients, institutionalization following formal rehabilitation occurred in four of 83 patients younger than 50.[53] The common feature of each of these four cases was severe disabling strokes occurring in association with poor social supports. In contrast, Adunsky et al., in their study of 30 stroke patients younger than 40 who underwent rehabilitation, noted that all patients went home but their average length of rehabilitation stays were long.[2] The patients achieved relatively high levels of functional independence at discharge compared to elderly stroke patients, which the authors attributed to a relative absence of previous and coexisting medical problems and "organic intellectual impairment."[2]

Return to Work

For elderly stroke patients, vocational concerns are rarely an issue because most of them are retired at the time of their stroke. For younger patients vocational issues are important. Monga has noted:

> [The] "rehabilitation community has devoted only limited effort to the task of defining what is meant by the phrase *return to work*, to develop measures of vocational function, to applying these measures to patient populations, and to tracking return to work as a measure of rehabilitation outcome. . . . In the published studies, the investigators do not all mean the same thing by "work"; for example, some include homemaking and study but others only competitive employment, and some restrict it to former employment but others do not specify it at all. The age ranges of groups studied differ widely, with some studies including persons 65 years old and older and others considering only patients younger than 30 or 45 years of age. Additionally, sample sizes differ greatly, and a few involve large cohorts.[39]

In their study of patients younger than 30 with ischemic strokes, Bogousslavsky and Regli found at 46-months follow-up that only seven of the 37 patients (18.9%) remained disabled by severe neurologic deficits, with an inability to resume their previous activities. However, 30 patients (81.8%) did well; 11 had no disability and 19 had returned to work and were fully employed despite a persisting mild neurologic deficit. In this study most patients did return to work, which was related to the degree of neurologic deficits.

Coughlan and Humphrey found that only 30% of male stroke survivors younger than 65 at follow-up were in paid employment, most of whom had reduced their hours or changed the nature of their work.[15] This study is different than Bogousslavsky and Regli's study in that many of the patients were older and more likely to retire in the face of neurologic deficit.[15] In Kapelle's study of young patients with ischemic stroke, only 42% of patients had a job and, of these, 23% required an adjustment in their occupation.[27]

Black-Schaffer and Osberg studied 79 patients age 21–65 who were employed at the time of stroke, had experienced a first stroke, and were discharged from rehabilitation at least 6 months before follow-up and were available for a telephone questionnaire.[6] Work was defined as full-time and part-time competitive employment, homemaking, and full-time university studies; 39 (49%) of the patients reported returning to work by time of follow-up a mean of 3.1 months after discharge from the rehabilitation program. Factors that had a negative impact upon success of return to work included aphasia, a longer rehabilitation stay, a decreased Barthel index, and prior alcohol consumption. Of patients returning to work, data were available on 34, 11 of whom had returned to work the same number of hours as before their stroke and 23 of whom had returned to work at an average reduction of 17.4 hours per week. However, 16 maintained full-time work, but at least five reduced their hours despite working full-time.[6]

The same authors noted: "The picture of the rehabilitated work that emerges from our descriptive results is an individual who has geared down his or her work activities after the stroke."[6] It was the impression of the authors that changes at work involved a reduction in the number or complexity of tasks. Age was a significant factor in predicting return to work. The authors also reported that "nearly half (48%) of the previously full-time workers returned to work only part-time after the stroke; two-thirds of the 39 who returned to work reduced their hours (some of them continued to be full-time by the 40 hours per week criterion), and over half (58%) of the 39 who returned to work acknowledged that their jobs required modifications because of changes in their abilities due to the stroke."[6]

Hindfelt and Nilsson found that of 62 surviving young stroke patients, 39 reported working full-time (mean age 46.6 years), seven part-time, and 17 were retired (mean age 52.5 years).[23] Only eight of the 17 retired stroke patients had moderate or severe neurologic handicaps. Seven of the patients needed continuous help from another person for daily activities; however, most of their needs were minor, and only one patient required institutionalization.[23]

Black-Schaffer and Lemieux reported: "A recurring theme in studies that look for predictive factors regarding return to work is interest in the educational level of the patient before the stroke and in the category of employment to which the patient will return."[7] They then noted that patients with higher educational levels and white-collar positions were more likely to return to work after a stroke than those with little education and blue-collar positions.[4,7,25,51] In their study of 35 young stroke patients who returned to work, 15 went back to secretarial/clerical positions and 17 to professional/technical positions.[7] They attributed the higher success regarding return to work for white-collar workers to better education, work conditions, pay, and less physically demanding jobs.[7] The authors noted that these jobs were more attractive, that workers had more work autonomy, or that fellow employees and employers were more likely to accommodate these individuals at work. Howard et al. reported that age, occupation, degree of disability, race, and side of lesion were significant factors influencing return-to-work potential.[25] Patients age 55 or younger were found to be the most likely to return to work poststroke. Managers represented the group most likely to return to work. Similarly, Sacki et al. reported that stroke survivors were more likely to return to work if they had limited residual muscle weakness, white-collar occupations, and no apraxia.[46]

The side of hemiplegia has not been consistently associated with the ability to return to work with either right- or left-sided weakness.[6,21,25,29,57] However, a distinct negative correlation between aphasia, considered apart from the side of hemiplegia, and return to work has been demonstrated.[6] Weisbroth et al. found that among left hemiplegics, those with better upper extremity use, ambulation, and abstract reasoning were more likely to return to work; however, among right hemiplegics those with milder communication and cognitive deficits also had better vocational outcomes.[57] Therefore, significant aphasia, cognitive problems, or severe hemiparesis/hemiplegia were most likely to preclude return to work.

Cognitive deficits following a stroke are being increasingly recognized as an important factor in determining return to work. However, many of these cognitive deficits are subtle or not readily apparent on general examination.[7] In such cases neuropsychological testing may be required to accurately delineate the extent of cognitive problems and determine how they might affect eventual return to work.[31,32] Intelligence and memory deficits, indifference, anosognosia, depression, and emotional lability have been shown to reduce the likelihood of returning to work poststroke.[29] Mercier et al. found that neuropsychological testing predicted return to work best out of a variety of factors they studied.[7,37]

Black-Schaffer and Lemieux[7] note: "Several studies have shown, not surprisingly, that higher functional performance on ADL and mobility indices at discharge from rehabilitation or at a post rehabilitation follow-up point correlates with greater likelihood of return to work[6,21,25]; in one study, ability to return to driving was strongly linked to return to work as well."[6]

Other studies show that stroke survivors tend to not return to their previous employment.[12,15,25,26] Brooks et al. found that only 29% of stroke survivors returned to work after a 7-year period.[12] Issac et al. studied 29 stroke patients, 11 of whom had full-time employment and eight of whom had full household duties prior to stroke onset.[26] Following discharge, none of the patients returned to any form of employment, one returned to full household duties, and two returned to partial duties. Sjogren noted in one study that 47 of 51 stroke patients were occupationally active until the day of their stroke.[50] However, following stroke only 17% of patients had returned to gainful employment and all of these had "part-time" work only. The inability to return to work frequently leads to emotional and financial hardships for stroke survivors and their families.[13]

FUTURE NEEDS

Hartke and Brashler reported on 100 young stroke survivors who responded to a questionnaire.[20] The patients were an average of 44 years old (range 21–57) and 4 years following stroke onset (range 1–21). A total of 78% of the survivors lived with another person, usually a spouse or other family member, and 22% lived alone. A total of 89% reported a substantial level of ambulation, 71% were independent in self-care, 74% reported making daily trips into the community, 27% were driving a car, and 27% were engaged in some form of employment, school attendance, or job training. When asked what programs they felt would be most helpful at that time, the patients chose, in order of importance: (1) exercise/fitness programs, (2) education/information programs, (3) individual counseling, (4) stress management programs, and (5) recreation/social programs. Vocational counseling was prioritized, as was recreation/social programs in high-functioning survivors. Other programs identified as important included family counseling, support groups, and sexual adjustment counseling.

Physicians, who also were questioned, valued, in order of importance: (1) education/information programs, (2) individual counseling, (3) sexual adjustment counseling, (4) vocational counseling, and (5) family counseling. Although regarded as generally important, patients rated exercise/fitness programs as far more important than did physicians, and physicians prioritized sexual adjustment counseling more.[20]

Hartke and Brashler noted that with the young stroke survivors:

the programs most frequently valued did not necessarily parallel development issues prescribed to be pertinent to a younger age group. Only vocational counseling was frequently chosen as valuable among the high-functioning survivors. Interventions concerning sexual functioning, parenting, and dating/interpersonal relationships were chosen relatively less frequently, although they might be assumed to be developmentally salient at a younger age. Instead, the programs most highly valued might be viewed as actually nonspecific to age. . . . In comparing the high- and low-functioning respondents, it is not surprising to observe the high-functioning survivors more frequently valuing vocational counselling and low-functioning survivors ranking family counselling higher. The high-functioning subgroup might be in pursuit of ambitions to return to work. In contrast, the low-functioning subgroups may have been expressing greater concern over family strain due to their dependence.[20]

CONCLUSION

Stroke is a disorder of older people, but a small but significant number of stroke patients are younger. Although the rehabilitation of younger and older stroke patients is similar, there are some unique differences. Strokes in young patients are characterized by a faster and more complete neurologic recovery. Apart from strokes due to premature atherosclerosis, stroke recurrences are uncommon. Social problems are common. Caregiving is often complicated by child care issues. Rates of return to work are generally low and are determined as much by socioeconomic factors as by neurologic deficits. Institutionalization occurs much less than in elderly stroke patients.

REFERENCES

1. Abu-Zeid HAH, Choi NW, Nelson NA: Epidemiologic features of cerebrovascular disease in Manitoba: Incidence by age, sex and residence, with etiologic implications. Can Med Assoc J 113:379–384, 1975.
2. Adunsky A, Hershkowitz M, Rabbi R, et al: Functional recovery in young stroke patients. Arch Phys Med Rehabil 73:859–862, 1992.
3. Barinagarrementeria F, Figueroa T, Huebe J, Cantu C: Cerebral infarction in people under 40 years. Cerebrovasc Dis 6:75–79, 1996.
4. Bergmann H, Kuthmann M, von-Ungern-Sternberg A, Weinman V: Medical, educational and functional determinants of employment after stroke. J Neural Transm 33(suppl):157–161, 1991.
5. Bevan H, Sharma K, Bradley W: Stroke in young adults. Stroke 21:382–386, 1990.
6. Black-Schaffer RM, Osber JS: Return to work after stroke: Development of a predictive model. Arch Phys Med Rehabil 71:285–290, 1990.
7. Black-Schaffer RM, Lemieux L: Vocational outcome after stroke. Top Stroke Rehabil 1:74–86, 1994.
8. Bogousslavsky J, Regli F: Ischemic stroke in adults younger than 30 years of age. Arch Neurol 44:479–482, 1987.
9. Bonita R, Beaglehole R, North JDK: Evidence, incidence and case fatality rate of cerebrovascular disease in Aukland, New Zealand. Am J Epidemiol 120:236–243, 1984.
10. Bonita R: Epidemiology of stroke. Lancet 339:342–344, 1992.
11. Boxell J, McKercher G: Needs of caregivers of elderly attending day hospital. Can Fam Physician 36:45–49, 1990.
12. Brooks N, McKinley W, Symington C, et al: Return to work within the first seven years after head injury. Brain Inj 1:5–19, 1987.
13. Churchill C: Social problems post stroke. Phys Med Rehabil State Art Rev 7:213–223, 1993.
14. Colerick EJ, George LK: Predictors of institutionalization among caregivers of patients with Alzheimer's disease. J Am Geriatr Soc 34:493–498, 1986.
15. Coughlan A, Humphrey M: Presenile stroke: Long-term outcome for patients and their families. Rheumatol Rehabil 21:115–122, 1982.
16. Falconer JA, Naughton BJ, Strasser DC, Sinacore JM: Stroke in patient rehabilitation: A comparison across age groups. J Am Geriatr Soc 42:39–44, 1994.
17. Feigenson JS, McDowell FH, Meese P, et al: Factors influencing outcome and length of stay in a stroke rehabilitation unit. Stroke 8:651–656, 1977.
18. Ferro JM, Crespo M: Young adult stroke: Neuropsychological dysfunction and recovery. Stroke 19:982–986, 1988.
19. Gresham GE, Fitzpatrick TE, Wolf PA, et al: Residual disability in survivors of stroke. The Framingham study. N Engl J Med 293:954–956, 1975.
20. Hartke RJ, Brashler R: Assessment of the needs of the young stroke survivor. Top Stroke Rehabil 1:15–24, 1994.
21. Heinemann A, Roth E, Cichowski K, Betts H: Multivariate analysis of improvement and outcome following stroke rehabilitation. Arch Neurol 44:1167–1176, 1987.
22. Hindfelt B, Nilsson O: The prognosis of ischemic stroke in young adults. Acta Neurol Scand 55:123–130, 1977.
23. Hindfelt B, Nilsson O: Long-term prognosis of ischemic stroke in young adults. Acta Neurol Scand 86:440–445, 1992.

24. Horowitz A: Family caregiving to the frail elderly. Annu Rev Gerontol Geriatr 5:194–246, 249–282, 1985.
25. Howard G, Till JS, Toole JF, et al: Factors influencing return to work following cerebral function. JAMA 253:226–236, 1985.
26. Isaacs B, Neville Y, Rushford I: The stricken: The social consequences of stroke. Age Ageing 5:188–192, 1976.
27. Kapelle LJ, Adams HP, Heffner ML, et al: Prognosis of young adults with ischemic stroke. Stroke 25:1360–1365, 1994.
28. Kinsella GJ, Duffy FP: Psychosocial readjustment in the spouses of aphasic patients. Scand J Rehabil Med 11:129–132, 1979.
29. Kotila M, Waltimo O, Neimi J, et al: The profile of recovery from stroke and factors influencing outcome. Stroke 15:1039–1044, 1984.
30. Link K: A synthesis of studies on stroke rehabilitation. J Chronic Dis 35:133–149, 1982.
31. Lindberg M, Angquist K, Fodstad H, et al: Self-reported prevalence of disability after subarachnoid hemorrhage, with special emphasis on return to leisure and work. Br J Neurosurg 6:297–304, 1992.
32. Ljunggren B, Sonesson B, Saveland H, Brandt L: Cognitive impairment and adjustment in patients without neurological deficits after aneurysmal SAH, and early operation. J Neurosurg 2:673–679, 1985.
33. Love BB, Biller J: Stroke in the young—cardiac causes. Stroke Clin Updates 1:13–16, 1990.
34. Mackay A, Nias BC: Strokes in the young and middle-aged: Consequences to the family and to society. J R Coll Physicians Lond 13:106–112, 1979.
35. Mayo NE, Goldberg MS, Levy AR, et al: Changing rates of stroke in the province of Quebec, Canada: 1981–1988. Stroke 22:590–595, 1991.
36. Mayo NE: Epidemiology of recovery. Phys Med Rehabil State Art Rev 7:1–25, 1993.
37. Mercier P, LeGall D, Aubin G, et al: Value of the neuropsychological evaluation in cerebral arterial aneurysms surgically treated. Neurochirurgie 37:32–39, 1991.
38. Meyer JR, Oreneia AJ, Biller J: Etiology and diagnosis of stroke in the young adult. Top Stroke Rehabil 1:1–14, 1994.
39. Monga T: The young stroke: Meeting the needs of the inpatient and outpatient recreational, vocational, and sexual needs of young stroke patients. Proceedings of the 59th Annual Assembly of the American Academy of Physical Medicine and Rehabilitation. Atlanta, November 13–16, 1997, pp 347–350.
40. Ostfeld AM: A review of stroke epidemiology. Epidemiol Rev 2:136–152, 1980.
41. Petitti DB, Sidney S, Bernstein A, et al: Stroke in users of low-dose oral corticosteroids. N Engl J Med 325:8–15, 1996.
42. Qureshi AT, Safdar K, Patel M, et al: Stroke in young black patients. Stroke 26:1995–1998, 1995.
43. Robins M, Baum H: The National Survey of Stroke. Incidence. Stroke 12(suppl 1):I45–57, 1981.
44. Rohr J, Kitlner S, Feeser B, et al: Traditional risk factors and ischemic stroke in young adults: The Baltimore-Washington cooperative young stroke study. Arch Neurol 53:603–607, 1996.
45. Rozenthul-Sorokin N, Ronen R, Tamir A, et al: Stroke in the young Israel. Stroke 27:838–841, 1996.
46. Sacki S, Ogata H, Okubo T, et al: Factors influencing return to work after stroke in Japan. Stroke 24:1182–1185, 1993.
47. Schuman JE, Beattie EJ, Steed DA, et al: Geriatric patients with and without intellectual dysfunction: Effectiveness of a standard rehabilitation program. Arch Phys Med Rehabil 62:612–618, 1981.
48. Shah SK, Bain C: Admissions, patterns of utilization and dispositions of cases of acute stroke in Brisbane hospitals. Med J Aust 150:256–260, 1989.
49. Silverstone B, Horowitz A: Issues of social support: The family and home care. In Dunkel RZ, Schmidley JW (eds): Stroke in the Elderly. New York, Springer, 1987, pp 169–185.
50. Sjogren K: Leisure after stroke. Int Rehabil Med 4:80–87, 1982.
51. Smolkin C, Cohen B: Socioeconomic factors affecting the vocational success of stroke patients. Arch Phys Med Rehabil 55:269–271, 1974.
52. Snyder BD, Ramirez-Lassepas M: Cerebral infarction in young adults. Long-term prognosis. Stroke 11:149–153, 1980.
53. Teasell RW, McRae MP, Finestone HM: Social issues in the rehabilitation of younger stroke patients [abstract]. 1998 Canadian Association of Physical Medicine and Rehabilitation Scientific Meeting.
54. Tobin SS, Kalys R: The family in the institutionalization of the elderly. J Soc Iss 37:145–157, 1981.
55. Tompkins CA, Schulz R, Ran MT: Post-stroke depression in primary support persons: Predicting those at risk. Consult Clin Psychol 56:502–508, 1988.
56. Weinfeld FD: National survey of stroke. Stroke 12(suppl 1):I1–90, 1981.
57. Weisbroth S, Esibill N, Zuger R: Factors in the vocational success of hemiplegic patients. Arch Phys Med Rehabil 52:441–486, 1971.

STEPHEN D. BAGG, MD, MSc, FRCPC

OUTCOME PREDICTORS AND THE EFFECTIVENESS OF STROKE REHABILITATION

From the Department of
  Rehabilitation Medicine
Queen's University
Kingston, Ontario
Canada

Reprint requests to:
Stephen D. Bagg, MD
Director, Stroke Rehabilitation
  Program
St. Mary's of the Lake Hospital
Kingston, Ontario K7L 5A2
Canada

The influence of intensive interdisciplinary stroke rehabilitation on functional outcome has been the subject of numerous studies over the past 20 years. In these times of economic restraint, it is essential that the provision of rehabilitation services is "evidence-based." Specifically, it is becoming increasingly important to identify which patients benefit from what specific rehabilitation interventions, in what setting, at what intensity, and for how long. Furthermore, the cost-effectiveness of these services must be determined. Rehabilitation programs are expensive, but the cost of stroke related to acute management and long-term disability is also tremendous, as are the major psychosocial consequences of stroke-related impairment and disability.

This chapter reviews the evidence regarding the effectiveness of stroke rehabilitation and discusses factors and tools that have been found useful in predicting outcome.

PATTERN OF RECOVERY AFTER STROKE

To predict outcome after stroke or to assess the effectiveness of a specific intervention to minimize stroke-related disability, one must understand how stroke-related impairments generally recover. Most stroke patients survive; the 30-day mortality rate is about 20%.[14] Most stroke survivors improve physically and functionally to some degree in a somewhat predictable pattern, but the rate and completeness of recovery is difficult to predict during the first few weeks after the onset of the stroke.

PHYSICAL MEDICINE AND REHABILITATION: State of the Art Reviews—
Vol. 12, No. 3, October 1998. Philadelphia, Hanley & Belfus, Inc.

581

In 1951, Twitchell reported the distinct pattern of motor recovery following stroke.[65] Typically, flaccid hemiparesis is followed by return of muscle stretch reflexes and onset of spasticity and then a return toward normal tone. Recovery of motor control typically starts proximally, at the trunk, shoulder and pelvic girdles, and moves into more distal limb muscles with time. Additionally, initial motor control occurs in a synergistic pattern (typically of flexion in the upper extremity and extension in the lower extremity). As recovery continues, active selective control of specific muscle groups is regained. Because most strokes occur in the middle cerebral artery territory, lower extremity functional recovery is usually more complete than in the upper extremity. Fewer than 10% of stroke survivors will have permanent severe impairment in the lower extremity, and one third of all stroke survivors will have no functional recovery in the upper extremity (one third will use the arm and hand functionally and one third will use the hand to assist or stabilize objects).[47,67]

It is generally agreed that most recovery occurs during the first 3 months after the onset of stroke,[6,36,37,47,52,56,67] but further functional recovery is still possible.[3,4,12,44,45,47] Hence, most of the published "stroke recovery curves," which plot physical or functional recovery over time, typically are most steep during the first month, have clearly started to plateau by 3 months, and have leveled out by 6 months. Although further neurologic recovery is highly unlikely after 6 months,[10,36] late adaptation and recovery as long as a year after stroke also has been reported.[45,63,67] For example, Tangeman et al. reported significant gains in the measures of weight shift, balance, and activities of daily living (ADL) scores after a 1-month rehabilitation program for 40 stroke patients at least 1 year after stroke onset.[63] This apparent discrepancy in the literature may be in part related to variability in the severity of patients included in different studies. The plateau in the recovery after a few months also may be a reflection of measurement tools that are insensitive to small but significant amounts of functional improvement, or they may be due to a "ceiling effect" (insensitivity to improvement at the upper level of function).[69] Hence, rehabilitation services clearly should not be provided for an arbitrary duration or withdrawn until the functional recovery has reached a plateau. Furthermore, rehabilitation services may need to be reactivated long after discontinuation of the initial services to maintain an individual at his maximal level of functional independence.[44]

EFFECTIVENESS OF REHABILITATION

In the past, the effectiveness of stroke rehabilitation programs in improving outcome has been unclear and controversial. This was related to several factors, including the heterogeneity of the patients involved in the initial studies, failure to stratify for severity of stroke, variety of treatment settings, differences in resources allocated to the management of stroke, quantity and quality of treatment settings, differences in resources allocated to the management of stroke, quantity and quality of treatments, lack of baseline information, and poor quality of data collected.[33] Over the past two decades, however, several well-designed randomized case-control studies and meta-analyses have demonstrated the definite benefits of rehabilitation.

Comparing the functional outcome for elderly patients with acute stroke randomized to a stroke unit or to medical units, Garraway et al. reported in 1980 that a higher proportion of patients in the stroke unit group regained functional independence. This difference in functional outcome, however, was no longer apparent at 1-year follow-up.[22]

In 1981, Smith et al. performed a randomized controlled trial on 133 patients, varying the intensity of outpatient rehabilitation therapy.[57] They reported significantly greater improvements in functional independence in ADLs with more intensive therapy.[57] One year later, Smith et al. randomized 121 acute stroke patients into three groups: intensive therapy (4 full days of therapies per week), conventional therapy (3 half days per week), and no therapy.[58] Some functional gains were made in the no treatment group, and they were simply related to spontaneous recovery. However, additional gains were reported in the conventional therapy group, and the greatest gains were achieved in patients receiving the intensive therapy.

In 1985, Sivenius et al.[56] reported the results of 95 stroke patients who were randomly assigned to either an intensive physiotherapy program on a rehabilitation unit or to a control group that received less intensive physiotherapy on a general medical unit. Patients were followed for 1 year, and the authors reported greater and more rapid recovery of motor and ADL functional scores in the group participating in the more intensive treatment program.

A prospective controlled trial was also reported by Kalra et al., who randomized 245 stroke patients (stratified into three prognostic groups using the Orpington Prognostic Score) to either a stroke rehabilitation unit or general medical ward.[33] Outcome measures included functional abilities, discharge location, and length of stay. Patients with good prognosis—mild disability—had comparable outcomes in both treatment settings. Severely disabled patients with poor prognosis showed higher mortality and longer hospital stay on the general wards, but functional outcome was similar in the two treatment settings. More physiotherapy was provided on the general wards, but over a longer time, suggesting that the efficiency of stroke rehabilitation in this setting is suboptimal. Patients with intermediate prognosis had better outcome on the stroke unit, including greater functional independence at discharge, shorter length of stay, and more patients discharged home.

The term *middle band* was introduced by Garraway.[23] The upper band referred to stroke patients with little or no motor deficit who typically were able to function independently in their homes. The lower-band stroke patients were defined as being unconscious at stroke onset and having severe hemiparesis and were felt to be unlikely to achieve functional independence regardless of treatment. Generally speaking, middle-band stroke patients are conscious at onset of stroke, have moderate impairment and disability, and are most likely to benefit from intensive rehabilitation efforts. Kalra randomized 146 such middle-band patients to management in a stroke unit or a general medical ward.[34] Functional recovery was significantly greater in the patients managed on the stroke rehabilitation unit. Furthermore, functional recovery was achieved at a faster rate in the rehabilitation unit (reaching a plateau at 6 weeks compared to 12 weeks on the general ward) without any additional physiotherapy or occupational therapy. The average length of stay was 6 weeks on the rehabilitation unit versus 20 weeks on the general medical unit. It was proposed that this significant difference in both effectiveness and efficiency of the specialized stroke rehabilitation setting may at least in part be related to the closer liaison between the patient, caregivers, and the professionals in this setting.

In 1995, Kalra and Eade reported a randomized controlled study of 76 stroke survivors with severe disability (Orpington Prognostic Score greater than 5) to a general medical ward or a stroke rehabilitation unit.[35] A trend toward increased median discharge Barthel Index scores was identified after the intensive rehabilitation. Furthermore, care in the rehabilitation units resulted in significantly lower mortality (21% versus 46%), higher discharge home rates (47% versus 19%), and shorter median length of hospital stay (43 days versus 58 days). These measures of improved outcome were attributed to a variety of factors, including specialist training, individualized rehabilitation programs, caregiver education and hands-on training, seamless professional collaboration, and innovative planning of postdischarge care.

Rønning and Guldvog compared the benefits of a hospital-based stroke rehabilitation program and a community-based program.[54] Average length of stay in the rehabilitation hospital was 27.8 days. Patients with moderate or severe disability (admission Barthel Index less than 50) reached a much greater level of functional independence after hospital-based rehabilitation (Barthel Index of 90 versus 73 in the community-based setting). Furthermore, treatment in the hospital rehabilitation unit resulted in fewer patients who were dependent (Barthel Index < 75) or dead (23% versus 38%) 7 months poststroke.

Several recent meta-analyses have been published to assess the effectiveness of inpatient rehabilitation. Ottenbacher and Jannell evaluated the results of 36 clinical trials, including 3,717 patients, and reported that the patients who participated in an individualized program of stroke rehabilitation performed better than 65% of those who did not.[51] Greater functional improvement was observed in younger patients and in patients with relatively short intervals between stroke onset and the beginning of rehabilitation.

In 1995, Evans et al. evaluated 11 studies published between 1980 and 1993 that met their stringent inclusion criteria.[17] Three of the papers, however, evaluated rehabilitation of individuals with disabilities other than stroke. Their analysis revealed that treatment on a rehabilitation unit resulted in greater odds of survival, higher rates of discharge to home and rates of remaining at home at 8–12 months of follow-up, and higher levels of functional ability at discharge. However, the differences in survival and functional independence had disappeared at the 12-month follow-up period, suggesting that many patients who are discharged from rehabilitation may deteriorate medically, physically, and functionally. This finding accentuates the need to assess the effectiveness of outpatient and home-based therapies after discharge from inpatient rehabilitation programs, as well as the role of maintenance therapy for individuals with stroke requiring long-term institutionalization.

The Stroke Unit Trialists' Collaboration systematically reviewed 19 randomized clinical trials that compared organized inpatient stroke care, including dedicated stroke units and mixed assessment/rehabilitation units, with conventional care that typically was provided in a general medical ward.[62] The distinctive features of the organized stroke units included coordinated multidisciplinary team care; nursing integration with team care; specialization of physicians, nurses, and therapists; education of staff and patients; and caregiver involvement. Stroke unit care was associated with a significant reduction in death at a median 1-year follow-up and the combined outcomes of death or dependency and death or institutionalization without an increase in length of stay.

Some authors suggest that most functional recovery after stroke is simply related to the spontaneous natural recovery from neurologic impairment.[16,42] However, Roth et al. recently assessed the relationship between impairment and disability after stroke in a prospective cohort of 442 patients consecutively admitted for rehabilitation.[55] Impairment was quantified with the National Institutes of Health Stroke Scale, and the Functional Index Measure (FIM) was used to measure disability. Statistically significant associations were demonstrated between impairment and disability at rehabilitation admission and discharge. However, only 2–36% of the variance in disability was explained by level of impairment; 85% of patients experienced no measurable reduction in impairment. Not surprisingly, the patient group that did demonstrate significant reduction in impairment (15% of the total group) also achieved significantly greater changes in the FIM motor and cognitive subscores than the patients with no measurable reduction in neurologic impairment. However, significant improvement in functional independence also occurred in the patients with no measurable reduction in impairment. Specifically, this group achieved a 38% (14.6-point) increase in the motor FIM subscore and a 22% (11.3-point) improvement in the cognitive FIM subscore. Hence, these results lend support to the observation that many factors other than impairment level can influence functional independence and also suggest that rehabilitation does have an independent role in improving function beyond that explained by spontaneous neurologic recovery.

Large-scale analysis of effectiveness of inpatient rehabilitation has been made possible since the development of the Uniform Data System for Medical Rehabilitation.[25] A total of 64,442 stroke survivors were included in the report of first admissions for 1996.[19] This analysis demonstrated significant, timely, and measurable functional improvement in patients undergoing stroke rehabilitation. Quality benchmarks in stroke rehabilitation were proposed, including number of days from stroke onset to rehabilitation admission (17), admission total FIM (63), discharge total FIM (87), FIM gain per week (7.7), length of stay (22 days), and percent discharged to the community (75). Similar benchmarks need to be established for stroke rehabilitation units in countries with different health care delivery systems than the United States. A typical stroke rehabilitation unit in Canada, for example, admits patients at a later stage of recovery (median admit FIM of 80), and length of stay is longer (averaging 64 days in 1993).[49]

While most papers assessing the effectiveness of stroke rehabilitation have focused on measuring improvements in impairment and disability, some investigators have attempted to quantify other outcomes related to quality of life, such as the ability of stroke survivors to return to work. Lawrence and Christie followed 45 stroke survivors for 3 years.[41] All patients were employed at the time of their stroke, 70% on a full-time basis, including full-time homemaking. After 3 years, only 20% of the men and 35% of the women were fully employed. Howard et al. reported that fewer than 20% of stroke survivors are able to return to work after stroke.[29] Neimi et al. found that 41% of stroke survivors younger than 65 were able to return to work, but 83% of them had not returned to their prestroke quality of life 4 years after stroke onset.[48] Black-Schaffer and Osberg studied 79 patients younger than 65 and reported that 49% had returned to work 6 months after discharge from rehabilitation.[8] About 90% were able to return to their prestroke employment and 10% needed to change jobs. However, only 32% of the patients who returned to work were able to do so on a full-time basis. Factors related to return to work included shorter length of stay, greater functional status on admission, and absence of aphasia. There clearly is a need for studies of the impact of rehabilitation on the stroke survivor's psychological well being and quality of life. The Rand 36-item Health Survey (SF-36 Questionnaire) appears to be used increasingly and should be helpful in addressing this area.[28]

MAINTENANCE OF GAINS AFTER REHABILITATION

Another important issue is sustaining levels of functional independence that were achieved during rehabilitation. Most studies report only short-term outcomes. Those that examine longer-term outcomes have reached mixed conclusions.[2,9,13,21,22,56,57]

Failure to maintain functional gains appear to underscore the need for continued practice after the patient returns home. The importance of encouragement and support by family and friends plus the need for the patient to accept responsibility for the maintenance of independent function cannot be overemphasized. Continued rehabilitation or inpatient or outpatient "tune-ups" may be indicated in some cases, but this needs to be justified by evidence of progress during treatment and deterioration in its absence.

PREDICTING OUTCOME

Early and accurate prediction of outcome after stroke is important for a variety of reasons. Stroke survivors typically want to know if they will walk again. Caregivers ask if their loved ones will regain continence or independence in self-care activities. Furthermore, as funding for health care services and rehabilitation decreases, the results of outcome studies are becoming critical in planning realistic short- and long-term rehabilitation goals, including functional independence in mobility and self-care activities as well as discharge planning. To address these concerns, we must rely on the results of studies assessing the outcome of cohorts of stroke patients.

Many investigators have attempted to identify the variables that best predict outcome, including discharge location, length of stay, and functional independence in mobility and self-care activities. Factors that have been reported to influence outcome include the following:

- Nature and severity of stroke (impairment)
- Functional abilities at entry into rehabilitation (disability)
- Age
- Cognitive impairments
- Perceptual deficits
- Depression
- Medical comorbidity
- Continence
- Presence of a supportive caregiver

Although these variables influence outcome after stroke, their relative importance in predicting outcome has been debated. Many studies have attempted to identify a small number of variables, which can be easily measured at the time of admission to rehabilitation, and accurately predict outcome.

Predicting discharge location is becoming increasingly important, particularly in light of the increasing demand for stroke rehabilitation services and the lengthy waiting lists for nursing homes. The Framingham study reported on 154 stroke patients who were followed for 1 year.[36] A total of 27% of the patients required long-term care in a nursing home or chronic care facility. Logistic regression analysis identified age, severity of impairment, and marital status as important variables influencing discharge location. DeJong and Branch reported that 85% of 84 middle-band stroke survivors remained at home at 1 year of follow-up.[15] Two variables, marital status and functional independence on admission, were reported to be extremely important in predicting the discharge living arrangement status. Living with a supportive caregiver clearly enhances the possibilities of a stroke survivor returning home. Furthermore, a person's marital status was more important for men than for women, a finding that was attributed to the traditional caregiving roles expected of women, especially for the age groups represented in the study sample.

Oczkowski and Barreca attempted to clarify the usefulness of the FIM as a prognostic indicator of outcome in 113 stroke survivors admitted to a Canadian rehabilitation unit a median of 52 days poststroke.[49] Average length of stay was 64 days, and 80 patients were discharged home; three patients died and the remaining 30 required long-term care in a nursing home or chronic care facility. The median FIM score was 80 on admission and 94 at discharge. Multiple logistic regression revealed that the best predictors of discharge location were the admission FIM score, admission postural staging, and age. The admission FIM score proved to be the most powerful predictor of discharge location. Three distinct groups of stroke survivors were identified. Patients with admission FIM scores of 36 or less showed minimal improvement, remaining severely disabled and typically requiring long-term institutionalization, particularly in the absence of an extremely supportive and healthy caregiver. Patients with admission FIM scores above 96 also tended to show relatively small FIM gains—perhaps related to a ceiling effect—and almost invariably were able to return home. Patients with admission FIM scores in the middle band, between 36 and 96, demonstrated the greatest overall FIM gains, but discharge destination was difficult to predict, presumably due to comorbidities, cognitive and perceptual impairments, and the presence or absence of a supportive caregiver.

Using a computerized neural network model design, Oczkowski and Barreca were able to predict discharge location with 75% accuracy.[50] Variables used to predict discharge location included patient age, time poststroke, motor recovery of the leg, motor recovery of postural control, visual field loss, sensory loss, neglect, admission FIM scores, and the presence of a supportive caregiver. Most errors in predicting discharge location occurred in the patient group with admission FIM scores between 37 and 96 (i.e., the group that seems to derive the greatest benefits from rehabilitation). This is not surprising when one considers that many of these patients must adapt to permanent impairment and disability, making the presence of a supportive caregiver, community resources, financial assets, and environmental factors important determinants in discharge location.

Ween and coworkers prospectively analyzed 536 consecutive stroke rehabilitation admissions in an attempt to identify the influence of preselected factors on functional improvement and discharge disposition.[68] Patients younger than 55 or with an admission FIM score above 80 almost always went home after rehabilitation. Conversely, patients admitted to rehabilitation with an FIM score less than 40 almost always required long-term care in a nursing home facility. An admission FIM of 60 or more was associated with a larger FIM improvement, but the absence of a committed caregiver at home increased the risk of nursing home discharge. This study also reported better outcome in individuals with small vessel strokes and fewer comorbid conditions. Patients recovering from intracerebral hemorrhages improved more than those with ischemic strokes but at a slower rate, and individuals with left hemispheric strokes had better outcomes overall than those with right hemisphere lesions.

The association of increasing age with poor outcome has been noted in numerous other studies.[34,46] Nakayama et al. reported that older patients made the same degree of neurologic recovery than younger patients but had a much lower functional gain.[46] It was suggested that the more elderly patients had less compensatory abilities than younger patients with comparable neurologic impairments. Kalra also reported that younger patients enjoyed greater functional recovery and higher rates of home discharge than elderly stroke survivors.[34] Alexander reported that stroke survivors younger than 55 almost always were discharged home regardless of stroke severity.[1] For patients older than 55, individuals with more severe strokes and/or of an older age tended to benefit less from rehabilitation in terms of functional recovery and discharge home.

Falconer et al. proposed that medical comorbidity associated with increasing age accounted for the negative influence of age on rehabilitation.[18] However, when Borucki et al. excluded patients with comorbid conditions, no difference in discharge Barthel Index scores was identified between patients younger than 70 and older stroke survivors.[9] This suggests that cognitive and perceptual impairments plus social factors such as the presence of a supportive caregiver may be more critical than medical comorbidity in adversely influencing discharge disposition.

The negative impact of cognitive, perceptual, and behavioral problems on stroke outcome have been confirmed in several recent studies. Tatemichi et al. reported significant cognitive impairment in 35% of stroke survivors, including impairments in attention and concentration, memory, orientation, and language.[64] Galski et al. demonstrated that cognitive impairment after stroke (affecting abstract thinking, comprehension, judgment, and short-term verbal memory) resulted in increased length of stay and increased requirements for outpatient and home-based services after discharge from rehabilitation.[20]

Stineman et al. presented the concept of the Functional Independence Measure–Function Related Groups (FIM-FRGs).[60] A total of 12,276 stroke patients were separated into five FIM-FRGs according to patient age and admission motor FIM subscores.[61] Mean, median, 25th and 75th quartile motor FIM gains, and length of stays were reported for each FIM–FRG. This information could be used to provide clinicians and administrators with reasonable outcome targets, but the authors recommended against using FIM–FRG systems to predict individual patient outcomes, stating that they were designed primarily to characterize differences among groups of patients.

A comprehensive and critical review of prognostic studies of stroke patients was reported by Kwakkel et al.[38] A total of 142 prognostic studies were initially reviewed, but only eight cohort studies met all the criteria for internal and statistical validity. An analysis of these studies demonstrated the ability of a number of determinants to predict functional recovery after stroke, including disability on admission, urinary incontinence, degree of motor paresis, age, level of consciousness within first 48 hours poststroke, orientation in time and place, status following recurrent stroke, sitting balance, and level of perceived social support.

Predicting outcome based on computed tomography (CT) can be difficult. Hertanu reported that the lesion size did correlate with disability but was not necessarily associated with ultimate discharge location.[30] Chaudhuri suggested that individuals with CT-proven bihemispheric infarcts had increased risk of institutionalization.[11] Valdimarsson et al.[66] indicated that stroke survivors were more likely to be severely disabled and have a poor outcome if the acute CT scan identified a large lesion, a mass effect, right parietal lobe lesion, or a deep lesion affecting the internal capsule. Beloosesky et al. reported greater functional independence in patients with lacunar infarctions than those with cortical strokes, where infarct size also correlated inversely with rehabilitation potential.[7] This most likely relates to the aphasia, apraxia, and cognitive and perceptual impairments that can result from large cortical infarctions.

Several recent studies have evaluated the ability to predict outcome after ischemic stroke using positron emission tomography (PET), which quantifies cerebral metabolic rate outside the area of infarction. Marchal et al. identified three patterns on PET scanning in 18 patients after middle cerebral artery territory infarcts.[43] Individuals with extensive hypoperfusion (indicative of severe and irreversible damage) had poor outcome at 2 months. Stroke survivors with moderate to large reductions in perfusion (a pattern suggestive of continuing ischemia) had variable 2-month outcomes. Patients with hyperperfusion on PET scan typically had excellent functional recovery at 2 months. Heiss et al. reported that the left hemispheric glucose value of the resting PET scan had significant value in predicting outcome from aphasia after an ischemic stroke.[27]

The ability to predict motor recovery after stroke using electromagnetic stimulation of the motor cortex also has been reported. Heald measured the central motor conduction times (CMCT) in stroke survivors during the first week postonset.[26] The absence of response to CMCT indicated poor functional recovery at 12 months. Conversely, patients with normal CMCT had higher scores in all outcome measures, including functional recovery at 12 months. Patients with delayed CMCT had outcomes between those of the first two groups.

The predictive ability of somatosensory evoked potentials (SSEPs) was reported by LaJoie et al. in 1982.[39] Only six of 60 individuals with profoundly abnormal SSEPs but seven of 12 stroke survivors with normal SSEPs were competent in basic areas of self-care at the time of discharge from rehabilitation. Zeman and Yiannikas reported that patients with an abnormal SSEP within the first 2 weeks poststroke had longer length of stay in hospital and decreased functional independence at the time of discharge from rehabilitation.[70]

CONCLUSION

The effectiveness of intensive, coordinated inpatient rehabilitation services for stroke patients has been clearly established in the scientific literature regarding rehabilitation. Benefits of stroke rehabilitation include decreased morbidity and mortality and improved functional independence in self-care activities and mobility. Many studies have provided further insight into the predictive value of physical, perceptual, and psychosocial factors.

With decreasing funds being allocated to health care services, rehabilitation teams are experiencing increasing pressure to decrease length of inpatient stays to minimize the overall cost of rehabilitation. However, a decrease in inpatient rehabilitation services must be complemented by a significant increase in outpatient and home-based rehabilitation programs. But, prior to making this change, the effectiveness of specific programs and interventions for specific stroke-related impairments and disabilities need to be quantified to develop the most efficient and cost-effective rehabilitation programs for individuals recovering from stroke-related disabilities. Additionally, there remains a great need to assess the long-term effectiveness of stroke rehabilitation, not only for the middle-band stroke survivors but also for the more severely disabled stroke survivors who require long-term care in institutions and typically do not receive ongoing maintenance therapies. Finally, a clear need exists to address and quantify the effect of rehabilitation on the quality of life of stroke survivors, their caregivers, and family members.

REFERENCES

1. Alexander MP: Stroke rehabilitation outcome, a potential use of predictive variables to levels of care. Stroke 25:128–134, 1994.
2. Anderson E, Anderson T, Kottke F: Stroke rehabilitation: Maintenance of gains. Arch Phys Med Rehabil 58:345–352, 1977.
3. Andrews K, Brockelhurst JC, Richards B, Laycock PJ: The rate of recovery from stroke—and its measurement. Int Rehabil Med 3:155–161, 1981.
4. Andrews K, Brockelhurst JC, Richards B, Laycock PJ: The influence of age on the clinical presentation and outcome of stroke. Int Rehabil Med 6:49–53, 1984.

5. Astrom M, Asplund K, Astrom T: Psychosocial function and life satisfaction after stroke. Stroke 23:527–531, 1992.
6. Bard G, Hirschberg GG: Recovery of voluntary motion in upper extremity following hemiplegia. Arch Phys Med Rehabil 46:567–572, 1965.
7. Beloosesky Y, Streifler JY, Burstin J, Grinblat J: The importance of brain infarct size and location in predicting outcome after stroke. Age Ageing 24:515–518, 1995.
8. Black-Schaffer RM, Osberg JS: Return to work after stroke: Development of a predictive model. Arch Phys Med Rehabil 58:345–352, 1990.
9. Borucki S, Volpe BT, Reding M: The effect of age on maintenance of functional gains following stroke rehabilitation. J Neurol Rehabil 6:1–5, 1992.
10. Carroll D: The disability of hemiplegia caused by cerebrovascular disease; serial study of 98 cases. J Chronic Disord 15:179–188, 1961.
11. Chauduri G, Harvey R, Sulton L: Computerized tomography head scans as predictors of functional outcome of stroke patients. Arch Phys Med Rehabil 69:496–502, 1988.
12. Chen Q, Ling R: A 1 to 4 year follow-up study of 306 cases of stroke. Stroke 16:323–327, 1985.
13. Davidoff GN, Keren O, Ring H, Solzi P: Acute stroke patients: Long-term effects of rehabilitation and maintenance of gains. Arch Phys Med Rehabil 72:869–873, 1991.
14. Dennis MS, Burn JPS, Sandercock P, et al: Long term survival after first ever stroke: The Oxfordshire Community Stroke Project. Stroke 24:796–800, 1993.
15. DeJong G, Branch LG: Predicting the stroke patient's ability to live independently. Stroke 13:648–655, 1982.
16. Dobkin BH: Focused stroke rehabilitation programs do not improve outcomes. Arch Neurol 46:701–703, 1989.
17. Evans RL, Connis RT, Hendricks RD, Haselkorn JK: Multidisciplinary rehabilitation versus medical care: A meta-analysis. Soc Sci Med 40:1699–1706, 1995.
18. Falconer JA, Naughton BJ, Strasser DC, Sinacore JM: Stroke inpatient rehabilitation: A comparison across age groups. J Am Geriatr Soc 42:39–44, 1994.
19. Fiedler RC, Granger CV: The uniform data system for medical rehabilitation—report for first admissions for 1996. Am J Phys Med Rehabil 77:69–75, 1998.
20. Galski T, Bruno RL, Zorowitz R, Walker J: Predicting length of stay, functional outcome and aftercare in the rehabilitation of stroke patients: The dominant role of higher-order cognition. Stroke 24:1794–1800, 1993.
21. Garraway WM, Akhtar AJ, Prescott RJ, Hockley L: Management of acute stroke in the elderly: Preliminary results of a controlled trial. BMJ 280:1040–1043, 1980.
22. Garraway WM, Akhtar AJ, Hockley L, Prescott RJ: Management of acute stroke in the elderly: Follow-up of a controlled trial. BMJ 281:827–829, 1980.
23. Garraway WM, Whisnant JP, Drury I: The changing pattern of survival following stroke. Stroke 14:699–705, 1983.
24. Gowland C: Predicting sensorimotor-recovery following stroke rehabilitation. Physiother Can 36:313–320, 1984.
25. Granger CV, Hamilton BB: UDS report—the uniform data system for medical rehabilitation. Am J Phys Med Rehabil 71:108–113, 1992.
26. Heald A, Bates D, Cartlidge NE, et al: Longitudinal study of central motor conduction time following stroke. Brain 116:1371–1385, 1993.
27. Hiess WD, Kessler J, Karbe H, et al: Cerebral glucose metabolism as a predictor of recovery from aphasia in ischemic stroke. Arch Neurol 50:958–964, 1993.
28. Hobson P, Bhowmick B, Meara J: Use of the SF-36 questionnaire in cerebrovascular disease. Stroke 28:464–465, 1997.
29. Howard G, Till JF, Toole YS, et al: Factors influencing return to work following cerebral infarction. JAMA 235:226–232, 1985.
30. Hurtanu JS, Denopoulos JT, Yang WC: Stroke rehabilitation: Correlation and prognostic value of computerized tomography and sequential functional assessments. Arch Phys Med Rehabil 65:202–512, 1984.
31. Jeffery DR, Good DC: Rehabilitation of the stroke patient. Curr Opin Neurol 8:62–68, 1995.
32. Johnston MV, Kirschbaum S, Zorowitz R, Shiflett SC: Prediction of outcomes following rehabilitation of stroke patients. Neurol Rehabil 2:72–97, 1992.
33. Kalra L, Dale P, Crome P: Improving stroke rehabilitation: A controlled study. Stroke 24:1462–1467, 1993.
34. Kalra L: The influence of stroke unit rehabilitation on functional recovery from stroke. Stroke 25:821–825, 1994.
35. Kalra L, Eade J: Role of stroke rehabilitation units in managing severe disability after stroke. Stroke 26:2031–2034, 1995.

36. Kelly-Hayes M, Wolf PA, Kase CS, et al: Time course of functional recovery after stroke: The Framingham Study. J Neurol Rehabil 3:65–70, 1989.
37. Kotila M, Waltimo O, Niemi ML: The profile of recovery from stroke and factors influencing outcome. Stroke 15:1039–1044, 1984.
38. Kwakkel G, Wagenaar RC, Kollen BJ, Lankhorst GJ: Predicting disability after stroke—a critical review of the literature. Age Ageing 25:479–489, 1996.
39. La Joie WJ, Nanjappareddy MR, Melvin JL: Somatosensory evoked potentials: Their predictive value in right hemiplegia. Arch Phys Med Rehabil 63:223–229, 1982.
40. Langhorne P, Williams BO, Gilchrist W, Howie K: Do stroke units save lives? Lancet 342:395–397, 1993.
41. Lawrence J, Christie D: Quality of life after stroke: A three year follow-up. Age Ageing 8:167–172, 1979.
42. Link K: A synthesis of studies on stroke rehabilitation. J Chronic Disord 35:1323–1349, 1982.
43. Marchal G, Serrati C, Rioux P, et al: PET imaging of cerebral perfusion and oxygen consumption in acute ischemic stroke: Relation to outcome. Lancet 341:925–927, 1993.
44. Mayo NE: Epidemiology and recovery. Phys Med Rehabil State Art Rev 7:1–24, 1993.
45. Mayo NE, Korner-Bitensky NA, Becker R: Recovery time of independent function post-stroke. Am J Phys Med Rehabil 70:5–12, 1991.
46. Nakayama H, Jorgenson HS, Rassachou HO, Olsen TS: The influence of age on stroke outcome. The Copenhagen Stroke Study. Stroke 25:808–813, 1994.
47. Newman M: The process of recovery after hemiplegia. Stroke 3:702–710, 1972.
48. Niemi ML, Laaksomen R, Kotila M, Waltimo O: Quality of life 4 years after stroke. Stroke 19:1101–1107, 1988.
49. Oczkowski WJ, Barreca S: The functional independence measure: Its use to identify rehabilitation needs in stroke survivors. Arch Phys Med Rehabil 74:1291–1294, 1993.
50. Oczkowski WJ, Barreca S: Neural network modeling accurately predicts the functional outcome of stroke survivors with moderate disabilities. Arch Phys Med Rehabil 78:340–345, 1997.
51. Ottenbacher KJ, Jannell S: The results of clinical trials in stroke rehabilitation research. Arch Neurol 50:37–44, 1993.
52. Prescott RJ, Garraway WM, Akhtar AJ: Predicting functional outcome following acute stroke using standardized clinical examination. Stroke 13:641–647, 1982.
53. Reding MJ, Potes E: Rehabilitation outcomes following initial unilateral hemispheric stroke. Life table analysis approach. Stroke 19:1354–1358, 1988.
54. Rønning OM, Guldvog B: Outcome of subacute rehabilitation: A randomized controlled trial. Stroke 29:779–784, 1998.
55. Roth EJ, Heinemann AW, Lovell LL, et al: Impairment and disability: Their relation during stroke rehabilitation. Arch Phys Med Rehabil 79:329–335, 1998.
56. Sivenius J, Pyörälä K, Heinonen OP, et al: The significance of intensity of rehabilitation of a stroke— a controlled study. Stroke 16:928–931, 1985.
57. Smith ME, Garraway WM, Smith DL, Akhtar AJ: Therapy impact on functional outcome in a controlled trial of stroke rehabilitation. Arch Phys Med Rehabil 63:21–24, 1982.
58. Smith DS, Goldenberg E, Ashburn A, Kinsella G: Remedial therapy after stroke: A randomized controlled trial. BMJ 282:517–520, 1981.
59. Stallones RA, Dyken ML, Fang HCH, et al: Epidemiology for stroke facilities planning. Stroke 3:360–371, 1972.
60. Stineman MG, Escarce JJ, Goin JE, et al: A case-mix classification system for medical rehabilitation. Med Care 32:366–379, 1994.
61. Stineman MG, Hamilton BB, Goin JE, et al: Functional gain and length of stay for major rehabilitation impairment categories: Patterns revealed by function related groups. Am J Phys Med Rehabil 75:68–78, 1996.
62. Stroke Unit Trialists' Collaboration: Collaborative systematic review of the randomized trials of organized inpatient (stroke unit) care after stroke. BMJ 314:1151–1159, 1997.
63. Tangeman PT, Banaitis DA, Williams AK: Rehabilitation of chronic stroke patients: Changes in functional performance. Arch Phys Med Rehabil 71:876–880, 1990.
64. Tatemichi TK, Desmond DW, Stern Y, et al: Cognitive impairment after stroke: Frequency, patterns, and relationship to functional abilities. J Neurol Neurosurg Psychiatry 57:202–207, 1994.
65. Twitchell TE: The restoration of motor function following hemiplegia. Brain 74:438–480, 1951.
66. Vladimarsson EB, Samuelsosn K: Prognostic significance of cerebral computed tomography results in supratentorial infarction. Acta Neurol Scand 65:133–136, 1990.
67. Wade DT, Hewer RL: Functional abilities after stroke: Measurement, natural history and prognosis. J Neurol Neurosurg Psychiatry 50:177–182, 1987.

68. Ween JE, Alexander MP, D'Esposito M, Roberts M: Factors predictive of stroke outcome in a rehabilitation setting. Neurology 47:388–393, 1996.
69. Wellwood I, Dennis MS, Warlow CP: A comparison of the Barthel Index and the OPCS disability instrument used to measure outcome after acute stroke. Age Ageing 24:54–57, 1995.
70. Zeman BD, Yjannikas C: Functional prognosis in stroke: Use of somatosensory evoked potentials. J Neurol Neurosurg Psychiatry 52:242–246, 1989.

INDEX

Entries in **boldface type** indicate complete chapters.